Health care provision

To Dr Nicola Valentine

My married daughter who, as a
general practitioner in North London,
has a special interest in health care.

Health care provision

Past, present and into the 21st century

SECOND EDITION

Audrey Leathard
Visiting Professor of Interprofessional Studies, South Bank University

T

First edition published by Chapman & Hall in 1990
Second edition published in 2000 by Stanley Thornes (Publishers) Ltd

Reprinted in 2001 by:
Nelson Thornes Ltd
Delta Place
27 Bath Road
CHELTENHAM
GL53 7TH
United Kingdom

01 02 03 04 05 / 10 9 8 7 6 5 4 3 2

A catalogue record for this book is available from the British Library

ISBN 0 7487 3354 X

Typeset by Acorn Bookwork, Salisbury, Wiltshire
Printed and bound in Great Britain by T.J. International Ltd, Padstow, Cornwall

CONTENTS

FIGURES

TABLES

PREFACE

The National Health Service celebrated its 50th birthday in July 1998 but, by 1999, was poised to move into the twenty-first century. A unique moment in time has been presented to assess past endeavours and future prospects. However, what about the health care system prior to the National Health Service in the pre-war years? How and why did Britain ever set up a National Health Service (NHS)? How was health care provision organized under the NHS and what have been the key outcomes over half a century? What can be foreseen as the NHS moves into the next century? This publication sets out to investigate these questions, amongst others, in the context of broader social policy developments.

The purpose of this book is to provide a considered account of the events for a wide range of health and welfare workers, students and general readers. For doctors, nurses, health visitors, midwives and district nurses, space has been given to show the professional issues involved in the provision of health care. Health educators, social workers, psychiatrists, physiotherapists, occupational therapists, dentists, those in professions allied to medicine, sociologists, managers, administrators and politicians all come into the account of events but also all need an acquaintance with the development of the health services in Britain which this book seeks to map out. In recent years, trends in health and social care have emphasized the need for many of these groups to work together, so particular attention has been given to collaborative developments between a wide range of health and welfare professionals alongside the place of patients, users and clients.

For all readers, the plan has been to present an account of health care provision in Britain, but more particularly in England and Wales, from 1900 to the year 2000, together with a twentieth-century vision of the twenty-first century. Up to the mid-1990s, points of interest and relevance to Scotland and, more briefly, to Northern Ireland, have been included. Certain tables also refer to all four parts of the United Kingdom. The analysis has focused on England and Wales because the organization of health care has differed significantly from that of Northern Ireland. Here different traditions have prevailed under a Parliament in Stormont which has exercised considerable autonomy, with direct rule from Westminster for 20 years until 1998, when a new directly elected Assembly was introduced. One notable difference dates from 1973, when the Province was organized into four Health and Social Services Boards which were accountable to the Secretary of State for Northern Ireland. The provision of health and social services was therefore combined. As the problems associated with the structural division of health and social care have escalated in Britain, the pathway in Northern Ireland seemed to contain a solution. Chapter 12 looks in further detail at the various options and proposals for integrated services in England and Wales, together with some reasons for their rejection. In Northern Ireland, health and social services teams have tended to be loyal to professional groups which has somewhat reduced the potential for integration.

By 1997, New Labour's approach, to the health and social services structural faultline in Britain, sought to emphasize joint working and partnership, as Chapter 14 explores. However, under New Labour's proposal for devolution, significant changes have taken place; therefore consideration has been given in Chapter 14 to the particular implications for the provision of health care in England, Wales, Scotland and Northern Ireland. More fundamentally, as devolution takes shape in the twenty-first century (Webster, 1998: 213), the opportunity has begun to open up for all four health care systems to diverge according to the wishes of the respective electorates. The question then remains as to whether divergence could undermine the basic principles of the NHS.

Appendix 2 sets out briefly the earlier background on the NHS organizational developments in Scotland and Northern Ireland. The further reading section provides a relevant list of publications. *Health and Welfare States of Britain: An Inter-Country Comparison*, a comparative study by Arthur Williamson and Graham Room, published by Heinemann in 1983, is helpful for those who wish to pursue the topic of the health services across the UK, as is Ruth Levitt, Andrew Wall and John Appleby's updated book *The Reorganized National Health Service*, published in 1999.

The present account opens with a review of the pre-war health care. A wider social policy perspective is then set out to show how and why the NHS emerged amidst the post-war Welfare State outcomes. Looking at the key issues which subsequently dominated the NHS, the background to a seemingly ongoing financial crisis is traced. Was there an alternative way forward? Has there been a more financially effective way to provide health care services? Importantly, health care systems abroad are reviewed at two stages, first with a mid-way assessment by the end of the 1980s (Chapter 7), then with a later overview by the end of the 1990s (Chapter 11), together with a look at the implications of Britain's involvement with the European Union.

The key NHS reforms are charted where matters of management (Chapter 5) and quality (Chapter 10) are featured. The increasing recognition of the place of service users is considered in Chapter 10 and with the wider perspective of caring in the community in Chapter 12. By the early 1990s, the theme of health promotion and preventative policies assumed a significantly wider role which is acknowledged in Chapter 13. The whole of Chapter 14 is devoted to the widespread changes under New Labour as the momentum into the twenty-first century is brought into focus in Chapter 15, where the place of health care professionals for the present is discussed together with the significant factors for the future. Key NHS issues that are likely to make a major impact at the start of the twenty-first century in Britain are then lined up. To understand the wider background of trends, changes and events, a social policy context is provided to set the developments in health and welfare alongside broader socio-economic issues. Four social policy models are explored in Chapter 16, to assess the advantages and disadvantages of different approaches to health care provision over the twentieth century.

Special thanks are due, for speedy help, to Chris Baker at the Audit Commission; Rebecca Rees at the Research Council for Complementary Medicine; Dr David Peters at the Centre for Community Care and Primary Health, University of Westminster; Irene Lambeth at the Department for Education and Employment; and Paul Simpson, Chief Executive of the Health and Social Services Executive, at the Department of Health and Social Services, Northern Ireland. From the experience of 7 years at Hull University and 20 years at South Bank University, this book has sought to convey sharing with students the interest, challenge and lively debate surrounding health care provision and social policy. Overall, my intent is to provide easy reading, to inform, to interest, and above all, to enjoy.

Audrey Leathard
Visiting Professor of Interprofessional Studies, South Bank University
Autumn 1999

ACKNOWLEDGEMENTS

The author and publisher would like to thank the following for permission to reproduce previously published material:

Audit Commission; Austin, David; Blackwell Publishers Inc.; Breeeze, Hector; Calman, Claire and Stephanie; Daily Telegraph (Telegraph Group Limited) and DT Matt; Department of Health; Djordjevic, Jovan; Evening Standard and Jak; Family Policy Studies Centre; Health Service Journal; Her Majesty's Stationery Office (crown copyright material reproduce with the permission of the Controller of Her Majesty's Stationery Office); King's Fund; Macmillan Press Ltd; Office for National Statistics; Office of Health Economics; Organisation for Economic Co-operation and Development; Punch (Punch Limited) and Illingworth; The Independent (Independent Newspapers (UK) Limited) and Nicholas Garland; The Times and The Sunday Times (News International Syndication) © Pugh/Times Newspapers Limited, 12/12/96 and 8/12/98; © Newman/Times Newspapers Limited, 25/5/97, 8/2/98, 14/6/98, 7/1/99 and 10/1/99.

Every attempt has been made to contact copyright holders and we apologise if any have been overlooked. Should copyright have been unwittingly infringed in this book, the owners should contact the publishers who will make corrections at reprint.

1 HEALTH CARE IN BRITAIN: PRE-WAR PROVISION, 1900–1939

Evolution, not revolution, has been the key factor in health care provision in Britain. Throughout the twentieth century transformations in health care have tended to unfold over time. The two world wars might have brought about abrupt change but even war only accelerated, rather than innovated, health care developments. This evolutionary change has also been markedly influenced by historical legacies. In order to trace past developments, the opening section provides a broad picture of how the nation set about caring for the health of its citizens before the Second World War and before the advent of the National Health Service in 1946.

THE PUBLIC HEALTH MOVEMENT

The most important area of state involvement in the provision of health services during the nineteenth century, in terms of the impact on people's health, was the enactment of public health legislation. Crisis situations, such as the cholera and typhoid outbreaks, posed a major threat to health at this time.

The main reason for the decline in infectious diseases and unsanitary conditions was not the advances in medical science but the developments in the system of public health, initiated by the first *Public Health Act* in 1848. The 1848 legislation enabled Local Boards of Health to be set up, with permissive powers to provide adequate water supplies, drainage, sewerage and street paving. Improvements were also due to Edwin Chadwick (and his supporters) who, as Secretary to the Poor Law Commission, was instrumental in establishing, by 1848, the General Board of Health to control the sanitary work of local authorities. Chadwick's public health campaigns were furthered by John Simon, Medical Officer to the Medical Department of the Privy Council, which succeeded the General Board in 1858. Developments were reinforced by the report of the Royal Sanitary Commission (1869–1871), which led to the formation of the Local Government Board in 1871, which was made responsible for the Privy Council's Medical Department. The Local Government Board both strengthened central and local administration and united the agencies concerned with problems of disease and poverty. One notable omission from the 1869–71 Commission's report was the field of occupational health, which remained outside the scope of mainstream health care policy throughout the next century.

A series of *Public Health Acts* from 1848 culminated in the comprehensive 1875 act, which brought together existing legislation on the sanitary conditions of life – from sewerage disposal and water supplies to street cleansing, food inspection and the provision of hospitals. Of particular importance, the preceding Act (in 1872) created sanitary authorities, who were obliged to provide public health services and, significantly, to appoint a Medical Officer of Health

(MOH), a sanitary inspector and a surveyor. In the years to come, the MOH was to play a key part in local authority health provision.

Of historical significance was the major contribution that improved environmental conditions made towards better health. However, the emphasis on public health was then to subside until the emergence of a new public health movement nearly 100 years later. By the end of the nineteenth century the state, particularly at local authority level, had taken on widespread responsibilities for public health measures, which were more to protect the community than to aid the sick individual.

THE DEVELOPMENT OF PERSONAL MEDICAL CARE

In contrast, the first half of the twentieth century saw the increasing assumption by the state of responsibility for the provision of health care for the individual. The driving factors included the following.

- Alarm at the poor physique of so many of the volunteers for the Boer War (1899–1901) triggered action.
- By 1904, the recommendations of an Interdepartmental Committee on Physical Deterioration led to the 1906 *Education (Provision of Meals) Act* and a school health service in 1907.
- The school health service, promoted by the reforming Liberal government elected in 1906, formed part of the government's wider social policy reforms, including the provision of non-contributory old age pensions in 1908.

All these elements acted as a precursor to the Welfare State legislation some 40 years later.

An important element of these Liberal reforms was Lloyd George's *National Insurance Act* in 1911. This legislation, which included some provision for general practitioner (GP) services, created an even greater precedent in state action. To understand its radical nature one has to appreciate that, at the beginning of the twentieth century, the development of public, voluntary and private health care was haphazard: need was dealt with as it was identified – piecemeal and according to financial means.

The background to health care

Rich people used the services of eminent or fashionable doctors whose income came largely from private practice, which had therefore to be nurtured. Although medical and surgical specialisms were growing in the teaching hospitals, the doctors in these fields were frequently used by their patients as GPs.

At the other end of the social scale, reinforced by the 1834 *Poor Law Amendment Act*, the Poor Law dominated the treatment of poor people until its abolition in 1948. At the beginning of the twentieth century, the Poor Law still rested on the assumption that public expenditure should be severely restricted and, if possible, reduced. Health care reformers therefore faced opposition to the demand for state-supported activity in preventive and curative medicine to reduce pauperism. Public health and personal medical activities were kept deliberately apart. Under the Poor Law, the destitute sick could be seen at home by the medical officers of the Board of Guardians but, owing to the prevailing principles of economy and deterrence, the service was often inadequate or too late. Outpatient advice and treatment were available to the needy who could present themselves at hospitals, charity clinics and public dispensaries without referral from family doctors.

In between the rich and the poor, most people were cared for by general practitioners for a fee. Owing to lack of specialized care, GPs often undertook surgical operations on their patients. Patients could choose their doctor; doctors were free to charge what they wished, but many had difficulty in extracting even small payments in poor areas. The problem of payment, especially when income was reduced by sickness, put a burden of decision on families about priorities: the wage earner and children came first in line for treatment, the housewife and aged members second. Some workers' friendly societies and provident clubs were formed to ensure that money would be available for members to cover medical costs when necessary.

The 1911 National Insurance Act introduced a radical change. For the very first time in medical care, the state entered into a contractual relationship with the individual through a compulsory national insurance scheme. The 1911 act provided for:

- free care from GPs for certain groups of working people earning under £160 per annum;
- income during sickness and unemployment;
- innovatively, the contractual nature of the scheme was based on contributions from the workers, the employer and the state.

Lloyd George had to push the 1911 Act through, in the face of opposition from the medical profession who were ever fearful of state control of their work and the financial consequences to themselves. These two issues have remained key factors in the medical mind throughout the subsequent history of health care in Britain. Doctors were persuaded into the scheme when the government agreed that payment should be based on the number of patients on a doctor's list – the capitation system, which preserved the GPs' independence – rather than on a salary (a method strongly rejected by GPs).

The 1911 compulsory national insurance scheme was to be administered, not by local authorities, but by 'approved societies' – as independent insurance committees or 'panels' – drawn from the insurance companies, friendly societies and trade unions, who had played a key part in cover against ill health. The GPs who chose to participate were known as 'panel' doctors; choice thereby safeguarded professional freedom. The financial fears of the profession were assuaged by generous levels of payment and by the exclusion of higher income groups, who thereby created a useful source of extra income for GPs.

At the start, national health insurance covered about one-third of the population. Following extensions to coverage, by the early 1940s more than half were covered, by which time about two-thirds of GPs were also taking part. One of the scheme's limitations was that it was available to insured workers only and not to their families, the self-employed, most of the unemployed nor to those engaged in non-manual occupations. This scheme was therefore designed specifically for employed members of the working class; the middle and upper classes were almost entirely excluded. Furthermore, the scheme did not provide a comprehensive range of benefits: for instance, no hospital nor specialist care was included. The Approved Societies varied in their resources and benefits (such as help with dental care and spectacles) and the whole system of health insurance proved cumbersome and costly. Nevertheless, the 1911 Act represented a major step forward in the involvement of the state in health care provision.

In the wake of the 1911 *National Insurance Act* and developments in hospital provision, the separation between general practice and hospital provision continued, however, particularly in urban areas, although rural GPs retained access to surgical facilities in the cottage hospitals. Alongside GP services, the delivery system for medical care was conducted through two further outlets: hospital and domiciliary provision, in both of which local authorities and voluntary bodies played a part. The divisions and patterns that had emerged by the inter-war years were to leave their own legacy to the National Health Service in the mid-1940s.

THE THREE MAIN SECTORS OF HEALTH CARE PROVISION

Table 1.1 provides a simplified map of the main sectors which provided health care, dating from the 1911 legislation which introduced national insurance for a limited section of the population. The pattern of provision remained along similar lines until 1948. It is significant that the services had already formed a pre-war tripartite pattern which was to evolve into the NHS.

Table 1.1 Health Care Provision in Britain: 1911–1948.

General practitioners	Local authorities	Hospitals
Private doctors	Domiciliary care	Municipal (run by local authorities from 1929)
Panel doctors under the National Health Insurance scheme	Care of elderly, mentally ill and mentally handicapped people	Teaching
		Voluntary

HOSPITAL SERVICES: PUBLIC PROVISION

The Poor Law had dominated the public provision of hospitals. The Poor Law principle of 'less eligibility' depended on the creation of a workhouse so unattractive as to discourage the poor from seeking relief.

Under the Poor Law, the destitute sick were treated or housed in infirmary wards or separate infirmaries under the Board of Guardians. Hospitals were partly founded to treat destitute sick and poor people but also to protect the community from the spread of infection. By 1905, most sick poor people received minimal medical care in unclassified institutions (often workhouses), where 'nursing' was still done by pauper inmates. However, the number of more modern purpose-built infirmaries with salaried medical staff, trained nurses and the latest hospital equipment was increasing, although such hospitals were ceasing to be regarded as a Poor Law service.

The 1929 *Local Government Act* marked the beginning of the end of the Poor Law. The act resulted in the transfer of the responsibility for workhouses and infirmaries to the local authority's health departments, which were under the control of the Medical Officer of Health – as were the public health services. The intention was to develop municipal general hospitals for sick people. By this time, qualified medical and nursing personnel were available and the standard of these hospitals became very high, but progress in their development up to the Second World War remained uneven. By the end of the 1930s there were about 1750 local authority hospitals of all types, including specialized hospitals for infectious diseases and tuberculosis (Ministry of Health, 1944). Local authorities generally levied charges for hospital services, fixed according to ability to pay: almost everywhere, it was possible for poor people to obtain the services free of charge or at purely normal rates. The facilities of these municipal hospitals were available to everyone, regardless of means, but the 1929 *Local Government Act* failed to remove the aura of the Poor Law or the class character of the system. Upper-income groups zealously avoided municipal hospitalisation whenever possible.

Institutional care therefore developed along several different unco-ordinated lines which tended to cater for different sections of the community. There was no form of central (or even local) planning. The municipal hospitals took over the treatment predominantly of the poor and lower-income groups. As medical techniques advanced, this feature somewhat diminished but was never relinquished. Voluntary hospitals, complemented by local authority provision, were the mainstay of hospital care.

VOLUNTARY HOSPITALS

The voluntary hospitals were the core of the hospital system in Britain before the National Health Service. As many local authorities were largely indifferent to their hospital responsibilities, the voluntary hospitals did most of the complex medical work, furnished virtually all the teaching facilities and contributed the major part of nurses' training. On the one hand, the upper-income groups were drawn to the best facilities that the hospital system had to offer. On the other hand, although the municipal hospitals were required by law to take in anyone needing treatment, excluding patients – other than on medical grounds – ran counter to the spirit of the voluntary system. Specialist treatment of lower-income groups was consequently financed by inordinately high charges to patients of middle and upper income groups. Enforced medical charity was therefore one method of funding voluntary provision.

It was, however, the means of financing the voluntary hospitals that increasingly proved to be the key problem in this sector. Income was derived from a variety of sources:

- some voluntary hospitals were endowed in medieval times, others in the eighteenth century;
- some became great medical teaching centres with unpaid specialist and consultant services;
- some were provided by trade unions for their members;
- others were small cottage hospitals serviced by local GPs.

Financed by voluntary donations, charitable input, endowments and later from patient's payments and insurance sources, the voluntary hospitals tended to treat acute conditions. The teaching hospitals encouraged the admission of interesting cases (for teaching material); the public hospitals were therefore left to receive the chronic sick and aged infirm.

Meanwhile, at a political level, in 1919 the Ministry of Health was established, which took over the Local Government Board's health functions. Christopher Addison, a doctor and Lloyd George's Minister of Reconstruction, became the first Minister of Health in 1919, although the powers of his new ministry were directed to a far broader span of administration than the health services, which were still in effect left to the doctors. As well as their role in the public hospitals, doctors played a key part in the voluntary hospitals.

Voluntarism was, however, increasingly in peril. In a period of rising costs following the First World War, the voluntary hospitals ran into severe financial difficulties. In 1921 a well connected committee of investigation, headed by Viscount Cave, recommended that £1 million should be allotted as a one-time subvention to assist voluntary hospitals. The government provided only half this sum and refused to make up the deficit. The future of voluntary hospitals looked bleak. By 1944 the thousand or more voluntary hospitals varied greatly in size, age, function, distribution and the services available. The proportion of patients being treated in the voluntary sector rose from 25% in 1921 to 36% by 1938, while the role of the public sector had dropped proportionately (Abel-Smith, 1964: 385). Nevertheless many voluntary hospitals – at least one-third according to a PEP (1937) report – faced bankruptcy.

HOSPITAL PROVISION FOR MENTAL ILLNESS AND MENTAL DEFICIENCY

In the nineteenth century, mentally ill people who needed care tended to be put into workhouses or in prison, if they could not pay for care in a private madhouse (although poor people were increasingly housed in county asylums, following legislation as early as 1808 – made mandatory in 1845). Mental illness was largely associated with stigma and destitution.

Legislation

Under the *Lunacy Act* of 1890, local authorities had a duty to provide hospitals for those of unsound mind or mental subnormality. The 1890 Act was concerned with the legal status of the patient and the regulations governing admissions, detention and discharge. Personal care, attention and treatment were curtailed by shortage of staff, the large numbers needing admissions and the slow development of psychiatry.

The 1913 *Mental Deficiency Act* was passed following the recommendations of the 1908 Royal Commission on Mental Deficiency. The 1913 Act defined mental deficiency primarily as a social condition (in terms of idiots, imbeciles, feeble-minded and moral defectives). The 1913 definitions marked, at this stage, a measure of achievement as, with some agreed degree of exactitude, greater discussion and recognition of the problems led to further social and medical research.

The 1913 legislation also set up a Central Board of Control (superseding the Lunacy Commissioners). The Central Board of Control made possible the expansion and development of provision through the work of local authority Mental Deficiency Committees.

By 1920, a new era of interest in mental illness had begun. Psychoanalysis was helping a limited number of neurotic patients and clinical psychiatric teaching started slowly to develop when, in 1907, the Maudsley teaching hospital was endowed for this purpose. A few other voluntary hospitals, such as St Thomas' in London, started psychiatric outpatient clinics.

By the 1930s, psychiatry had begun to provide more effective treatment. In 1930, the *Mental Treatment Act* strengthened the Board of Control, abolished outmoded terminology and encouraged people to seek early treatment by allowing for voluntary admission to mental hospitals and for public hospitals to have outpatient clinics. By 1944, the government estimated that some 100 public hospitals were caring for 130 000 mentally ill patients, but that there were also about 125 000 persons of unsound mind in other local authority hospitals and public assistance institutions (Jones, 1960: 119).

Overall, the development of mental health services was both divided and uneven. Some local authorities had developed services for mentally ill people but had neglected those with mental deficiency; some had neglected both. The dichotomy between these two aspects of provision persisted, while community services – outpatients clinics, domiciliary social work visits and occupational centres – assumed increasing importance. The Ministry of Health exercised little central control, apart from a financial overview; the initiative remained with the more energetic local authorities. Between 1914 and 1939, ideas gradually changed about the care of mentally deficient and mentally ill people. There had been a swing away from the concept of permanent detention towards the growth of care in the community (Jones, 1960).

STAFFING THE HOSPITALS: THE TRAINING OF DOCTORS AND NURSES

Medical training

Until the twentieth century, hospitals were rather dangerous places to be in, largely due to fear of infection. Only in extreme cases could patients be persuaded to enter hospitals. For those who could afford it, illness was treated in the home, as hospitals had little to offer. Rapid developments in medical science and staff training changed this picture.

The *Medical Act* of 1858 secured the registration of doctors. The Act also established the General Council of Medical Education and registration, which laid down minimum requirements for qualifications and kept a register of practitioners. However, while the qualified doctor was identified and standards of training were supervised, the standard of care was often limited by the patient's financial means. Furthermore divisions in practice persisted. The physicians and surgeons had access to the hospital beds and undertook all the clinical teaching of students, while general practitioners worked in the community. To represent their interests, maintain standards and create exclusive powerful groups, separate Royal Colleges were developed (of Physicians in 1518, of Surgeons in 1800 and of General Practitioners, much later in 1952).

Nurse training

Although the 1902 *Midwives Act* regulated registration for midwives, it was not until 1919 that nurses succeeded in winning registration by Acts of Parliament. Developments were spearheaded by the newly formed College of Nursing (supported by the nurse training schools), which set out in 1916 to promote the better education and training of nurses and the advancement of nursing as a profession. Three *Nurses Registration Acts* in 1919 led to the establishment of the General Nursing Councils in England, Wales and Scotland. These Acts secured major gains for nursing: the concept of registration was finally acknowledged and enshrined in statute; training was guaranteed by legislation; and the responsibility for exercising these powers was vested in bodies, most of whose members were elected by the professionals. Nevertheless, this did not mean that all women acting as nurses were trained to the General Nursing Council standard and registered: many were assistant nurses with little but practical experience.

The 1919 legislation was influenced by what had happened in the nineteenth century. In an attempt to make nursing a respectable career for women, reformers tied it to the ideal of Victorian womanhood, supervised within a closed institution and subordinated to the male profession of medicine. However, at the insistence of Florence Nightingale – whose own training school was started in 1860 – the profession was under the control of trained matrons. Embodying the 'virtues' of servility and loyalty in return for little financial reward but potential prestige and stable employment, nursing entered the twentieth century as an underpaid occupation with long hours of work and a comparatively short working life. Despite parliamentary modifications to the restrictive plans and attitudes held by the professionally conscious lady nurses, the outcome of the 1919 legislation was educational standards that were too strict to yield enough nurses to meet all demands (Abel-Smith, 1960: 242).

The College of Nursing also identified the need for post-basic education for nurses. The College therefore set up its own education department to develop courses beyond the limits of basic nurse training. In 1928, the College was incorporated by Royal Charter and, by 1939, had been granted the title 'Royal'.

THE DEVELOPMENT OF DOMICILIARY CARE

Nursing care in the home: the district nurse

When, in 1919, the battle to secure state registration for nurses had finally been won, against a background of rampant snobbery and militant feminism (Abel-Smith, 1960), it was anticipated that district nurses – or Queen's Nurses as they were then known – would register. However they did not and nursing care in the home developed along its own lines.

The pioneering work of William Rathbone in Liverpool led, in 1859, to the emergence of the first professional community nursing service (Stocks, 1960). In 1887, the Queen Victoria Jubilee Institute for Nurses was founded, using money donated to celebrate the Queen's Jubilee, to further district nursing and domiciliary work nationally. In 1925, the name was changed to the Queen's Institute of District Nursing.

The Institute co-ordinated the work of the local voluntary nursing committees and sought to maintain the high standards of training and practice. Indeed, the Charter of the Institute in 1928 stated the objects as being the training, support, maintenance and supply of women to act as nurses for the sick poor. Gradually the service extended to all sick people in their homes. By 1947, men were able to train as district nurses. Although local authorities had the power to provide home nurses – usually only for expectant or nursing mothers, children or patients suffering from infectious diseases – most home nursing services were provided by voluntary district associations funded by donations.

The care of mothers and infants: the role of the midwife and the health visitor

As maternal mortality remained high and the infant mortality rate continued unchanged at 150 per 1000 live births throughout the nineteenth century, from the start of the twentieth century, state concern increased for the health of mothers and young children. Pressure from the Midwives Institute (founded in 1881 and later to become the Royal College of Midwives) and the belief that the lack of midwifery skills was a causal factor in the high infant and maternal mortality rates resulted in legislative change in 1902.

Primarily for the protection of the public, the 1902 *Midwives Act* therefore laid down standards for training; established a Central Midwives Board to oversee registration; ensured a minimum of three months' professional training; and prohibited untrained women from practising. Qualified midwives worked either as private practitioners or for voluntary nursing associations. The local supervision of registration was the responsibility of the Medical Officer, whose office was becoming increasingly powerful.

The trend was reinforced by the 1907 *Notification of Births Act*, one aim of which was to develop health visiting as a local authority service. Local authority employment and training of health visitors in maternal guidance and education and the preventive health care of children had until then been haphazard. The 1907 Act enabled progressive Medical Officers of Health to obtain early information about the birth of a child by arranging for a home visit by a responsible health department officer. Some of these visitors were trained nurses, others were regarded as qualified for this work through their experience as 'social workers', but they all became known as health visitors. By 1918, the number of health visitors employed by local authorities had increased to 3038 (Frazer, 1950: 412).

Several schools for health visitors were established in the first 20 years of the century, but the standards of training varied. In 1925, the Ministry of Health became responsible for training, the Royal Sanitary Institute (later renamed the Royal Society of Health) was appointed as the central examining body and health visitors became a recognized body of trained women. In 1929, the Local *Government Act* required the issuing of statutory rules setting out the qualifications of health visitors. The first major steps towards becoming a profession had been taken: the provision of qualifications and standard training.

Meanwhile, spurred on by the 1918 *Maternity and Child Welfare Act*, local authorities began to provide a further range of services for expectant and nursing mothers and children under five. These included antenatal clinics, infant welfare centres, maternity homes, employment of health visitors and theregistration of midwives. The 1918 *Midwives Act* went on to authorize local authorities to make grants available towards the training of midwives.

Furthermore, in the face of massive opposition to birth control (largely on religious grounds), concerted pressure group action from various elements of the birth-control movement finally persuaded the Ministry of Health in 1930 to concede, through Memorandum 153/MCW, that local authorities could give birth control instruction to mothers whose health would be injured by further pregnancy. Surrounded by controversy, clinic instruction and information was largely undertaken by a voluntary body, the National Birth Control Association, renamed the Family Planning Association in 1939 (Leathard, 1980).

In contrast to fertility control, maternal mortality was perceived as a major health issue. Continuing concern about the high rate of maternal deaths, revealed in the 1930 and 1932 reports of the Departmental Committee on maternal mortality and morbidity, led to the expansion of antenatal clinics and, after the 1936 *Midwives Act*, to the development of a local authority salaried midwifery service, of which most self-employed midwives became a part.

Overall, developments in domiciliary care took place on a piecemeal basis, involving both local authority and voluntary bodies, largely prompted by the concern with maternal and child health.

DENTAL CARE

Apart from extractions, dental care was almost unknown among the working population. Little was done to improve matters except in the maternity and child welfare services and in the School Health Service. Started in 1907, the School Health Service was a direct result of the discovery of the poor standards of health and fitness of army recruits for the Boer War. The army medical examinations for the First World War continued to confirm the widespread effects of lack of dental care. However, popular indifference, shortage of trained staff and their uneven distribution in a fee-paying service combined to keep dental services minimal. There was little charitable provision for dental care apart from the teaching hospitals. Dental education and dental care were still lacking, by the mid-1940s, when the National Health Service inherited a legacy of need – especially for dentures – that was far greater than imagined.

DOMICILIARY CARE FOR MENTALLY ILL AND MENTALLY DEFECTIVE PEOPLE

Progress was slow. Unsystematic and inadequate provision was hampered by a lack of knowledge of the causal factors and effects of mental deficiency. There was a need for institutional care other than in workhouses and for training and special educational facilities. In 1913, the *Mental Deficiency Act* set up mental deficiency committees in local authorities to provide institutional care, supervision, guardianship, training and occupation. In 1929, these committees took over responsibility for pauper defectives from the Poor Law Board of Guardians. Legislation in 1927 further stressed the duties of local authorities under the 1913 Act, as many were still evading their responsibilities for provision, because much of the legislation was permissive rather than mandatory.

Many voluntary agencies were founded to offer inpatient care, training, aftercare and supervision and to whom local authorities often delegated their community care work. The Central Association for Mental Welfare was the most widely known voluntary agency which not only carried out statutory supervision but also ran occupation centres and employed home teachers. Overall, however, the quality of domiciliary care was variable and unevenly distributed.

PRE-WAR LEGACIES

Up until the outbreak of the Second World War the provision of health care in Britain gently evolved in a piecemeal fashion. The First World War produced no revolution, no radical break with former patterns, but revealed deficiencies in the organization of the nation's health services. Failings in the health of the people were also revealed. The high proportion of men rejected for active service had established the need for better preventive and promotive services. The war had also provided a severe test for the administration of the country, both central and local, and the machinery of local government had been found inadequate. Despite subsequent reform, in both health care organization and local government, the stigma of the Poor Law remained, regardless of the higher standards in the public infirmaries. Hospital policy was based on two classes of patients: the private patient who paid the whole cost and the ward patient who paid what could be afforded.

While the policy of the Poor Law was to deter, the principle of public health services was to prevent. In the nineteenth century, sanitation, personal cleanliness and environmental ordering had reduced the incidence of cholera, typhus and other infectious diseases. In the first half of the twentieth century, the communal care of mothers and children and medical inspection of schoolchildren sought to raise standards of health and physical fitness in the community. However, although in a variety of ways responsibility for the provision of health care had been increasingly taken over by the state, developments had produced a pattern of unco-ordinated, inadequate and unevenly distributed services, delivered by a variety of bodies. The Second World War was to speed up events and confront these shortcomings and legacies.

2 THE CREATION OF THE NATIONAL HEALTH SERVICE: THE ROAD TO 1946

The National Health Service came into existence on 5 July 1948. Over the previous 100 years the battle against ill health in Britain had been fought on four main fronts and in overlapping phases.

- Initially, attention focused on environmental improvement and preventive public health measures.
- Advances in medical science then turned concern to the treatment of the sick.
- A more personal approach evolved for the protection and improvement of maternal and child welfare.
- By 1911, legislation had increased state responsibility for individual health insurance and access to health services.

This process culminated in the creation of the National Health Service.

The developments that led up to the 1946 NHS legislation can be more fully understood by looking at three key issues: the wider background of the Welfare State, the health care systems in 1939 and the specific proposals for health service reform.

THE BACKGROUND TO THE WELFARE STATE

Widespread legislation was passed in the 1940s that laid the foundation of the post-war Welfare State, although the process and pressure for reform had been evolving for decades. In the mid-nineteenth century, rationalism of the Benthamite tradition advocated state action to promote the greatest happiness of the greatest number: the principle of utility. 'Utilitarianism' favoured radical reform in political justice, health and education.

Meanwhile, differing philosophies and value systems sought to make an impact.

- Rationalist philosophers opposed unnecessary suffering; evangelical Christians believed in a God of love. Both philosophies had an essential humanitarian element.
- Individualistic philosophy, characteristic of Protestant religious leaders and free thinkers alike, opposed government control and collective action.
- The Tories believed in the value of paternalism.
- The working-class movement believed in the effectiveness of collective action.

Throughout the nineteenth century, each of these elements struggled for expression in legislation, set against three prevailing doctrines.

- Individualism contended that poverty was the fault of the individual.
- Laissez-faire stemmed from a deterministic economic theory which stressed the inability of government action to change the position of poor people.
- A market economy approach left the flow of goods and services to forces of the market.

Gradually the humanitarian elements were reinforced by the pressure of events. The Victorian origins of the Welfare State and British collectivism could be traced back to the response to the squalor, ill health and disease in the overcrowded towns, coupled with the administrative reforms in central and local government, the emergence of an efficient civil service and the introduction of inspectors in factories, mines, public health and education. These developments contained a dynamic which led inevitably to the extension of state intervention.

At the start of the twentieth century, the concept of utility began to be replaced by the concept of collective action in social welfare reform. Collectivism had been spurred on by the growing strength of the working-class movements: the development of the trade unions, the extension of the Parliamentary franchise to working class men in 1867, the emergence of Labour MPs in 1906 and the permeating influence of the reformist Fabian Society. The rise of British socialism called for collective action rather than individual solutions to overcome the inefficiency and injustice of a free market capitalist economy.

Public shock at a series of issues also prompted stirrings for social reform.

- The surveys of Booth in London in 1889 (Booth, 1903) and Rowntree in York in 1899 (Rowntree, 1901) had decisively shown that the greatest causes of poverty were low wages and interrupted earnings due to sickness, unemployment and old age.
- The idea that most poor people were responsible for their own condition was therefore no longer tenable.
- The poor level of physical health and nutrition among the (1899–1901) Boer War recruits.

A Royal Commission was set up in 1904 to consider the operation of the Poor Law. In 1909, the Commission produced a majority report which recommended retention of the Poor Law with modifications. However, a minority report that reflected the views of the influential Fabians, Sidney and Beatrice Webb, significantly proposed breaking up the Poor Law and the institution of various services such as a unified health service run by local authorities. Modified, the views of this minority report prevailed in the long run.

The immediate outcome of these pressures was that the 1906 Liberal government produced a programme of welfare legislation. Despite these advances, gaps in the assistance required, to meet the needs, remained. Subsequent legislation attempted to improve on measures of help, but the inter-war years were overshadowed by the problem of unemployment, which at times reached 20% of the population. The industrial depression curtailed resources for social services and weakened the power of the Labour party and trades unions to bring about further reform. However, mass unemployment revealed the inadequacy of the Poor Law to deal with the problem of poverty.

Furthermore, the assumptions underlying the provision of social services were being questioned. Economic growth by itself was seen as no solution without a redistribution of wealth; charity could only touch the fringe of the problem of needy and deprived people; and encouraging individuals to be thrifty was a long process unlikely to succeed for those on low incomes. It was increasingly felt that the only really effective way forward was for the state to commit itself to dealing with the socio-economic problems and, where possible, to try to prevent them.

The Second World War accelerated rather than initiated the process of change. As Richard Titmuss (1950) recognized, in his history of wartime social policy, it required the war experience to transform the whole mood, if not the pattern of interests, which sustained Britain's existing health services. The methods of meeting the needs of citizens, exposed to total war and its levelling effect, profoundly influenced the outcome of post-war provision. In the climate of sharing risks, resources and austerity, radical measures became more readily acceptable.

Wide-reaching legislation in the 1940s fundamentally altered the whole social welfare perspective by rationalizing and nationalizing services. The main features are set out in Table 2.1. Overall, these social service measures, largely introduced by the Labour government in the early post-war years, contained similar aims throughout. The measures included, in varying degrees, a move towards rationalized, comprehensive, universal social services in which the state accepted increasing responsibility for the welfare of its citizens, underpinned by a full employment policy. However, two types of welfare system were effectively introduced. Family allowances, education and health care were to be financed collectively through taxation and thus free at the point of use. The social security scheme introduced an alternative model of a partnership between the state/ employer and the individual to protect against loss of earnings through compulsory National Insurance.

The social security measures followed the recommendations of the widely acclaimed Beveridge Report in 1942 on *Social Insurance and Allied Services*, which were largely adopted under the 1946 *National Insurance Act*, the 1946 *National Industrial Injuries Act* (and the 1945 *Family Allowances Act* whose arrangements were not insurance based, see Table 2.1). Under the social security scheme, individual contributions and benefits were to be flat rate, regardless of size of income, and paid out at an adequate or subsistence level (a national minimum), as of right. The flat rate approach reflected the wartime levelling effect but, in seeking to alleviate poverty through providing financial cover for loss of earnings, the insurance system was based on a time-honoured work ethic, underpinned by gender assumptions about the role of the breadwinner. Financed by contributions from employer, employee and the State, the Beveridge scheme introduced three radical innovations: it was to be administratively unified, universal in coverage and comprehensive in scope (Beveridge Report, 1942). The

Table 2.1   Key elements of the Welfare State in Britain 1944–1949.

Legislation	Purpose	Principles and Organization
1944 *Education Act*	To combat ignorance	Free, universal education for children, according to their age, aptitude and ability, organized by Local Education Authorities at primary, secondary and further education levels, financed by taxation and headed by Ministry of Education
1945 *Family Allowances Act*	To alleviate child poverty	A universal system of payments for each child, after the first, up to leaving school. Financed by general taxation
1946 *National Insurance Act*	To attack want and to alleviate poverty	(1) Everyone of working age insured, except for some non-employed but including married women securing entitlement through their husband's contributions (2) Every contributor classified as employee, self-employed or non-employed (3) Entitlements provided to cover prime causes of need from the 'cradle to the grave' for maternity, sickness, unemployment, widowhood, retirement and death (4) State, employer and flat-rate employee contributions and benefits. Abolished the Poor Law
1946 *National Industrial Injuries Act*	To help loss of earnings	Financial cover for employees injured at work
1948 *National Assistance Act*	To alleviate poverty	Means-tested, taxation-based, to provide a financial safety net for those either inadequately or not covered by insurance. Local authorities to provide care, assistance and rehabilitation for elderly, mentally ill and disabled people together with a duty to provide housing for homeless people
1946 *National Health Service Act*	To combat disease	Universal, comprehensive services, free at the point of use and financed by taxation; National Insurance covered a small element
1946 *Housing Act*		General housing subsidies introduced largely to place the emphasis for building (council houses to let) upon local authorities
1947 *Town and Country Planning Act*		Enabled the government to control the physical environment
1949 *Housing Act*	To combat squalor	Local authorities empowered to make grants for property improvement or conversion. Council housing was no longer to be confined to 'the working class'

1948 *National Assistance Act* formally abolished the Poor Law and, through the newly established National Assistance Board gave means-tested assistance, financed by taxation, to those in poverty.

In many respects, the new social services were a natural development of the past. The services were an extension of policies that had evolved piecemeal and had been accepted. Previous institutions and methods were therefore used. Two key new elements arose. First, the universal character of the provision – covering the whole population – received support partly from the sense of national unity which persisted for a time after the war. Secondly, the acceptance by the state of a much fuller responsibility for the determination of social policy. It was acknowledged that social and economic planning would be needed and that the state could no longer simply fill in the gaps left by private enterprise in the market economy or by the voluntary bodies in social welfare provision. Overall, the concept of the Welfare State was to move away from the stigmatization and deterrence of the Poor Law towards the notion of a citizen's right to social services, to be claimed at the point of need and supported by collective action.

The Beveridge Report (1942) spoke of 'five giants' on the road of post-war reconstruction: disease, ignorance, squalor, idleness and want. The aim of the Welfare State legislation was to combat these evils. The *National Health Service Act* in 1946 therefore formed part of this wider process of social change and reform which specifically addressed the giant of 'disease'. Each element in the Welfare State contained its own historical impetus. To understand the build-up of pressure for reform in the health services, the positive and negative features of pre-war provision need to be summarized.

ACHIEVEMENTS AND SHORTCOMINGS IN HEALTH CARE PROVISION UP TO 1939

By the outbreak of the Second World War, successes in health protection included:

- virtual elimination of diseases such as cholera and typhus;
- significant reduction in deaths from other killer diseases, such as tuberculosis;
- maternal and infant mortality rates were falling (for example, from 151 per 1000 live births in 1901 to 46 per 1000 in 1939);
- fall in the overall death rate, from 17.1 per 1000 in 1900 to 12 per 1000 in 1939;
- increase in the average life span from 45 years in 1900 to 60 years or more by 1939

By 1948, the pre-war National Health Insurance system covered half the population who had a right to choose a GP and use the free drugs prescribed.

However, the first drawback was that more than half the population was not covered by this scheme – children, wives not in paid work, the self-employed, higher paid employees and many old people. Cumbersome and costly, the system contained marked variations and uncertainties about the insurance provision of additional benefits (e.g. dental and ophthalmic care). Entitlement depended on where you lived and your health history. Worst of all, it excluded hospital and specialist treatment.

Secondly, specialist and GP services were unevenly distributed. As most of a GP's total earnings came from private patients, practitioners were heavily concentrated in the more affluent neighbourhoods. Fee-paying also encouraged a two-tier system: some GPs had separate waiting rooms for 'panel' patients and private fee-paying patients.

Thirdly, adequacy and efficiency in the local authority health services varied considerably. On paper the range of services was impressive. To a widely varying extent, local authorities provided antenatal and postnatal clinics, welfare centres and health visitors to give advice in the home. Midwives were employed either by local authorities or by voluntary organizations. Local authorities also had other major functions, including overall care and treatment of mental illness and mental handicap, clinics for venereal diseases and hospital care (largely for the chronically sick, for infectious diseases and tuberculosis). By 1939, local authorities provided about four-fifths of all the hospital beds in Britain. However, marked disparities were due to differences in resources, the multiplicity and division of local government and division of authorities, the enterprise of the local councils and the interpretation of permissive legislation. Overall, there was little cohesion or co-ordination.

Finally, the hospital services were also unevenly distributed because they depended on the existence of fee-payers and on local authority and voluntary effort (street collections and charity), the overall outcome of which was both unreliable and unco-ordinated. The most glaring deficiency in the hospital service was the shortage of beds, aggravated by an understaffed nursing force. Although the supply of nurses was increasing, it did not keep pace with demand. Hospital waiting lists were long and abuses occurred, ranging from queue-jumping to the failures of GPs to call in consultants soon enough. Furthermore, there was much unfriendly rivalry between the municipal and voluntary hospitals. No effort was made either to integrate facilities or develop them to serve the needs of the people. In the light of the medical knowledge at the time and the state of the national economy, Powell's (1997: 37) evaluation of health care before the NHS was that institutions ranged from good to scandalous.

The drawbacks of the pre-war system could be summarized under five headings.

1 Shortage of facilities and trained staff.
2 Inequitably distributed services, both geographically and functionally.
3 Uneconomic use of services arising from irrational organization.
4 Lack of adequate funds, making any significant expansions impossible.
5 The persistence of unsatisfactory clinic conditions.

Overall, the administrative structure of the existing health services was complex, ineffective and lacking in central organization and planning. It was, however, the money barrier that lay at the root of consumer anxiety. Doctors' bills generated by serious illness could be financially catastrophic for middle-class patients, who had incomes that were likely to be above the entitlement to free services, but who were not necessarily covered by the barely developed private insurance schemes. On the other hand, while free or partly free services of varying quality were available to lower income groups, there was a deep-seated reluctance to use the 'Poor Law' service. Many health conditions deteriorated due to inadequate medical services and delay in seeking treatment. Reports increasingly drew attention to all these deficiencies and strengthened the case for a National Health Service.

THE BUILD-UP TO THE NATIONAL HEALTH SERVICE

A series of reports in the inter-war period called for the co-ordination and conso-lidation of service provision. Set up to make proposals to the Ministry of Health for improving health care organization, the Dawson Committee (1920) recom-mended the provision of comprehensive medical, preventive and curative services in a network of primary and secondary health centres, administered by a single authority in each locality. However, these far-sighted recommendations stopped short of a free national health service. The 1926 Royal Commission on National Health Insurance (1928), the 1937 Sankey Commission on Voluntary Hospitals, the report on the *British Health Services* from PEP (1937), and the British Medical Association's (BMA) (1929 and 1938) published views, all pointed to the shortcomings in the existing patterns of services. Their proposals for change included:

- the need for the greater co-ordination of hospitals on a regional basis;
- the extension of health insurance to other groups in the population;
- the possibility of funding the health service from general taxation rather than based on the insurance principle (suggested by the Royal Commission but opposed by the BMA).

The BMA, speaking from knowledge and experience, but also with an entrenched corporate interest, proposed no basic changes but put the family doctor in the centre of the delivery system.

The Second World War gave new momentum to reforms hitherto fiercely resisted. The idea of a fully fledged state health service was increasingly being promoted by individuals and groups: the Fabian Society, the Labour party and a group of doctors who formed themselves into the Socialist Medical Association (SMA) in 1930.

- The SMA pressed for medical services to be administered by local authorities, free of charge, with full-time state-employed doctors, health centres and large district hospitals (SMA, 1933).
- The Labour party's (1943) proposals, drawn up in close association with the SMA, were along similar lines.
- The BMA was more cautious: GPs disliked the idea of a salaried service;

specialists were afraid that a state medical service might threaten their private practice. By 1942, the BMA's Medical Planning Commission argued for a centrally planned comprehensive public health service, a regionalized hospital service and general practice organized in health centres, but the BMA remained wedded to the idea of extending health insurance cover to excluded groups.

The outbreak of the Second World War found the hospitals unable to cope with new and urgent demands. The government met the crisis by creating, in 1939, an Emergency Medical Service for war casualties (financed by the Exchequer) which had the power, under the control of the Ministry of Health, to direct all hospitals to secure widespread rationalized regionally based provision. From the experience of planning on a nation-wide uniform basis, there was no question of a return to the pre-war inadequacies.

The first major statement of post-war policy was contained in the Beveridge Report in 1942. Though dealing primarily with social security, the report drew attention to the need for a national system of health services. Although no details were given for the prevention and cure of disease, the report placed health policy in the context of general social policy. The government's attention consequently turned from hospitals to the planning of a general health service. The Beveridge Report caught the public's imagination; the coalition government was therefore increasingly committed to action; the principle of a NHS was virtually accepted. The question was now one of form.

The movement for change gathered momentum. In March 1943, the Ministry of Health presented a draft plan for a unified service. In 1944, a revised plan appeared in the White Paper *A National Health Service* (Ministry of Health, 1944), which outlined the public provision of a comprehensive medical service, available to all, democratically controlled through Parliament and elected local authorities but which took account of professional views. By now, most agreed on the principles of the new service which reflected recognition of the need for change. However, putting these principles into practice embroiled the government and the medical profession in four years of conflict and contention.

Prolonged negotiations over control and organization therefore preceded the start of the service. A Gallup poll in the summer of 1944 revealed that most doctors were opposed to the White Paper which, they believed, would make medicine less attractive as a profession and would reduce the quality of health care. GPs were anxious to preserve their professional freedom and were opposed to any idea of a salaried service. Hospital doctors and specialists accepted payment by salary but fiercely resisted local government control. Doctors feared municipalization more than nationalization

It was the Conservative Minister of Health, Henry Willinck, who had to face the first attacks and acrimonious feelings. Difficulties about pay, suspicions about their role and professional standards led to bitter clashes between the doctors and the subsequent Labour Health Minister, Aneurin Bevan, when he published his National Health Bill in 1946. As Asa Briggs (1978a: 386) has remarked: 'The road to 1946 lay straight through the general election of 1945'.

THE OUTCOME OF THE NEGOTIATIONS

The NHS came into existence in 1948 but embodied various concessions. The medical profession was successful in winning many of its objectives: the independent contractor system of GPs; the option of private practice and access to pay beds in NHS hospitals for hospital consultants; a system of distinction awards for consultants; a major role in the administration of the service at all levels; and success in resisting local government control. By securing the support of hospital consultants through generous payments, Aneurin Bevan said that he had 'stuffed their mouths with gold' (Abel-Smith, 1964: 480).

The local authorities and voluntary bodies were less successful. They lost control of their hospitals, which were to be placed under a single system of administration, despite Labour Minister Herbert Morrison's advocacy of the local government viewpoint. One major reason was the unsuitability of local authority areas for hospital administration. Furthermore, the complex network run by Approved Societies and insurance committees were to be rationalized away. The service was to be funded mainly out of general taxation: state-run insurance contributions were to be kept to a minimum.

The groups with skills to offer, particularly the medical profession, therefore did best (Willcocks, 1967). The groups with property to offer – local authorities and voluntary hospitals – lost their powerful position once the decision was made to nationalize their property. No organized group represented the users or potential users of the service: the one person therefore not to be represented in the negotiations was the patient.

The 1946 *National Health Service Act* provided a broad plan for merging all the various elements of the personal health services but excluded any form of industrial medical service (nor did it incorporate the armed forces' medical services which retained their own control). The intention of the Act was to uproot as little as possible but to extend all necessary services to those who wished to use them, irrespective of financial means. In the event, parliamentary debate was of less importance in policy formation than the influence of the major pressure groups and agencies. Overall, the attitude of the doctors played the most significant part in determining the final structure of the service.

The outcome of the NHS negotiations was essentially evolutionary: Bevan took over much of what had gone before. A tripartite structure was created from two previous systems (local authority and GP services), but one new feature was added: the transfer of the ownership of hospitals to introduce a nationalized hospital service. By then, the idea of unification had been abandoned. Political realities had overcome idealism. While embracing new developments, the National Health Service therefore represented a stage in an evolutionary process which expressed values and embodied traditions of long duration.

THE STRUCTURE OF THE NATIONAL HEALTH SERVICE IN 1948

The tripartite structure of the NHS (see Figure 2.1) was strongly shaped by historical legacy. The closest link was within the general practitioner services,

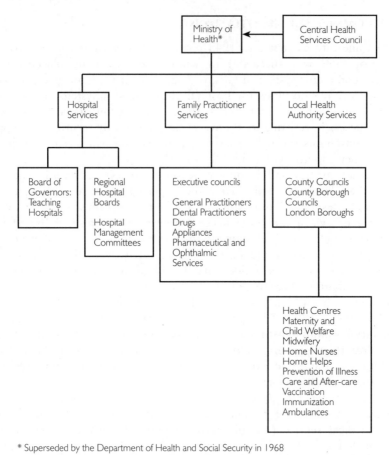

* Superseded by the Department of Health and Social Security in 1968

Figure 2.1   Structure of the National Health Service (England and Wales), 1948–1974.

along with services of dentists, opticians and pharmacists, which were administered by 134 Executive Councils who took over from the old insurance
committees. Funded directly by the Ministry of Health, the services were
provided by individual practitioners, paid under contract, on a capitation basis.

Still closely linked with the previous system, Local Health Authorities, at
county and county borough level, became responsible for a range of environmental and personal health services (as displayed in Figure 2.1). The key local
officer continued to be the Medical Officer of Health. Funding was partly
provided by central government grants and partly by local rates.

The hospital system was, however, to be administered by completely new
bodies: 14 (15 in 1959) Regional Hospital Boards (RHBs) in England and Wales
(each being associated with a university medical school and teaching hospital)
were to plan, provide and supervise services in the region. Under the RHBs were
some 400 Hospital Management Committees (HMCs) to undertake the day-to-

day administration. The HMCs were appointed by the RHBs who were, in turn, appointed by the Minister of Health. Special status was given to teaching hospitals: they retained their elite nature and were organized under Boards of Governors in direct contact with the Ministry of Health through the RHBs. Consultants and doctors were to be salaried although they could undertake some private work. Patients were to be referred to the hospitals by general practitioners.

Lastly, general control of the NHS rested with the Ministry of Health, advised by a Central Health Services Council and responsible to Parliament.

THE AIMS AND PRINCIPLES OF THE NATIONAL HEALTH SERVICE

The services were to be comprehensive in provision, universal in population coverage and free of charge at the point of use. The intention was to integrate, plan and distribute services more effectively, to enable equality of access to health care. Freedom of choice was upheld by doctors, who could choose or refuse patients, by patients who could change doctors, and by private practice, which was permitted so that neither patients nor doctors could complain.

The NHS started out with three operational objectives.

1 Adequate and rational public financing of services.
2 Rational control of service distribution.
3 Appropriate planning and co-ordination of workloads and service delivery, based on an effective doctor–patient relationship.

The NHS therefore came into being, not only to improve the distribution and volume of services to patients, but also to improve the services themselves.

In 1948, the NHS represented the values of rationality, efficiency and national equity which fundamentally contradicted the values of localism (responsiveness, differentiation and self-government) expressed through local government control. In Klein's (1983) view, these inherent contradictions were to bedevil the subsequent history of the NHS.

For Aneurin Bevan, however, on presenting the *National Health Service Bill* to the House of Commons on 30 April 1946, the intention was to 'universalize the best', to divorce the ability to secure the best health service and treatment from the ability to pay.

Above all, the 1946 *National Health Service Act* contained a vision of optimum standards of service. In contrast to the social security legislation of the time, which provided for a basic minimum, the new National Health Service aimed 'to secure improvement in the physical and mental health of the people and the prevention, diagnosis and treatment of illness' (Merrison Report, 1979: 8). The service was designed to meet health needs wherever and whenever they arose, although the NHS did not undertake an occupational health service or comprehensive family planning provision. *NHS was lacking!*

The question for the future was how far Bevan's vision of the optimum could be sustained.

3 THE FIRST 30 YEARS: DEVELOPMENTS IN THE NHS
1948–1976

Popular response to the National Health Service was overwhelmingly favourable. Shortly after the appointed day, 5 July 1948, some 97% of the population had been accepted by NHS doctors. Despite the fierce controversies over the preceding negotiations, up to 98% of GPs, 94% of dentists and virtually all pharmacists joined the scheme. Two major issues, however, dominated the newly formed NHS for the next three decades: finance and effective organization.

FINANCIAL RESOURCES

From the start, offering 'the best' was a challenging concept but an open-ended one. The running costs of the NHS were difficult to predict: health economics was then an unknown science. The health service was further hampered by financial restrictions and adverse economic conditions. Successive governments felt that expenditure had to be kept within proper boundaries. A decade of slow progress followed: with the building of few new hospitals; arguments about doctors' pay which encouraged their migration; and in the failure to allocate adequate resources to areas of deprivation (Briggs, 1978b).

The NHS estimates for the first full year of operations were well below the actual cost of £433 million (Table 3.1). Revised (increased) estimates were justified on the basis of the backlog; overwhelming demand for dentures and spectacles had been unforeseen. Actual costs seemed to increase alarmingly, in part due to the unexpected popularity of a comprehensive, free (of direct charge) health service but even more due to inflation.

In post-war Britain the basic economic problem was to provide adequate resources for the Welfare State. Straightened circumstances caused by the war and the subsequent 'cold' war, which required greatly accelerated military spending, adversely affected social services and health services in particular. Successive governments gave priority to the construction of houses and schools rather than hospitals. To supplement NHS income, charges were introduced for dentures and spectacles in 1951. Aneurin Bevan, along with Harold Wilson and John Freeman, resigned from Atlee's government in disgust. In 1952, charges for prescriptions and dental treatment, exemptions apart, were brought in. Professional and popular reaction to the charges was unfavourable because they threatened two of the basic NHS principles: universality and deployment of resources according to medical need.

While the problems remained, the paradoxes continued. The proportion of the gross domestic product absorbed by the NHS fell from 4.21 to 3.41 in the mid-1950s (Table 3.1). Further, it was the middle classes (and working-class wives) who actually benefited more in financial terms than any other section of the community. They had done the least well out of the pre-war services.

Table 3.1   NHS expenditure and gross domestic product, UK, 1949–1977.

			£ million			
Calendar year	NHS current	NHS capital	NHS other†	NHS total	GDP at factor cost	NHS total as percentage of GDP at factor cost
1949	414	15	4	433	10969	3.95
1950	458	16	4	478	11346	4.21
1951	476	17	6	499	12617	3.95
1952	476	15	6	497	13889	3.58
1953	500	16	5	521	14881	3.50
1954	515	18	4	537	15730	3.41
1955	555	20	4	579	16873	3.43
1956	609	20	4	633	18270	3.46
1957	655	26	4	685	19377	3.54
1958	694	29	5	728	20206	3.60
1959	750	34	4	788	21260	3.71
1960	819	37	5	861	22642	3.80
1961	879	44	5	928	24231	3.83
1962	909	55	7	971	25294	3.84
1963	968	60	7	1035	26894	3.85
1964	1047	76	7	1130	29255	3.86
1965	1176	91	8	1275	31237	4.08
1966	1290	102	9	1401	33139	4.23
1967*	1423	125	10	1558	34925	4.46
1968	1540	143	10	1693	37411	4.53
1969	1626	137	10	1773	39450	4.49
1970	1860	151	13	2024	43445	4.66
1971	2104	181	14	2299	49264	4.67
1972	2413	223	14	2650	54963	4.82
1973	2706	277	30	3013	63946	4.71
1974	3622	296	16	3934	73722	5.34
1975	4903	366	30	5299	92507	5.73
1976	5788	425	23	6236	109499	5.70
1977	6477	393	27	6897	123353	5.59

*Up to 1966 NHS current expenditure includes an imputed rent element; from 1967; this is replaced by a charge for non-trading capital consumption.
†Includes current grants to the personal sector and abroad and capital grants to the personal sector and to companies.

Source: Merrison Report (1979: 431).

Nevertheless, the main concern of the 1950s remained that of rising costs. Set up in 1953, the Guillebaud Committee was asked to look into the cost of the National Health Service. The Committee's report, published in 1956, did much to allay public anxiety. Using research carried out by Richard Titmuss and Brian Abel-Smith, the Committee concluded that there was no evidence of extravagance nor inefficiency in the NHS. The Committee felt that more money, not less, should be allocated to the health service, particularly to make up for the lack of capital building (Abel-Smith and Titmuss, 1956).

Throughout the next 20 years concern over the mounting costs of the NHS

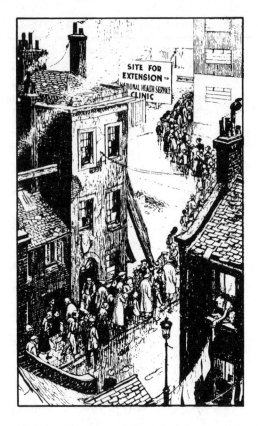

Illingworth on the tough economic choices. The caption read: 'Prevention is better ... (estimated additional expenditure on NHS for 1950, £129 m; proposed reduction in expenditure on housing for 1950, £24 m).'

Source: Punch 1950.
Reproduced by kind permission of Punch.

continued. One of the assumptions in the Beveridge Report (1942) was that there was a fixed quantity of illness in the community which the NHS would reduce. It was therefore expected that expenditure on health care would decline once the backlog of ill health had been eradicated. This assumption proved false. Far from declining, expenditure increased steadily (Table 3.1). By 1977, total NHS expenditure had risen to £6897 million. Various factors contributed to the potentially limitless demand for health care.

- A long-term tendency for demand to increase as public expectations rose.
- Post-war developments in pharmaceutics and medical science further increased the costs of drugs, equipment and medical treatment.
- Expanding medical technology opened up new areas, such as heart surgery and hip replacements, which were not feasible at the start of the NHS.
- As the service was labour intensive, staff numbers had to increase to meet rising needs and demands. The total numbers of nurses, midwives and health

Table 3.2   Growth in numbers of doctors: Great Britain 1949–1978.

		Whole-time equivalents				
	1949	1974	1975	1976	1977	1978
*Hospital Doctors**						
England	} 11 735	25 618	26 922	27 686	28 397	29 293
Wales		1 472	1 528	1 648	1 705	
Scotland	1 900†	4 417	4 509	4 591	4 737	–
General Medical Practitioners‡						
England	} 18 000§	21 531	21 752	22 015	22 327	22 651
Wales		1 354	1 370	1 362	1 394	1 418
Scotland	2 000§	2 959	3 006	3 041	3 089	3 148
Community and School Health Services						
England	–	2 347	2 565	2 681	2 745	2 782
Wales	–	176	193	205	209	204
Scotland	–	307	417	436	452	–

*Excludes locum staff, (except in 1949), and GPs holding hospital appointments.
†1948. Excludes honorary staff.
‡Numbers rather than whole-time equivalents.
§*Estimated.*
– Figures not available.

Source: Merrison Report (1979: 209).
Crown copyright material is reproduced with the permission of the Controller of Her Majesty's Stationery Office.

visitors in England rose from 272 630 in 1971 to 335 081 in 1977 (Merrison Report, 1979: 194). Table 3.2 shows the growth in the numbers of doctors in Great Britain from 1949 to 1978.

- The rising number of elderly people, who made the heaviest demands on the health and community services, also created one of the major problems facing the NHS. By 1978, those aged 65 and over in England and Wales had increased in numbers to represent 14% of the total population (DHSS, 1978a).

RESOURCE PRIORITIES

A key issue in the financing of the NHS was the question of resources. In 1968, the Department of Health and Social Security (DHSS) superseded an amalgamation of the Ministry of Health and the Ministry of National Insurance. The Secretary of State for Social Services was therefore responsible to Parliament for the central administration of health, the personal social services and social security. The DHSS had then to face both persistent inflation and the mounting economic crisis of the 1970s which forced the NHS to adjust to a lower rate of growth of current expenditure – from an average annual rate of 3.5% (1970–1973) to around 0.5%.

By the mid-1970s, despite increased National Insurance contributions and

Table 3.3   NHS sources of finance*: percentage of total by year, Great Britain 1949/50–1983/4.

Financial year	Consolidated fund	NHS contributions	Charges	Miscellaneous
1949/50	87.8	9.8	0.7	1.7
1950/51	87.6	9.4	0.7	2.3
1951/52	88.3	9.2	1.8	0.7
1952/53	87.6	8.0	4.0	0.4
1953/54	86.5	8.3	5.0	0.2
1954/55	86.9	7.9	5.0	0.2
1955/56	87.6	7.1	5.0	0.4
1956/57	88.7	6.4	4.7	0.2
1957/58	85.0	9.5	5.3	0.3
1958/59	80.3	14.4	5.0	0.3
1959/60	80.4	14.5	4.9	0.3
1960/61	81.9	13.3	4.5	0.2
1961/62	77.7	16.5	5.6	0.2
1962/63	77.1	17.2	5.5	0.2
1963/64	77.9	16.4	5.4	0.3
1964/65	79.6	15.0	5.1	0.4
1965/66	83.8	13.3	2.6	0.2
1966/67	84.8	12.4	2.4	0.3
1967/68	86.5	10.9	2.3	0.3
1968/69	84.8	11.8	3.1	0.3
1969/70	85.9	10.3	3.5	0.3
1970/71	85.8	10.8	3.2	0.3
1971/72	85.7	10.3	3.6	0.5
1972/73	87.0	9.0	3.6	0.4
1973/74	88.1	7.9	3.5	0.5
1974/75	91.3	5.7	2.6	0.4
1975/76	89.2	8.5	2.0	0.3
1976/77	88.0	9.7	2.1	0.2
1977/78	88.0	9.6	2.1	0.3
1978/79	88.0	9.6	2.1	0.3
1979/80	88.0	9.5	2.2	0.3
1980/81	89.1	8.2	2.4	0.3
1981/82	87.8	9.4	2.5	0.3
1982/83 (estimated)	85.8	11.2	2.7	0.3
1973/84 (estimated)	85.8	10.9	3.0	0.3

*Excludes local authority health expenditure before 1974.

Source: Social Services Committee (1984: 45). Public Expenditure on the Special Services. Fourth Report, Session 1983/84, London: HMSO.
Crown copyright material is reproduced with the permission of the Controller of Her Majesty's Stationery Office.

extended charges, the Consolidated Fund (general taxation) still formed the major source of funding for the NHS (Table 3.3), a method which facilitated resource planning.

The process of planning priorities was started by a DHSS consultative document *Priorities for Health and Personal Social Services in England* (DHSS, 1976) and continued with revised guidance in *The Way Forward* (DHSS, 1977a). The main thrust of the plans in both England and Wales was to give a much greater emphasis to preventive services and community care. Priority was to be

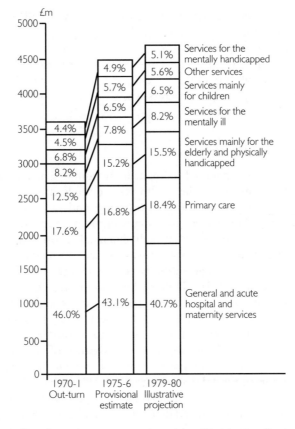

Figure 3.1 Expenditure by programme as a percentage of total expenditure: current and capital expenditure in millions of pounds (November 1974 prices).

Source: DHSS (1976).
Crown copyright material is reproduced with the permission of the Controller of Her Majesty's Stationery Office.

Table 3.4 The outcome: spending on health and personal social services 1975–76 and 1979–80 as percentage of net current and capital expenditure.

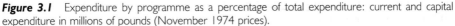

	1975–76	**1979–80**[*]
Primary care	18.3	19.0
General and acute hospital and maternity services	40.5	39.2
Elderly and physically handicapped	14.1	14.2
Mentally handicapped	4.4	4.4
Mentally ill	7.6	7.5
Children	5.3	5.5
Other	9.9	10.2
Total (£million: 1980 prices)	**8618**	**9003**

*Provisional figures

Source: New Society (19 November 1981)

given to the development of services for children, mentally ill, mentally handi-capped, physically handicapped and elderly people (Figure 3.1). The key to achieving the planned switch in resources was to get better value out of allocated money. The most expensive branch of the NHS was the hospital and specialist services, despite careful economy. It remained to be seen whether resource priorities could be realigned but progress was slow, as the outcome in Table 3.4 shows.

FINANCIAL REVIEW 1948–1978

In retrospect, politicians invented a financial treadmill when they created the NHS. Initially, the financing of the health service made little allowance for the correction of inherited problems (maldistribution and deficiency in standards; Webster, 1988: 398). There were no inbuilt curbs on expenditure: the whole point of the NHS was to eliminate all financial considerations by giving treatment according to need. The patient was to meet no financial barriers at the point of access; the doctor was given the freedom to do the best for their patients regardless of cost (Klein, 1983). While seeking an elusive concept of adequacy, the NHS continued its own dynamic to generate costs and new demands. By 1978, Bevan's vision of optimum standards had been sorely tested financially.

In 1976, a Royal Commission was asked to consider the best use and management of the financial and manpower resources of the National Health Service. By 1979, the Royal Commission reported that the NHS gave good value for money and endorsed the DHSS priorities, which emphasized prevention and community care (Merrison Report, 1979). Having considered and rejected alter-native methods of financing the NHS (insurance, charges and ear-marked tax revenue), the report concluded that NHS funds were being 'properly spent' although there was no 'right' level of NHS expenditure. The Commission encouraged both increased expenditure and the more efficient use of resources (Merrison Report, 1979: 346, 353).

EFFECTIVE ORGANIZATION

Set against a background of ongoing financial concern, the early years of the NHS laid down the organizational foundations. After an initial decade of recon-struction, re-equipment and consolidation, from 1960 to 1974 the NHS entered a period of innovation, expansion, development and strategic planning.

THE FAMILY DOCTOR AND PRIMARY CARE SERVICES

Effective organization in the general practitioner services was strongly linked with remuneration and significantly influenced by developments in group practice and health centres. The problem of the uneven distribution of doctors was partly overcome by the regulation procedures of the Medical Practices Committee and partly through financial inducements. However, the remuneration of GPs resulted in widespread dissatisfaction. By 1960, on the recommendations of the Pilkington Committee, a review body was set up in 1962, which led to major changes to reflect the individual doctor's services for patients and practice expenses. In turn, doctors' surgeries and services improved.

The outcome of this 'Family Doctors' Charter' by 1966, together with the more favourable economic climate, prompted rapid growth of health centres. During the 1950s, some Medical Officers of Health had started to attach health visitors and district nurses to doctors' practices; group practices also developed. These experiments were so successful that a widespread movement began to attach health visitors, district nurses, midwives and sometimes social workers to GPs' surgeries.

Asked to produce 10-year plans for the development of their services, Local Health Authorities (LHAs) showed wide variations in service intentions (Ministry of Health, 1963). During the 1960s, however, the LHA services became more closely co-ordinated with the family doctor services. Health centres were a way forward.

In 1974, one GP in six was working single-handed; many were attached to a group practice and over three-quarters of GPs worked with district nurses and health visitors. From 1965, the number of health centres expanded rapidly, from 28 to 953 in 1979, by which time 23% of all GPs were working in a health centre designed to accommodate a basic primary care team (Ham, 1982).

LOCAL HEALTH AUTHORITY SERVICES IN THE COMMUNITY

Maternity and child welfare

The introduction of health centres meant that facilities for mothers and children could be provided on the same premises as the family doctor services. However, the organizational context was changing. Home midwifery was on the decline. From the late 1960s, the policy was to make it possible for all births to take place in hospitals: in 1960, 34% of confinements were at home but by 1974 only about 6% of children were born at home (Abel-Smith, 1978). The major work of domiciliary midwives therefore became antenatal and postnatal care of women in the community.

Amongst the wide range of medical, supportive and community preventive services, the maternity and child welfare centres included welfare foods, antenatal and postnatal clinics, child welfare clinics and the advisory services of health visitors.

Family planning and abortion

The maternity and child welfare centres also provided (on medical grounds only) family planning services, which had been pioneered by the Family Planning Association (FPA). Nevertheless, the provision of family planning remained an anomaly: it was neither free nor comprehensively covered by the NHS. Almost a quarter of LHAs tended to subcontract this work to the FPA – a specialist voluntary body – which by 1969 was still running 90% of the family planning clinics in England and Wales.

With the arrival of the contraceptive pill, four factors directly led to legislative change in 1967.

1 The interest of the medical profession in hormonal contraception.
2 The marked change in public attitudes towards widespread acceptance of birth control provision.
3 The increasing popularity of the pill which radically altered the patterns of contraceptive use.
4 The consequent accelerating demand for contraceptive advice and facilities.

At this point the inadequacy of NHS provision was revealed. Under the *National Health Service (Family Planning) Act* of 1967, LHAs were enabled to extend family planning services to unmarried women and to those who needed them on non-medical grounds (for whom a charge could be made for prescription and supply at LHA discretion).

The legal advance in family planning was greatly helped by the simultaneous passage of the controversial legislation on abortion, which drew major pressure-group fire in Parliament. After fiercely contended debates in both houses, the 1967 *Abortion Act* legalized abortion under strict medical safeguards. By 1974, again following immense pressure-group action and parliamentary controversy, free family planning on the NHS was finally secured (Leathard, 1980).

Domiciliary health care in the community: health visitors

Developments in the training of staff, the clarification of their role and the hand-over process from voluntary bodies to the NHS were amongst the key elements in the organization of domiciliary health care in the community.

The 1946 *NHS Act* required LHAs to provide a health visiting service. Early in the 1960s, not only was there a shortage of health visitors but a clearer under-standing of their role was needed to meet the changing health scene.

Sir William Jameson's Working Party, set up to advise on the proper field of work, recruitment and training of health visitors, considered that training should seek to integrate the elements of student nurse training and state registration, midwifery, social studies and public health, to provide a clear understanding of family health and welfare services. The health visitor was described as a health educator and social adviser to families and individuals in the community, more especially to mothers, their young children and to old people (Jameson Committee, 1956).

Following the recommendations of the Jameson Report in 1956, the Council for the Training of Health Visitors was set up under the *Health Visiting and Social Work (Training) Act* 1962. The name was amended to the Council for the Education and Training of Health Visitors (CETHV) in 1971. The CETHV played an important part in initiating a new approach to training and education and to setting high training standards. By the 1970s, the health visitor's role was perceived by the CETHV as promoting personal health, preventing mental, physical and emotional breakdown, identifying needs and mobilizing resources.

District nurses

The district nursing service was also an LHA statutory responsibility. Under the NHS, district nursing was made available, free at the point of use, to all persons who needed nursing in the home. By 1960, about four-fifths of LHAs made direct provision; others shared the service with, or left it exclusively to, voluntary associations with whom agreements were negotiated (Lindsey, 1962). Before the NHS, direct nursing was left almost entirely to voluntary organizations. The slow handover was yet another indication of the evolutionary process of health care in Britain.

Much of the increase in demand for home nursing was attributed to elderly patients, who accounted for 60% of all visits by the late 1950s. The number of district nurses in whole-time equivalents consequently rose from about 7100 in 1960 to 11 700 in 1974 (Abel-Smith, 1978).

On the recommendations of the Working Party on District Nurses' Training in 1955, a panel of assessors was established in 1959 to ensure adequate and standardized training procedures. In 1968, the panel took over full responsibility, from the Queen's Institute, for the training, syllabus, examinations and the award of the National District Nursing Certificate (UKCC, 1984).

By the mid-1970s, the government's policy on priorities emphasized the importance of both health visitors and district nurses. The aim was to avoid the need for hospital admissions by enabling people to remain in the community with appropriate help from community-based staff.

Midwives

The domiciliary midwifery service was well rooted in the pattern of local health services before 1948. The statutory basis was not changed by the 1946 *National Health Service Act*, but charges were abolished. Initially apprehensive about their role and status under the NHS, domiciliary midwives soon found their work was complementary to that of obstetricians and general practitioners, rather than in competition as in the pre-NHS era. The NHS therefore improved relations and co-operation between these former rivals (Lindsey, 1962).

Midwifery training and examination were under the control of the Central Midwives Board. Midwifery had long been a female preserve but, under the 1975 *Sex Discrimination Act*, midwifery training was opened up to men. By the end of the 1970s, however, the training programme was to be significantly strengthened overall (Allan and Jolley, 1982).

Effective organization in the domiciliary services was therefore strongly influenced by the need to standardize, improve and advance the training of health visitors, district nurses and midwives. A further trend stressed the shift in priorities towards the provision of care in the community in which domiciliary health care played an important part.

Dental, ophthalmic and pharmaceutical services

Once the initial backlog of demand had been met, these services settled down to a steady level of annual provision. Apart from a shortage of dentists, one organizational issue was the rising costs, which were counteracted by various forms of charges:

- from 1956, NHS lenses could be put in new private frames, thus extending consumer choice;
- in 1971, flat-rate ophthalmic charges were replaced by cost-related charges, but were re-introduced in 1976;
- the 1951 dental charges (children and certain other community members exempt) were geared to restorative treatment;
- dental charges were increased in 1968 for treatment and, in 1969, for dentures.

Nevertheless, the pattern of dental work had changed dramatically. Pre-war National Health Insurance dentists largely extracted teeth; NHS dentists increasingly concentrated on filling teeth where possible. Furthermore, the greatest increase in the use of the general dental service was by children, who were encouraged to take part in preventive dental treatment (Abel-Smith, 1978).

The early demand for free drugs seemed excessive so, in 1952, prescription charges were brought in, abolished in 1965, reintroduced in 1968 and increased in 1971. The cost of drugs remained a vexed issue. Many of the drugs prescribed were produced commercially by pharmaceutical companies whose costs covered the expense of research and promotion but the feeling persisted that drug companies were making excessive profits at the expense of the NHS.

Although the cost of the pharmaceutical service seemed high, it returned dividends in better health. Drugs lowered the mortality rate, eased suffering and shortened recovery periods. Many patients, who previously would have been sent to hospital, were treated at home and inpatients were released much earlier. The relationship between the NHS and the pharmaceutical industry therefore remained controversial and problematical.

Effective organization in the dental, ophthalmic and pharmaceutical services was inhibited largely by financial issues, although the delivery system (organized by the 134 Executive Councils) experienced fewer problems than did other aspects of health care provision.

Mental illness and mental handicap

The organization of care for mentally ill and mentally handicapped people attempted to reassess policy and standards and to transform the nature of service provision. Mental illness was now regarded as a largely curable or self-correcting condition, which could range from mild depression to violent psychopathy. Mental handicap, in contrast, resulted from retarded development of mental powers (from simple-mindedness to severe subnormality), which could not be cured but could be helped through care and training.

The Local Health Authorities were responsible for a number of services in the field of prevention, illness and after-care under the 1946 *NHS Act*. The Act was important because it stated that health care provision was to secure improvement in physical *and* mental health and was to seek prevention as well as integrated care and treatment in both.

This viewpoint was made explicit by the Royal Commission on Mental Illness and Mental Deficiency (1957). Many of the Commission's recommendations were enacted in the *Mental Health Act* 1959. The 1959 legislation marked a turning point, in seeking to transform NHS services from the traditional source of hospital treatment towards community-oriented provision. LHAs were urged to develop their services, including the provision of hostels, group homes, social work support and day centres. These developments were facilitated by changes in public and staff attitudes and by the therapeutic advances in new drugs.

The 1959 *Mental Health Act* established:

- a less stigmatizing terminology: four categories of patient were to be recognized (mentally ill, severely subnormal, subnormal and psychopathic);
- that Mental Health Tribunals were to be introduced into each hospital region to protect the liberty of the individual and to deal with any complaints from compulsory admissions;
- that hospitals were to be regarded as places of treatment rather than of custody;
- that an open-door policy was to be encouraged whereby people could attend for voluntary provision through informal admission.

The policy shift to community care was confirmed by the 1962 Hospital Plan, which forecast that the number of beds allocated to mental illness would be almost halved by 1975 (Ministry of Health, 1962). However, faced with limited finance and a lack of knowledge of what needed to be done, LHAs tended to give more attention to extending those services for which they were solely responsible than to developing community care services to replace hospital provision. The outcome of the 1959 *Mental Health Act* did not therefore significantly extend the range of community facilities, although it remained the major piece of mental health legislation for the next 23 years.

Community provision for mentally ill people still remained inadequate. For some the 'open door' policy became a 'revolving door' as patients returned to hospital if community facilities were not available. In 1974, only about one-sixth of the day centre places and one-third of the residential care places estimated to be needed were available (Abel-Smith, 1978).

By 1975, the White Paper *Better Services for the Mentally Ill* set out a comprehensive long-term programme to improve the quality of services. The policy again advocated a shift in the balance of care and treatment away from hospitals towards local community services by decreasing inpatient services and increasing day hospitals, outpatient facilities, day centres, homes, hostels and nursing provision in the community (DHSS, 1975). In a government review of the *Mental Health Act* of 1959 some 20 years later, amendments were proposed to the hospital admission procedures but the review did little to shift care away from the legal and medical model, embodied in the 1959 Act and towards a social approach (DHSS, 1978b).

Policies for mentally handicapped people underwent a significant change following a report on the Ely hospital 'scandal' in Cardiff, which revealed major deficiencies in the standard of patient care (Ely Report, 1969).

New policies were then set out in the 1971 White Paper *Better Services for the Mentally Handicapped*. The main objectives were:

- to reduce, by about half, the number of hospital beds provided for mentally handicapped people;
- to expand local authority places in residential homes, training centres, foster homes and lodgings;
- to establish a Hospital Advisory Service to visit long-stay hospitals;
- to advise on the management of patient care (DHSS, 1971a).

Despite these initiatives, further hospital scandals came to light following reports on conditions at other long-stay hospitals, including Whittingham, South Ockenden, Farleigh and Normansfield. The process of change demonstrated that significant improvements were slow to occur and difficult to achieve.

By 1979, only about half of the adult training and occupation places estimated to be needed in the community had been provided, and about one-third of the residential homes; there were still some local authorities who made no provision at all (Abel-Smith, 1978). Overall, the concept of community care sought to enhance the quality of life, while seeking to reduce expensive hospitalization. However, appropriate forms of care evolved slowly (Webster, 1988: 395) and their organization proved less than effective due to under-resourcing in the Community Health Services.

THE HOSPITAL SERVICE

The amalgamation of local authority and voluntary hospitals in 1948 brought better use of resources. Further, the grouping of hospitals on a district basis under the control of a Hospital Management Committee, underpinned by regional planning, helped to rationalize the delivery system. However, the problems of accommodation shortage and waiting lists persisted.

In 1962, the Ten-Year Hospital Plan envisaged the nation-wide provision of district general hospitals with some 600 to 800 beds, each to serve a population of 100 000 to 150 000 (Ministry of Health, 1962). The plan was intended to concentrate resources, lay down uniform criteria and enable a team approach to treatment. After years of restraint, the hospital building programme underwent significant expansion. However, in 1975, the government announced public expenditure cuts, which curtailed any further building of large district hospitals: smaller hospitals were to be developed instead. The overall result was that 60% of beds remained in pre-First World War hospitals.

Four issues surrounded the effective organization of hospital provision up to the late 1970s: resource priorities (already outlined), the controversy over pay beds (to be discussed in the next section), staff shortages and, above all, the reorganization of the whole structure of the NHS.

NHS STAFFING AND STRUCTURES

Doctors

Shortage of doctors and nurses bedevilled NHS provision. The Willink Committee's mistaken policy on medical education in 1957 had not helped: medical training was consequently reduced. Medical staffing structures provided further unrest: junior doctors considered themselves underpaid and overworked; registrars and senior registrars were unable to secure consultant posts. The Ministry of Health was reluctant to increase NHS costs by increasing the number of consultants. However, following the Royal Commission on Medical Education in 1968, the Government announced plans to increase the numbers of students entering medical school in Great Britain (from 2400 in 1965 to 4000 by 1980), to expand existing medical schools and to create new ones (Southampton, Leicester, Nottingham and Swansea were chosen; Todd Report, 1968).

Consquently, high priority was given to teaching hospitals in the hospital building programme. By 1974, the Government had agreed to a steady but significant expansion in consultant numbers. The relative pay of junior hospital doctors had by now improved; a 1972 circular also laid down off-duty entitlements. However, in 1979, the Royal Commission on the NHS still found the contracts for hospital doctors inappropriate for the needs of their profession and considered the career structure defective (Merrison Report, 1979).

Nurses

Changes were also introduced in the management of the nursing services. When the NHS came into being, the position of Matron in many hospitals was already beginning to change. Following the Salmon Report (1966), Chief Nursing Officers were appointed; these were responsible for the nursing services in each group of hospitals. Nurse administrators were given further training to help them exercise their management responsibilities. However, there was no place in this structure for matrons and deputy matrons working in the traditional way. Chief Nursing Officers had to become managers of numbered nursing grades, to adopt bureaucratic considerations and to apply fiscal rather than nursing values.

The Mayston Report (1969) was set up to apply the Salmon principles to LHA services. Directors of Nursing Services were therefore made responsible for community nursing and midwifery provision. The outcome of nursing staff restructuring, both in hospitals and in the community health services, was that nurses had the right to be heard on all nursing matters and were made clearly responsible for planning and administering nursing education and services.

Improvements in working conditions had gradually taken place. Weekly working hours fell from a recommended 48 in 1949 to 40 by 1972. Holidays were longer and equal pay was provided to male and female nurses. By the mid-1970s, nursing staff could no longer be dismissed on marriage; nor were the majority required to live-in (Abel-Smith, 1978).

The education and training of nurses became concentrated in fewer, larger, better-staffed and better-equipped schools. Schools of Nursing consequently reduced in number from 878 in 1949 to 308 in 1974. However, the 1948 *Nurses Act* allowed different types of experimental courses for basic training, which opened up the way for collaboration with higher education institutes and the evolution of degree courses from the late 1950s onwards (Owen, 1984).

In 1972, the Briggs Committee recommended some fundamental changes in nurse education and training. The main proposal was that all nurses should undertake the same basic 18-month study course, to be followed by a further 18 months of training for registration; further study could then lead to higher qualifications in specialist fields. New statutory bodies were also proposed to control the nursing, midwifery and health-visiting professions (Briggs Committee, 1972).

In a review of the position of nurses, midwives and health visitors, at the end of the 1970s the Royal Commission on the NHS was disappointed that more progress on the Briggs recommendations had not been made. Finding that considerable problems had been caused by the implementation of the Salmon (1966) and Mayston (1969) Reports, the Commission recommended improvements in the clinical career structure and pressed for the encouragement of flexibility in the way nurses worked (Merrison Report, 1979).

The concept of effective organization in the hospital services, whether concerned with staffing or structural arrangements, remained problematic. As Culyer (1976) has analysed, an assessment of meeting health needs was required in relation to a measurement of health outcomes. Furthermore, a sharp distinction had to be drawn between efficiency and effectiveness. In the mid-1970s these notions of health economics were well in advance of their time. Meanwhile, the major preoccupation of health care providers in Britain was with the reorganization of the delivery system.

THE REORGANIZATION OF THE NHS IN 1974

NHS structural reorganization reflected, once again, the evolutionary process of health care provision in Britain. The post-war tripartite arrangement had led to mounting criticism over the fragmented, unco-ordinated system, which had, in fact, been a pre-war problem which the NHS had inherited but failed to overcome. It had become evident that a divided service impeded a clear rationale for the allocation of resources. Local Health Authorities were not co-ordinated with one another (Webster, 1988: 395), nor did their own health services work together. Overall planning between the separate branches of the NHS was also poorly developed. Furthermore, the requirements for hospital accommodation depended on the priority local authorities gave to their community care services. Therefore, as the NHS services developed, so the case for unification grew.

The idea of an integrated service was not new. Dating back to the pre-war years, an ongoing series of proposals were put forward by varying committees and reports.

- The Dawson Committee (1920) favoured single health authorities.
- The Guillebaud Committee (1956), while reporting on NHS costs, identified the weakness of the NHS as the tripartite division between preventive medicine, general practice and hospital provision, with its most serious impact on maternity and child welfare services. Although structural change was considered premature, the need for greater co-operation was stressed.
- The Cranbrook Committee (1959), set up to investigate this alleged confusion in the maternity services, confirmed the need for greater co-ordination.
- The Gillie Report (1963) suggested that the health services should be co-ordinated through family doctors.
- The Porritt Report's (1962) proposals for local unified NHS administration, under Area Health Boards, came closest to the eventual outcome.
- The Seebohm Report (1968) and the Royal Commission on Local Government (Redcliffe-Maud Report, 1969) furthered the idea that local government should take over NHS responsibilities.

Reorganization went through a lengthy process of public discussion, negotiation and review. A 1968 Labour government Green Paper on the NHS administrative structure considered a single-tier system of 40–50 Area Boards, accountable to the Ministry of Health (Ministry of Health, 1968). This was opposed by doctors, who feared for their independence, and by those who criticised the Boards as liable to become remote from the public. A further Green Paper expanded the number of Health Boards to 90, to be co-ordinated by Regional Health Councils (DHSS, 1970). It was followed in 1971 by a consultative document of the new Conservative government which introduced an emphasis on managerial and administrative efficiency (DHSS, 1971b). In August 1972, the final proposals for unification were presented in a White Paper (DHSS, 1972) which became mainly incorporated into the *NHS Reorganization Act* of 1973.

THE NHS STRUCTURE IN 1974

The 1973 legislation provided the basis of the system which came into operation in April 1974. After almost 26 years, the NHS underwent a major organizational change.

Within the new structure (Figure 3.2), the DHSS was responsible to Parliament for the overall policy of the NHS, for central strategic planning, monitoring performance, obtaining, allocating and developing resources, finance, buildings, staff forecasting and training, statistics and research.

REGIONAL HEALTH AUTHORITIES

The second tier was taken over by 14 RHAs from the previous Regional Hospital Boards with slightly modified boundaries. Members of the RHAs were appointed

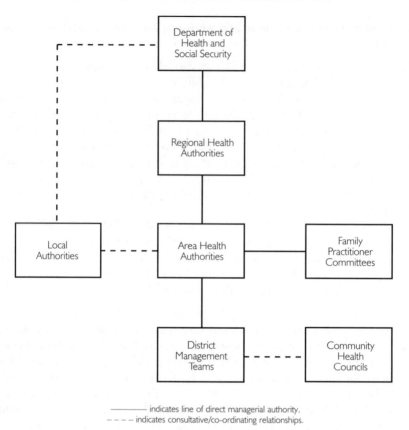

indicates line of direct managerial authority.
– – – – indicates consultative/co-ordinating relationships.

Figure 3.2 Structure of the NHS 1974–1982.

by the Secretary of State for Social Services. An RHA's main function was regional planning and prioritization. RHAs also had responsibility for major building projects, for postgraduate medical, dental and nurse training and for the allocation and monitoring of financial resources between lower tier health authorities.

In the absence of RHAs in Wales, the Welsh Office combined the functions of a central government department and a regional authority.

AREA HEALTH AUTHORITIES

Beneath the RHAs and responsible to them were 90 Area Health Authorities (AHAs) in England and Wales. Members were partly appointed by RHAs, partly by local authorities, universities and professional nominees, and partly by members of the non-medical and nursing staff. The AHA Chairman was appointed by the Secretary of State.

AHA duties included planning and management, study of the health needs of each area to find out where provision fell below required standards and all the functions of the Hospital Management Committees, Executive Councils and most of those under the former LHAs.

One of the most important AHA function was to develop services jointly with the now coterminous local authorities (i.e. whose boundaries matched).

Alongside each AHA was a Family Practitioner Committee (FPC), financed directly by the DHSS, which administered the contracts of GPs, dentists, pharmacists and opticians. FPC members were appointed by the AHA, local professionals and local authorities.

Most areas were split into health districts, whose day-to-day running was administered by District Management Teams, the lowest tier of the NHS. At each level of the management structure were strong professional advisory committees.

COMMUNITY HEALTH COUNCILS

The 200 or so Community Health Councils (CHCs) were an important innovation located at district level (one for each district). CHCs were introduced to represent the interests and views of the consumer and to monitor the health services. Though financed by AHAs, the CHCs were to be independent bodies whose members were to be nominated by local authorities (one-half), by RHAs (one-sixth) and by voluntary agencies (one-third). CHCs were created to compensate for the somewhat remote position of the AHAs.

THE AIMS OF THE 1974 REORGANIZATION

The NHS reorganization in 1974 had three main objectives. First, it was intended to unify health services by bringing them all under one authority at Area Health Authority level. By dovetailing the three arms of the NHS more efficiently, satisfactory patient care was to be ensured. Steps towards integration had indeed been taken: the teaching hospitals lost their independent status under Boards of Governors and were brought into the AHA structure. All local authority community health services were transferred to the NHS but local government retained an environmental health role. However, full unification was not achieved as GPs remained independent contractors. The functions of the Executive Councils, while under the AHAs, were run by Family Practitioner Committees, which reflected the GPs' successful assertion of their right to an element of independence. Nevertheless, unification might have been differently secured – alternatives had been considered but ruled out. One was for local authorities to take over the health services. This option would have found favour with local authorities but had been fiercely opposed by doctors (quite apart from the problems raised by having to change boundaries and resource capacities). In reverse, the local authority lobby would never have allowed the transfer of local government welfare services to the NHS (Klein, 1983).

Within the second aim, services were intended to be more effectively co-ordinated between health authorities and related local government services. The boundaries of the new AHAs were therefore made largely coterminous with those first-tier local authorities (County Councils, Metropolitan District Councils, London Boroughs) who provided the personal social services. In addition, Area Health Authorities were required to set up joint consultative committees to facilitate collaboration. Furthermore, the boundaries of the new AHAs had been planned in the context of the 1970 restructuring of local authority personal social services and of the reorganization of local government which came into effect on the same day as the reorganization of the NHS – 1 April 1974.

A third aim was to introduce better management through multidisciplinary management teams in which medical, nursing, financial and administrative staff provided health care based on 'consensus' management.

Another way of seeking to improve managerial efficiency was the introduction of a corporate planning system in 1976. The management aim, overall, was to delegate more responsibility to health authorities without undermining the Secretary of State's accountability to Parliament. The intention was summed up in the slogan 'maximum delegation downwards, maximum accountability upward'.

All these changes were devised to find more effective ways of pursuing national priorities at local level, to raise the level of performance through better management and to shift resources in favour of neglected groups (Ham, 1982).

The aims of the 1974 reorganization attempted to reconcile conflicting policies: to promote managerial efficiency but also to satisfy the professions; to create an effective administrative structure for establishing national policy but also to give delegated scope to those running the services at the far reaches of the NHS. Consequently, while the organizational outcome had the potential to unify the delivery system, it contained the seed-bed of further trouble. As Glennerster (1995: 131–2) commented, not only was the 1974 NHS structure the most Byzantine ever imposed on a UK public service but, unlike a large company or the armed forces, the lower tiers in the NHS were run by medical politics and no one was clearly charged with managing the change. Furthermore, the divisions between the NHS and local authority services had simply been shifted: a potentially divisive boundary line now ran between NHS health services and social care in the community under local government – a division which was to have repercussions over the next 26 years. Following reorganization, therefore, far from setting off into a period of consolidation with calm and steady progress, the National Health Service eventually moved, in the view of many participants, towards crisis and chaos.

4 HEALTH CARE AND CONTROVERSIES: NEW DIRECTIONS IN THE NHS, 1979–1987

On the return of the Conservative Government in the spring of 1979, a programme of curbs on public expenditure was immediately announced to defeat inflation and to enable the depressed economy to pay its way. These features underpinned a watershed in social policy and in the provision of State Social Services. The impact on the NHS was to impose cuts and efficiency savings. Furthermore, alternative methods of health care provision were encouraged through the private sector, the voluntary sector and informal caring by the family. Under Mrs Thatcher's Tory administration, a significant shift towards welfare pluralism therefore emerged. As new directions evolved, so controversies arose over NHS remuneration, inequalities and costs; these culminated in further reorganization and management restructuring.

PRIVATIZATION

Pay beds

One group of participants who sensed a mounting crisis in the NHS were those involved in the controversies over private practice. Confrontation between the medical profession and the government began to escalate in the mid-1970s when the Labour party sought, through the *Health Services Act* in 1976, to phase out pay beds (except for overseas patients). These were beds reserved for fee-paying patients to receive private treatment in NHS hospitals – the outcome of Bevan's concession to secure the consultants' support for the principle of the NHS. There were 5829 pay beds in England and Wales in 1956, but numbers had decreased to 4210 by 1976 (Merrison Report, 1979: 291). The 1976 Act set up the Health Services Board to regulate the phasing out of pay beds and introduced a licensing system for private nursing homes and hospitals.

Both for the medical profession and for the Labour party, the existence of private practice – as expressed by pay beds – was symbolic: it reflected, at a simplistic level, professional independence on the one hand and the perception of financial privilege on the other. The combination of the Labour government's commitment to phasing out NHS pay beds, loading contracts in favour of full-time consultants and an incomes policy, which squeezed pay differentials for all NHS workers, prompted industrial action amongst the junior hospital doctors in 1975. In response to the doctors' demands, the Labour Prime Minister (Harold Wilson) intervened by setting up a Royal Commission to enquire into the financing and organization of the NHS. The intentions of the incoming Conservative Government were made immediately clear when the *Health Services Act* in 1980 abolished the Health Services Board, relaxed controls over private hospital development and restored the Health Minister's discretionary power to allow pay beds.

The private sector

The private sector of the health services (a somewhat imprecise term) had always ranged more widely than pay beds, to include:

- commercial sales of medicines;
- sales of drugs and appliances in chemists' shops and supermarkets;
- private treatment by GPs and hospital-based specialists who also work for the NHS;
- private hospitals, nursing homes and clinics;
- private practice undertaken outside the NHS by dentists, medical practitioners, nurses, chiropodists, physiotherapists, osteopaths and chiropractors (the last two were rarely employed by the NHS).

Overall, the 1979 Royal Commission on the NHS estimated that private practice in relationship to the NHS was still small. The private sector accounted for 2% of all acute hospital beds, 6% of all hospital beds in England and about 3% of total expenditure on health care in the UK (Merrison Report, 1979).

Throughout the first half of the 1980s, the Conservative government pressed towards wider measures to encourage privatization. The New Right ideology was based on the view that the private sector had an important role to play: it increased available health care facilities, relieved pressures on the NHS, reduced the dangers of the NHS being a monopoly supplier and employer, increased consumer choice and enabled the provision of an alternative to the NHS (Le Grand and Robinson, 1984).

The private sector was subsequently boosted, in 1983, by the government's intention to further partnership between the public and private sector through treating NHS patients on a contract-out basis, sharing equipment, co-operating on training and selling surplus NHS property to private medical bodies complementary to the NHS (*The Health Services*, 1983). From 1983, the government insisted that NHS catering, laundry and cleaning services should be tendered to private contractors to secure cheaper contracts (DHSS, 1983a). The moves towards privatization embroiled the government in public rows with health authorities (Sheffield, Greenwich and Brent amongst others), who refused to comply – whereupon the government threatened court action. Health ministers argued that private firms could carry out services more cheaply and efficiently. Subsequent reports on private contracting maintained that standards had suffered (Thomas, 1985). By 1986, savings from competitive NHS tendering were diminishing as some firms were losing interest in bidding for contracts (Audit Commission, 1987).

The private sector was further extended by:

- the introduction of a limited NHS list of drugs, which required all patients to pay the full cost of any drug not on the NHS list;

- the regular increase of dental and prescription charges (exempt groups apart, children, pensioners, those on supplementary benefit and family income supplement (renamed income support and family credit, respectively under the *Social Security Act* 1986) which rose from 20p per item in May 1979 to £2.20 in April 1986);
- the phasing out of NHS spectacles and optical services (by July 1986), except for children and poor people (on a voucher basis). However, sight tests remained free.

As prescription charges went up, patients were deterred by the rising costs of seeking treatment (Ryan and Birch, 1988). Laurance (1986a) described the developments in primary health care as 'privatization by stealth'.

In the wake of this significant shift towards privatization in NHS policy, industrial action, uncertainty and protest ensued. Furthermore, as concern with NHS provision increased, so the growth of private insurance in the late 1970s rose sharply (Figure 4.1), aided by more aggressive marketing, tax relief on health insurance for all workers earning less than £8500 and by a change in the consultant's contract which enabled them to undertake more private work. The boom in the major non-profit-making provident associations – British United Provident Association (BUPA), which covered three-quarters of the market and the smaller companies (Private Patient's Plan (PPA), the Western Provident Association (WPA)) – reached a peak in 1981 with the coverage of some four million people, largely male professional workers and senior managers. These Associations found

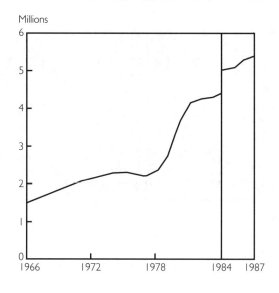

Figure 4.1 Private medical insurance: persons insured, UK.

Source: Central Statistical Office (1989: 131). Social Trends, 19, London: HMSO.
Crown copyright material is reproduced with the permission of the Controller of Her Majesty's Stationery Office.

they too had to face escalating costs (Laurance, 1983). Costs were aggravated by the very cause of the insurance companies' success – the rise in the schemes negotiated by trade unions on behalf of their workers, who were more sick than the typical subscriber and more inclined to use their insurance (Higgins, 1988). After 1981, the increase in the size of insurance premiums put a brake on growth. By 1986, the scale of the private sector still remained relatively small in relation to the NHS: only 13% of all hospital beds in England and Wales were in private hospitals and nursing homes. However, by 1987, 5.3 million people were covered by private medical insurance – some 9% of the population (CSO, 1989: 131).

The case for and against private health care

The existence of a private sector in health care remained problematical and highly controversial. Some argued in favour of private health care, that:

- NHS waiting lists were reduced by taking patients away;
- competition and a measure of standards were provided for the NHS;
- delays were overcome and special amenities provided (a single room, a telephone, access to a particular consultant);
- choice was offered to the public and greater freedom for doctors who might otherwise emigrate;
- a financial discipline was produced to curb abuse and time wasted with trivial complaints;
- above all, much needed revenue was raised.

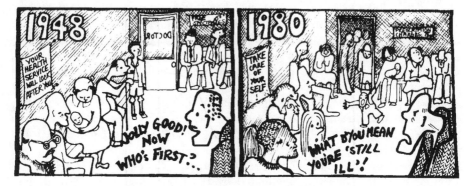

Source: Politics of Health Group (1981) Going Private: The Case against Private Medicine, London.

In contrast, there were those who argued, equally passionately, that the disadvantages of the private sector:

- encouraged withdrawal of resources (e.g. doctors) from the NHS;
- created a maldistribution of resources (private practice went to the areas where the money was);

- enabled the possibility of 'jumping the queue' by avoiding the NHS waiting list;
- deterred treatment for patients who could not afford the charges;
- could never provide comprehensive insurance cover for all health care needs (especially for dental care, childbirth, mental illness, long-term rehabilitation and geriatric care); and
- generated two standards of health care and access to provision: those who could afford private treatment and those who could not.

In 1979, the Royal Commission on the NHS found that issues such as which sector gained from or gave more to training, research, subsidy of equipment, resources and medical staff – or indeed over the extent to which taxpayers paid 'twice' (to the NHS and to the private sector) – were unquantifiable. Furthermore, because NHS facilities were inadequate, there remained two areas – abortion and the health care of elderly people – where the private sector made a significant contribution (Merrison Report, 1979). Nevertheless, those who stood against the expansion of the private sector rested their case principally on the basis that the NHS was created to provide a comprehensive, caring, health service, according to need, free at the point of use and available to all citizens regardless of financial means.

COMMUNITY SERVICES: PRIORITIES, VOLUNTARY SERVICES AND INFORMAL CARING

As the issues surrounding privatization became more complex, so the sharpness of the debate became more blurred, which was well illustrated by the increasing emphasis given to welfare pluralism. The importance the government attached to NHS collaboration with the private and voluntary sectors and informal carers was expressed in the consultative document *Care in Action* (DHSS, 1981a), which informed health authorities of the DHSS' priorities for the development of health and personal social services.

As a successor to the priorities documents of the 1970s, *Care in Action* (DHSS, 1981a) re-stated the emphasis on prevention of mental and physical ill health and on dependent groups such as elderly, mentally ill, mentally handicapped and physically handicapped people. Priority community services were widened to include primary care, maternity care and services for children. The focus on children reflected concern (highlighted by the Court Report (1976) on child health services, the Short Report (1980) on perinatal and neonatal mortality and the Black Report (1980) on inequalities in health) to reduce infant mortality, to tackle ill health and handicap amongst babies and children and to improve child health. However, unlike its predecessors, *Care in Action* (DHSS, 1981a) did not suggest (efficiency savings apart) how extra resources could be found for the priority services at a time of severe budgetary restraint.

A further major priority was to reduce public spending. Importance was therefore attached to the theme of NHS collaboration, not only with the private

Table 4.1   The value of care.

Hours per week	Percentage of carers*	Number of carers	Annual value of care at £4.00[†] per hour (£ thousands)
1–4	37	2 277 000	474 000 – 1 894 000
5–9	20	1 231 000	1 280 00 – 2 304 000
10–19	19	1 169 000	2 432 000 – 4 620 000
20–49	10	615 000	2 559 000 – 6 268 000
50+	14	861 000	8 954 000 – 8 954 000
Total	100	6 153 000	15 699 000 – 24 010 000

*Based on 1986 population estimates for Great Britain.
[†]Average hourly cost of providing local authority home helps in 1987 was £4.09.

Source: Family Policy Studies Centre (1989) Family Policy Bulletin, *Issue no. 6, winter, based on Green, H. (1988).*
Reproduced by kind permission of the Family Policy Studies Centre.

sector, but also with the voluntary services and informal caring from family, friends and neighbours (DHSS, 1981a).

At conferences in 1981, both the Prime Minister and the Social Services Secretary spoke of the voluntary services as being at the heart of the welfare movement. The voluntary sector was to be encouraged to make a far greater contribution than its previous complementary/supplementary role to state services.

Both voluntary and informal caring had already played an important part in care provision. In an attempt to reduce public spending, however, they were now being officially incorporated into the health care programme. There were costs involved. A DHSS research report on community care in 1981 drew attention to the costs to informal carers of providing unpaid care in the community (DHSS, 1981b); but the government's document *Care in Action* (DHSS, 1981a) made no comment on this issue. Various studies subsequently revealed the considerable emotional and financial costs incurred by (mostly) married women as informal carers (EOC, 1982; Nissel and Bonnerjea, 1982; Finch and Groves, 1983; Parker, 1985). However, the informal sector did provide economic gains for the Treasury: in 1984, the National Council for Voluntary Organizations showed that if only 1% of families caring for an elderly person refused to carry on doing so, and asked for their dependent relative to be placed in residential care, the cost to the state would increase overnight by 20% (Longfield, 1984).

It was subsequently estimated, from the 1985 *General Household Survey*, that the value of care from all six million carers (15% of women, 12% of men) ranged between £15 and £24 billion pounds per year (Table 4.1; Green, 1988).

MENTALLY HANDICAPPED PEOPLE

From 1971, despite a significant move away from hospital provision, the bulk of the services continued to be provided in a hospital setting. The 1979

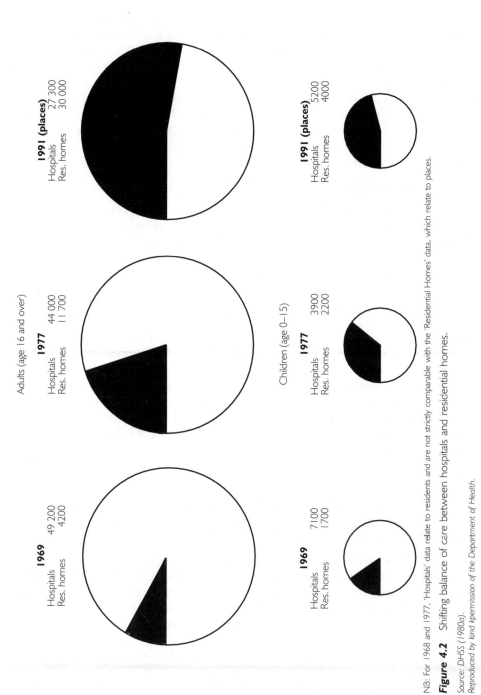

Adults (age 16 and over)

1969
Hospitals 49 200
Res. homes 4200

1977
Hospitals 44 000
Res. homes 11 700

1991 (places)
Hospitals 27 300
Res. homes 30 000

Children (age 0–15)

1969
Hospitals 7100
Res. homes 1700

1977
Hospitals 3900
Res. homes 2200

1991 (places)
Hospitals 5200
Res. homes 4000

NB: For 1968 and 1977, 'Hospitals' data relate to residents and are not strictly comparable with the 'Residential Homes' data, which relate to places.

Figure 4.2 Shifting balance of care between hospitals and residential homes.

Source: DHSS (1980a).
Reproduced by kind kpermission of the Department of Health.

Jay Committee recommended a model of care, based outside hospitals in small local units, to enable mentally handicapped people to live a normal life within the community (Jay Report, 1979). The Jay Committee was not unanimous in making this recommendation; debate therefore continued as to whether certain groups, especially adults with severe handicaps, required hospital care. Financial restraints made any rapid movement towards the Jay model unlikely.

A DHSS review of services for mentally handicapped people (DHSS, 1980a) indicated that progress had been made since the 1971 White Paper *Better Services for the Mentally Handicapped* (DHSS, 1971). The 1980 review showed that the number of adults in hospital had fallen (Figure 4.2), although at a slower rate than envisaged. Places in local authority training centres and residential homes had correspondingly increased, although the increase in residential provision for mentally handicapped children was much slower (DHSS 1980a).

The consultative document *Care in the Community* suggested that, by 1981, 15 000 mentally handicapped people – including 2000 children living in hospital (about one-third of the total) – could be discharged from hospital if community services were available. A number of proposals for transferring patients and resources from hospitals to the community were discussed (DHSS, 1981c).

MENTALLY ILL PEOPLE

Care in the Community also estimated that some 5000 mentally ill people would not need to be in psychiatric hospitals if suitable facilities existed in the community (DHSS, 1981c). However, following persistent pressure from the campaigning group Mind, the main development came with the *Mental Health (Amendment) Act* 1982 and the *Consolidation Act* of 1983. The new legislation changed the law relating to the compulsory admission of mentally ill people to hospital and their subsequent treatment. The legislation furthered many of the major mental health issues of the decade:

- automatic review by tribunal and the availability of legal representation;
- consent to treatment;
- guardianship (compulsory care in the community);
- a new Mental Health Commission to protect detained patients; and
- the right of voluntary patients to vote at elections.

The Act also established a fuller role for the approved social worker – a professional who was to be trained, approved and who would have a clearer statutory role concerning compulsory admissions. One controversial outcome was the problem faced by local authorities to train approved social workers without the resources to do so. In the view of the 1985 Social Services Select Committee on Community Care, a lack of resources held back improvements that were urgently needed to facilitate the switch of responsibility from hospital to community provision and to enable local authorities to play a greater role in the care of mentally ill and mentally handicapped people (Short Report, 1985).

By the mid-1980s, the Audit Commission (1985) had provided a comprehensive review of community care at work. In a nutshell, the policy was not working effectively. Services for elderly people were wastefully provided and inadequately managed; arrangements were ineffective regarding community nursing support and medical treatment for disabled elderly clients and co-ordination between health, housing and social services was inadequate.

For elderly, mentally ill, mentally and physically handicapped people, the policies of successive governments had been to promote community-based services to reduce long-stay hospital provision. Apart from very severely handicapped people, community care was generally considered not only better in most situations but more economical, according to the Audit Commission (1986). Although some local authorities had made worthwhile progress, care in the community was far from a reality. Funds to bridge the transition were inadequate; responsibility for community-based services was fragmented between agencies. The Audit Commission (1986) concluded that joint planning and community care policies were in disarray.

THE PLACE OF HEALTH VISITORS, MIDWIVES, NURSES AND HEALTH EDUCATORS

In seeking to promote an effective strategy for the prevention of ill health in the community, the government strongly supported the role of nurses, midwives, health visitors and health educators in health education and other preventive programmes (DHSS, 1976, 1977b, 1981a). The Royal Commission on the NHS, while acknowledging that preventive measures were by no means the exclusive responsibility of the NHS, recommended that health education should be expanded and funds increased for the Health Education Council – the government's central organization set up in 1968 to develop health education (Merrison, Report, 1979).

Following the recommendations of the Briggs Committee (1972), the *Nurses, Midwives and Health Visitors Act* in 1979 produced a notable, long-awaited contribution to nursing education. The 1979 Act provided for a single United Kingdom Central Council (UKCC), supported by powerful national boards in England, Wales, Scotland and Northern Ireland, which replaced the separate bodies responsible for the education and regulation of the profession. The Central Council had a duty to prepare and maintain a central register of qualified nurses, midwives and health visitors and to determine their education, training and standards (UKCC, 1984).

By the autumn of 1982, however, controversies had flared up: disputes raged over rejection by the Royal College of Nursing (RCN), one of the least militant health unions with its no-strike policy, of the government's pay offer. The matter was eventually settled in November 1982, but not before the united front of the health unions had mounted a one-day stoppage – which represented the first ever national strike in the NHS over pay. In contrast to the training and outlook of nurses in general, confrontation and the adversarial character of pay negotiations had become part of the controversies throughout the NHS.

The groups involved ranged from doctors to cleaners, caterers and launderers. In the climate of resource restraint, the disputes presented a seemingly ongoing crisis in the NHS as well as a threat to patient care (Laurance, 1982).

INEQUALITIES IN HEALTH CARE

Amongst other controversial issues was the continuing criticism of inequalities and variations in the provision of health care which undermined the fundamental NHS concept of equality of access to services. Both the Royal Commission on the NHS (Merrison Report, 1979) and, more particularly, the Black Report (1980) on *Inequalities in Health* showed how disparities in health and health services had persisted. The variations had three aspects.

First, hospitals continued to absorb up to 70% of NHS expenditure (Merrison Report, 1979). Furthermore, the resources were distributed unequally between client groups in hospitals: by and large, geriatric and mental patients tended to be in older hospital buildings, had more crowded conditions and far fewer beds in teaching hospitals.

Secondly, regional inequalities continued despite closer integration and planning. On the basis of a formula devised in 1976, which took account of population size, age and regional morbidity rates (amongst other factors), the Resource Allocation Working Party (RAWP) system attempted to identify 'health deprivation areas' and to allocate regional funds accordingly to allow differential growth (Merrison Report, 1979). Despite the RAWP mechanism, geographical disparities continued; one notable example was the wide variation in the provision of NHS abortion, sterilization or vasectomy services between NHS regions where facilities and their access were much influenced by the resources available and the views of the professionals involved in these potentially controversial matters (Leathard, 1985).

Thirdly, the Black Report documented the marked correlation between social class differentials and NHS inequalities. Morbidity and mortality statistics showed that social classes IV and V were among those most in need of care. For example, the death rate for unskilled workers was double that for professional people and, between 1949/53 and 1971/2, the discrepancy between social classes I and V had increased. Notwithstanding, the lower income groups appeared to receive fewer NHS resources in proportion to need. Inequalities were reinforced by geographical factors: semi-skilled and unskilled workers tended to be concentrated in the north and east, which received a lower average allocation of the NHS budget. Lower income groups tended to receive poorer quality services (more so in GP than in hospital provision). Furthermore, evidence suggested that lower income groups underused the services available, due to inadequate knowledge about illness and about the NHS machinery: the very structure of the health services was more suited to middle-class mores.

In documenting the extent of inequalities in health, the Black Report (1980) also speculated about their causes. Four types of explanation were listed.

1 *Artefactual*: the use of figures – directed more at the question of trends over time (which could be misleading).
2 *Selective*: the outcome of social mobility.
3 *Materialist*: the influence of material deprivation (e.g. affording a healthy diet).
4 *Cultural/behavioural*: health states which resulted from personal choices (e.g. smoking, drinking, taking exercise).

Overall, the explanations led to one key conclusion: that reducing health inequalities and reducing poverty must go together. To combat inequalities in health, a comprehensive anti-poverty programme was therefore outlined (Black Report, 1980). The government rejected the report: the Social Services Secretary estimated that the cost would amount to upwards of £2 billion a year and concluded such a sum was unrealistic (Townsend and Davidson, 1982).

The publication of the Black Report (1980) was not without controversy of its own. Finding little official favour, only 260 duplicated copies of the typescript were made publicly available in the week of August Bank Holiday. Townsend and Davidson (1982) then gained permission to publish a slimmed-down version to enable wider availability.

WIDENING INEQUALITIES IN HEALTH: POVERTY AND DEPRIVATION

Significant social class differences in access and health remained throughout the decade. In 1987, *The Health and Lifestyle Survey* showed that illness was linked to poor pay and deprivation. A third of unskilled manual workers, which included most of the unemployed, reported ill health, compared with 12% of those in professional and managerial jobs. The higher up the social ladder, the fitter people were, the better their diet and the less they smoked (Cox et al., 1987).

Also in 1987, the Health Education Council's report *The Health Divide* underlined how the serious social inequalities, discerned by the 1980 Black Report, had become clearer. Death rates at the bottom of the social scale were much higher than at the top at every stage of life: from birth, through to adulthood and well into old age (Whitehead, 1987).

The British Medical Association's (BMA) report *Deprivation and Ill-Health* also drew attention to the mass of evidence showing how deprivation, generated by unemployment and low pay, caused sickness and premature death. The wives of unemployed men had higher death rates than those married to wage earners; their babies suffered higher death rates; their children were shorter. The BMA called for government action against poverty (BMA, 1987).

UNEMPLOYMENT AND ILL HEALTH

All three 1987 reports on inequalities in health pointed to the strong correlation between unemployment and ill health. During the 1980s, numerous studies sought to prove (or disprove) that unemployment actually caused ill health but, owing to methodological and conceptual difficulties, few definitive results emerged, according to a review undertaken by Whiteside (1988). In contrast, Richard Smith's (1987) assembly of all the key research in Britain showed beyond reasonable doubt, in Laurance's (1986b) view, that unemployed people died earlier than those in work, especially by suicide, while suffering more physical and, particularly mental, ill health.

REGIONAL INEQUALITIES

The Health and Lifestyle Survey showed that inequalities in health between social classes and occupational status were further compounded by regional differences in health (Cox et al., 1987). *The Health Divide* also pointed out that the north–south divide was getting wider all the time. Early death rates were highest in Scotland, the north and north-west of England and lowest in the south-east (Whitehead, 1987).

RACIAL INEQUALITIES

Alongside other forms of inequalities in health, the interaction between healthcare provision and the needs of black people and ethnic minorities remained low on the agenda and largely marginalized.

Racism in the health service could be perceived by black and ethnic minorities, both as workers in the NHS and as consumers. As workers, studies had repeatedly shown how black nurses had had negative professional experiences in terms of access to training, promotion, recognition and encouragement (CRE, 1987; Baxter, 1988). Black nurses tended to work in the less prestigious geriatric and mental hospitals (McNaught, 1988). Consequently, in the face of overt and covert racism, fewer young black people were applying for nurse training (Alibhai, 1988). Ethnic minority workers were also concentrated in areas that tended not to attract indigenous labour (domestic staff, ancillary and maintenance staff; McNaught, 1988).

Discrimination against black and ethnic minority doctors began with applications to medical schools (CRE, 1988) which then continued with work rotas, job applications, staff selection, promotion and selection for in-service training (CRE, 1986; McNaught, 1988). Black doctors were also concentrated in less popular specialities, notably geriatrics, accident and emergency and psychiatry. Few reached consultant level (CRE, 1986).

MINORITY NEEDS AND HEALTH CARE PROVISION

In seeking to meet the healthcare needs of black and ethnic minority people, some attempts had been made by the NHS to improve access and to address language problems (Jofre, 1988) but the lack of awareness of cultural practice and principles persisted amongst some health professionals (Donovan, 1986; Mind, 1987). Where NHS ethnic advisers *had* been appointed, they had begun to step outside the stereotyping framework of perceiving the minority community as a 'problem' (McNaught, 1988). A few health authorities, such as Newham, had been treating equal opportunities as a serious issue (GLARE, 1987; Suppiah, 1989). However, as Larbie's (1985) study of maternity provision revealed, health care provision had not been formulated with ethnic minority needs in mind (Donovan, 1986). This situation was further reflected in the lack of black or ethnic minority people on health authorities or Community Health Councils or in NHS policy-making positions (BMA, 1987).

Overall, NAHA's (1988a) strategy report showed that most health authorities had ignored Department of Health advice on tackling racial inequalities in the NHS which had, in turn, failed to respond to the needs of Britain's black population. Even more fundamentally, as both Alibhai (1988) and McNaught (1988) pointed out, the whole approach in the NHS had been colour blind, as managers rejected allegations of racism. At root was the failure to recognize the effect of institutional racism – the organizational culture of the NHS – which remained immune to change (Conroy and Mohammed, 1989).

Alongside the (albeit marginalized) aspects of inequalities in health, the mounting number of studies increased pressure for action and change. Meanwhile, the crisis surrounding NHS resources provided a further focus of controversy.

HEALTH CARE AND ITS COSTS

The costs of the NHS continued to be highly controversial in the 1980s. In a determined effort to curb public expenditure, efficiency savings and cuts were variously imposed: charges were increased, contracting-out of support services encouraged and attempts were made to cut the drugs bill by limiting the list of drugs that doctors could prescribe on the NHS. Nevertheless, the funding base remained fairly intact. The NHS was still largely funded by taxation (Table 4.2). However, in an analysis of healthcare and its costs, the DHSS (1983b) claimed that the NHS was giving better treatment to more people at lower cost, despite the fact that advanced medical techniques and the escalating number of elderly patients put pressure on resources.

Meanwhile, somewhat paradoxically, funds for the NHS had substantially increased since 1979, under a government anxious to restrain public expenditure. The total cost of the National Heatlh Service in the UK rose from £9282 million in 1979 to £19 801 million in 1986 (Table 4.2). Furthermore, the NHS increased its share of the Gross National Product from 5.37% in 1979 to a new high of 6.29% in 1983, although the proportion fell back to 6.12% in 1986, by which time each sector of the NHS felt threatened by diminished resources (OHE, 1987: 16).

The paradox of increased NHS funds led a foremost commentator on the NHS, Professor Rudolf Klein, to ask whether the NHS really was in crisis. In a *New Society* article (November 1983), Klein argued that the NHS had been in a continual state of crisis: in the early 1950s it was the crisis of overspending; in

Table 4.2 Cost of the NHS 1949–1987.

Year	Taxation		National Insurance contributions		LHA		Patient payments		Total NHS
	£ million	% NHS	£ million	% NHS	£ million	% NHS	£ million	% NHS	(£ million)
1949	437	100.0	–	–	–	–	–	–	437
1950	477	100.0	–	–	–	–	–	–	477
1951	414	82.3	42	8.3	41	8.2	6	1.2	503
1952	422	80.2	42	8.0	44	8.4	18	3.4	526
1953	436	79.9	41	7.5	45	8.2	24	4.4	546
1954	451	80.0	41	7.3	47	8.3	25	4.4	564
1955	489	80.4	42	6.9	51	8.4	26	4.3	608
1956	539	81.2	41	6.2	56	8.4	28	4.2	664
1957	572	79.4	55	7.6	60	8.3	33	4.6	720
1958	567	74.2	99	13.0	65	8.5	33	4.3	764
1959	608	73.6	113	13.7	71	8.6	34	4.1	826
1960	671	74.4	118	13.1	77	8.5	36	4.0	902
1961	706	72.0	142	14.5	87	8.9	46	4.7	981
1962	718	70.0	163	15.9	95	9.3	49	4.8	1025
1963	772	70.7	165	15.1	104	9.5	51	4.7	1092
1964	854	71.8	169	14.2	113	9.5	54	4.5	1190
1965	981	75.1	166	12.7	127	9.7	32	2.5	1306
1966	1102	77.0	166	11.6	134	9.4	30	2.1	1432
1967	1207	77.6	164	10.5	153	9.8	32	2.1	1556

1968	1310	76.6	178	10.4	168	9.8	54	3.2	1710
1969	1416	78.8	186	10.4	131	7.3	64	3.6	1797
1970	1635	79.9	209	10.2	135	6.6	67	3.3	2046
1971	1862	80.2	232	10.0	154	6.6	75	3.2	2323
1972	2179	81.3	236	8.8	178	6.6	88	3.3	2681
1973	2499	82.3	239	7.9	204	6.7	96	3.2	3038
1974	3610	91.0	235	5.9	–	–	103	2.6	3968
1975	4737	89.4	451	8.5	–	–	108	2.0	5296
1976	5546	88.3	605	9.6	–	–	128	2.0	6279
1977	6147	88.1	676	9.7	–	–	151	2.2	6974
1978	7072	88.4	761	9.5	–	–	166	2.1	7999
1979	8200	88.3	882	9.5	–	–	200	2.2	9282
1980	10587	88.9	1042	8.7	–	–	282	2.4	11911
1981	12027	87.7	1344	9.8	–	–	348	2.5	13719
1982	12484	86.2	1594	11.0	–	–	404	2.8	14482
1983	14170	86.5	1754	10.7	–	–	459	2.8	16383
1984	14898	86.4	1858	10.8	–	–	481	2.8	17237
1985	15801	85.9	2036	11.1	–	–	563	3.1	18400
1986#	16929	85.5	2252	11.4	–	–	620	3.1	19801
1987#	18189	85.0	2522	11.8	–	–	691	3.2	21403

All figures relate to calendar year. LHA = former Local Health Authority. From 1974 onwards, services provided by LHA were transferred to the NHS.
= estimated.

Source: OHE (Office of Health Economics) (1987), Table 2.8 (last column omitted).
Reproduced by kind permission of the Office of Health Economics.

the 1960s it was the crisis of underspending; in the 1970s it was the crisis of reorganization. Klein then identified a conflict of evidence: doctors, nurses, administrators and trade unionists were convinced that the NHS was heading for a disaster, but the government's own statistics appeared to demonstrate that the NHS had been improving every year. Amidst the rising costs and the tightening of the NHS budget, the paradox of the 1980s seemed to be explained by a shift of activity in the NHS from cure to care, from extension of life to the alleviation of misery and conditions which could not be cured – in line with an ageing population. The crisis of the NHS was a microcosm of the crisis in Britain. A sense of grievance, of relative deprivation, was generated by Britain's slide down the international economic league table in which the USA, Sweden and West Germany were wealthier and spent a high proportion of a relatively larger income on health care (Klein, 1983).

By 1986, the paradox was becoming even clearer, according to *New Society* analyst Jeremy Laurance (1987a). The government's repeated claim, that ever more was being spent on the NHS, was now challenged by figures published by the Office of Health Economics (OHE, 1987), which showed that, in cash terms, the health service's budget had indeed grown (Table 4.2). However, because the economy had grown faster, the NHS *share* of the national wealth had declined. The government's tight grip on public spending had not allowed the NHS to share in the country's growing prosperity. The pressure on the NHS budget had caused acute problems, especially in London, which had been hardest hit by the RAWP formula (under which resources were being progressively redistributed to the poorer regions of the north), despite a £13 million bridging fund made especially available to the four Thames regions late in the autumn of 1986 (Laurance, 1987a).

As the reality became clearer, so the apparent crisis deepened. By 1987 the various controversies were to lead to a political explosion.

5 REORGANIZATION AND THE SEARCH FOR BETTER MANAGEMENT: 1982 ONWARDS

THE BACKGROUND

Criticism had been mounting over the administrative structure brought into being in 1974, hardly before the new NHS system had had a chance to settle down. Problems centred on delays in decision-making, elaborate consultation procedures, structural complexity and a widespread feeling that too many tiers and too many administrators created excessive bureaucracy, duplication and waste. Research on the operation of the new structure revealed further issues, such as the high cost of reorganization and low staff morale (Brown, 1979). Resentment of central control contributed to low morale amongst the peripheral health authorities, while Parliament was dissatisfied with the lack of accountability.

Stress of organizational change and financial stringency in the 1970s had never enabled the hopes raised by the 1974 structure to be fulfilled. What *had* emerged from the 1974 reorganization was a somewhat cumbersome arrangement of regions, areas and districts; each tier had responsibilities but the whole reflected a compromise between conflicting interests. The 1974 model sought to reconcile a variety of policy aims, to preserve consensus but to avoid conflict and to placate everyone: professionals, civil servants, NHS managers and administrators (Klein, 1983). The outcome pleased no one. Furthermore, as the Community Health Councils (CHCs) opened up the way to making the NHS more responsive to the public through committee representation, public meetings and access to information, so these measures institutionalized criticism. The NHS therefore became politicized in a way previously unknown.

In 1979, the Royal Commission on the NHS endorsed the view that there was one tier of administration too many and recommended that there should be only one level of authority below the regional (Merrison Report, 1979: 376). Events then moved swiftly. In December 1979, the Conservative government's consultative paper *Patients First* announced agreement with the proposal that one tier of administration should be removed. Following criticism that Area Health Authorities were too small for proper planning and too large for delivery of services, *Patients First* suggested that they should be replaced by smaller District Health Authorities (DHAs) to combine the function of the existing areas and districts. This realignment, the government claimed, would save some 10% on management costs (DHSS, 1979).

Accordingly, the *Health Services Act* of 1980 enabled the Secretary of State to restructure the NHS. The government's final decisions on reorganization were then published in July 1980 (DHSS, 1980b). In the light of ongoing financial difficulties and constraints, a constant feature of the NHS has been for the government of the day to turn to structural reorganization as a solution. Once again, in 1982, the NHS underwent restructuring.

THE 1982 NHS REORGANIZATION

By April 1982, the Area Health Authorities (AHAs) had been abolished to be replaced by 201 new DHAs; nine in Wales and 192 in England (190 by 1989, following two amalgamations: Figure 5.1).

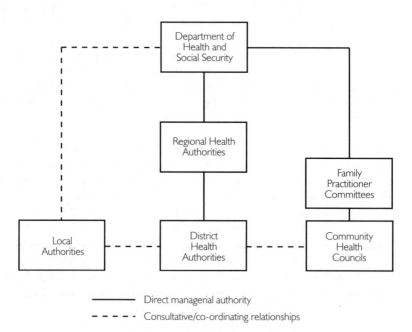

Figure 5.1   The structure of the NHS after 1982. Special health authorities were created under the NHS Act 1997 (which served largely to draw together previous legislation into a more comprehensive Act) to administer some 14 NHS bodies:

The Prescription Pricing Authority
The Health Service Supply Council
The Rampton Hospital Review Board
The Board of Governors for the Hospitals for Sick Children
The Board of Governors of the National Hospital for Nervous Diseases
The Hammersmith Special Health Authority
The Board of Governors of Moorfields Eye Hospital
The Bethlem Royal Hospital and the Maudsley Hospital
The Board of Governors of the National Heart and Chest Hospital
The Board of Governors of the Royal Marsden Hospital
The Welsh Technical Services Organization
The Central Blood Laboratory Authority
The NHS Training Authority
The Rural Dispensing Committee.

- The DHAs were made responsible for assessing local health needs, for the employment of medical and other staff and for the planning, administration and day-to-day management of the hospital and community services under guidance from the Regional Health Authorities (RHAs), whose responsibilities remained unchanged.
- Each DHA was to have a Chair, appointed by the Secretary of State for Social Services and normally 16 other members (four of whom were to be appointed by local authorities and the others by the RHA, who had to include one nurse or health visitor, a GP, a consultant and a nominee from a university medical school).
- In Wales, as most districts were too small to make satisfactory DHAs, the districts were abolished but the AHAs were retained and renamed District Health Authorities, under which a system of unit management was established.
- Overall, the responsibilities of the DHSS remained the same under the 1982 arrangements as in 1974.

The central feature of the 1982 NHS responsibilities was structural simplification: the central tier – the AHAs – had gone. Apart from the reduction in administration, a further significant change was the loss, in many parts of the country, of the principle of co-terminosity (similar boundaries) between health and local authorities, although the CHCs and the DHAs were to remain co-terminous. The Family Practitioners Committees (FPCs) also became increasingly separate bodies from the main line of NHS administration. Further, under the 1984 *Health and Social Security Act* FPCs became employing health authorities in their own right. These developments reflected the fact that the NHS had still not secured the full administrative integration of general practitioners whose FPC boundaries and finances now emerged entirely independent of DHAs.

The main differences between reorganization in 1974 and 1982 were:

1 Restructuring in 1982, unlike the extensive discussions that led up to 1974, did not derive from substantial documentation because the changes were originally envisaged as an adjustment rather than full-scale reorganization.
2 The 1974 change was influenced by consensus politics (where both major political parties agreed on the broad strategy for health care) and extensive debate, whereas the 1982 arrangements directly reflected the philosophy of Conservative Ministers who believed that much decision-making should be decentralized and left to the local level.
3 While the 1974 model emphasized administrative unification, central planning rationality and the values of efficiency, the 1982 reorganization stressed structural simplification, small size, the values of localism and decentralization – at the cost of co-terminosity and, some feared, at the cost of diluting technical expertise, scattered more thinly at DHA level (Klein, 1983).

There were, however, some similarities between the reorganizations of 1974 and 1982. Neither attempted to include occupational and environmental health services or the armed forces. Furthermore, although the 1974 reorganization aimed to present a unified and closely co-ordinated system, both structures remained administratively separate from housing, education and personal social services at local government level. The mechanisms to liaise and co-ordinate work between DHAs and local authority social services departments remained the same: joint-funded schemes, overlapping DHA membership and joint consultative committees.

Above all, the process of evolution in the NHS was exemplified by the 1982 restructuring which, according to Charles Webster's (1998) historical analysis, was seen as a piece of fine tuning rather than as a major shake-up. Only briefly between 1974 and 1982 had an attempt been made to unify the delivery system. Once again hospital and family practitioner services were to be administered separately. The community care services remained even more separately organized under the auspices of local government.

The sense of crisis in the NHS, which had been building up throughout the late 1970s, had been fuelled by the trend to assertive unionization, the tensions between the medical profession and the government, the growth in the demand for health services and the squeeze on public resources. By 1982, restructuring might even have been perceived as a scapegoat for other problems in the NHS. The outcome of the 1982 reorganization was less of a settled solution than seemed apparent on the surface (Webster 1998: 61).

THE SEARCH FOR BETTER MANAGEMENT: 1983 ONWARDS

As the 1982 model took shape, so the NHS went through a notably unsettled period. Disruptive effects had to be absorbed as the new structure was set up. In particular, many administrators had to re-apply for jobs. However, this reorganization had barely been put into motion when, in 1983 the NHS faced further change.

From 1979, the Conservative government had invoked an ideology of minimal government intervention (whenever possible), a commitment to reducing public expenditure and a return to the market economy. The National Health Service had been somewhat protected from this harsh new economic reality by the commitment of both major political parties in the 1979 election to give the NHS priority, by the vigilance of pressure groups and, above all, by the continuing popularity of and strong public support for the NHS (Taylor Gooby, 1985; Jowell et al., 1986). The positive public attitude made it difficult for the government in the early 19980s, which was attracted to the notion of dismantling the Welfare State, to abolish or replace the NHS by some form of privatized insurance-based alternative.

However, the government sought to control the health care cost 'explosion'. The strategy of welfare pluralism attempted to off-load as much as possible onto the private, voluntary and informal sectors. Following an overwhelming majority at the 1983 general election, the Conservative administration generated programmes for effective planning and resource use in the search for better management.

The appointment of Norman Fowler, as Secretary of State for Social Services, heralded an alteration in the government's approach to health policy. The emphasis began to move, from devolution of NHS decision-making down to district level towards ensuring the NHS's upward accountability to Parliament. In 1983, an independent inquiry was established to look into NHS management practices in England. This was to be conducted by Roy Griffiths, the managing director of Sainsburys.

The Griffiths Management Inquiry Team (MIT) decided to focus on matters primarily relating to hospital management and to recommend reforms that could be achieved within existing legislation. The Griffiths MIT diagnosed the central problem of the NHS as a massive and generalized failure of clearly defined management function. The Griffiths MIT therefore recommended a commitment to general management, which was to be extended above and below the level of health authorities. The proposals (summarized in Figure 5.2) were as follows.

1 At the DHSS, a Health Services Supervisory Board (HSSB) should be established to decide overall objectives, budgets and NHS strategy. The HSSB
   would be chaired by the Secretary of State and include the Minister of State
   for the NHS, the Permanent Secretary, the Chief Medical Officer, the
   Chairman of the Management Board and two or three non-executive
   members with general management skills and experience.
2 Accountable to the HSSB, an NHS Management Board should be set up to
   take overall responsibility for running the NHS. The Board was to be chaired
   by a relatively independent (i.e. non-NHS) individual (who would become a
   civil servant) to provide professional input and managerial direction and who
   would be the Secretary of State's deputy.
3 To strengthen management, all RHAs and DHAs should be asked to appoint
   their own general managers to take charge of services at regional (RGM) and
   district (DGM) management level from April 1984. Every unit at district level
   should also have a Unit General Manager (UGM).
4 Clinicians should be more closely involved in the management process
   through the introduction of resource budgeting (Griffiths Report, 1983).

Once again events moved at speed. It took less than two years from the publication of the Griffiths MIT report in October 1983 to the implementation of its
key recommendations.

By 4 June 1984, a DHSS circular required health authorities, by now punch-
drunk with continual upheavals, to establish a general management function and
to appoint general managers: at regional, then at district and finally at unit level
(DHSS, 1984a).

In line with the Griffiths MIT's concept of encouraging the appointment of
general managers from outside the NHS, on 1 January 1985, Victor Page,
Chairman of the Port of London Authority and Deputy Chairman of the recently
privatized National Freight Consortium, was appointed as the NHS's first
Managing Director (Hencke, 1984). On 3 April 1985, the Secretary of State
announced the membership of the NHS Management Board, which had been

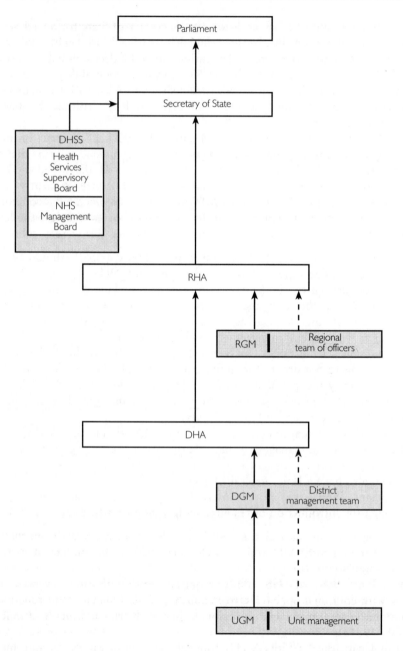

RHA: *Regional Health Authorities; RGM: Regional General Manager; DGM: District General Manager; UGM: Unit General Manager.*

Figure 5.2   Health authority management following the NHS Management Inquiry Team, 1983.
Source: DHSS (1984a).
Reproduced by kind permission of the Department of Health.

drawn from the NHS, the DHSS and the business world as the Griffiths Inquiry had recommended, together with a Chief Nursing Officer at the insistence of the House of Commons Social Services Committee (Social Services Committee, 1984).

By June 1985, most DGMs had been appointed. The final RGM posts were filled in July 1985. At this stage, fewer than 15% of the posts had been secured by staff from outside the NHS (Carrier and Kendall, 1986).

THE 1983 GRIFFITHS REPORT: REACTIONS AND OUTCOMES

The overall significance of the Griffiths model was the intention to promote and control change in a much more positive, centralized, manner. The purpose was to transform the NHS into a managed rather than merely an administered service.

A modification of consensus management was one clear outcome. The NHS had had a tradition of consensus management (Merrison Report, 1979: 314) in which a form of shared managerial responsibility, between doctors, nurses and administrators, had been based on perceived need and demand for considerable professional autonomy, especially for the hospital consultants. The Griffiths MIT saw consensus management as leading to 'lowest common denominator' decisions and to long delays in the management process (Griffiths Report, 1983: 17). Following the Griffiths proposals, a radically different model for NHS management emerged, in which shared management was to be replaced by a single general manager who would act as a chief executive and be responsible for a health authority's performance. By September 1986, the DHSS had announced a merit plan for NHS managers, in which they could be awarded up to 20% in bonus pay if objectives and goals were exceeded (DHSS, 1986a). The overall purpose was therefore to strengthen, even by incentives, the managerial approach to the distribution of resources, performance criteria and the account-ability of decision-makers.

Democracy and the place of health authority members

The shortness of the period for public consultation on the Griffiths recommenda-tions, as well as the lack of public discussion on the restructuring of the DHSS, was criticized by various sources. Indeed, the wider implications for democracy and the NHS were raised by Griffiths' perfunctory references to the public repre-sentative role of RHA and DHA members and the equally brief references to CHCs. The position of CHCs had already been threatened: *Patients First* (DHSS, 1979) had indicated that the need for separate consumer representation was not entirely clear, especially at a cost of £4 million a year. However, support from the health authorities and the general public persuaded ministers to retain the 'voice of the consumer', albeit on a reduced council membership basis.

Secondly, health authority members, having escaped the continuous refashioning of NHS management, remained largely peripheral to the debates about the 1982 reorganization. Haywood (1985) has suggested that such comparative stability was explained by their long tradition of public involvement in health care and, possibly, the political desirability of shared responsibility for rationing decisions. The Griffiths' changes were likely to transform the 'taken-for-granted' role of health authority members, pressing them into developing systems to assess the quality of care, to agree standards of acceptable performance and to review performance levels.

Former DHSS Minister Ray Whitney argued that the Griffiths' proposals had failed to solve the real problem of the NHS. The formula was inherently flawed, by being unable to create a satisfactory relationship between the general manager and the chairman at various levels or between a nationally funded organization with a service which was essentially local and directed towards the individual (Whitney, 1988: 79). In the view of the Association of Community Health Councils, the introduction of general management had led to a decline in the influence of health authority members and to a deteriorating relationship with CHCs, but changes in the consultation processes greatly depended on whether the DGM was 'autocratic' or enthusiastic about the consumerist spirit of the Griffiths Report (ACHCEW, 1988).

Internal tensions

A rather different, but vital, implication of the Griffiths Report was the extent to which the civil service should be involved in the management of the NHS. Halpern (1985) argued that there were distinct problems for civil servants as managers. Internal NHS tensions had already been compounded by competition between professional and other power groups, by the growing assertiveness of the trade unions and groups representing the consumer and by the NHS constitution in which the DHSS was staffed by civil servants rather than health service employees. The 1982 model left unresolved the basic dilemma, that had always haunted the NHS, of the relationship between the centre (the policy makers) and the periphery (the clinical decision makers). On this score, Griffiths was hardly revolutionary; the proposals represented no more than a further twist in the spiral of centralization (Petchey, 1986). Increased tensions became apparent early on, when the first Chair of the NHS Management Board (Victor Page, appointed as a second permanent secretary) suddenly resigned after only 18 months in office, following a disagreement with ministers over his right to manage. Frustration had mounted over priorities between management and politics. In October 1986 Tony Newton, then Minister of Health, was put in charge of the NHS Management Board, neatly side-stepping the underlying problems faced by a civil service manager.

The general managers

After the honeymoon period was over, it became clearer how the developments in the Griffiths' reorganization were shaping up. Analysis of the general manager posts (Table 5.1) showed that, by 1985, over 60% of all appointments went to NHS administrators.

Health authorities had been largely unsuccessful in attracting new blood, as

Table 5.1 Who got the jobs? Progress records on the posts of general managers 1985–1987.

1985 Analysis of all general manager appointments in UK				1985 Analysis of NHS all general managers by function				1985 Analysis of UK all general managers by sector		
Administrators	(same HA)*	120	54.8%	Administration	137	77.0%		NHS	178	81.3%
	(other HA)†	14	6.4%	Finance	19	10.7%		Military	13	5.9%
Treasurers	(same HA)	12	5.5%	Medical	17	9.5%		Other public sector	5	2.3%
	(other HA)	7	3.2%	Nursing	5	2.8%		Private sector	23	10.5%
Medical Officers	(same HA)	12	5.5%							
	(other HA)	2	0.9%	Total	178	100.0%		Total	219	100.0%
Nursing Officers	(same HA)	3	1.4%		—	—			—	—
	(other HA)	2	0.9%							
Unit administrators		3	1.4%							
Clinicians		3	1.4%							
Military		13	5.9%							
Other public sector		5	2.3%							
Private sector		23	10.5%							
Total		219	100.0%							
		—	—							

*Successful candidate came from within Health Authority.
†Successful candidate came from outside Health Authority.

Source: Alleway (1985).
Reproduced by permission of the Health Service Journal.

Table 5.2 December 1987: Background of postholders at regional, district and unit level by function.

Provenance	RGM	DGM	UGM	Total	%
Administrator	9	114	350	473	57.97
Treasurer		18	5	23	2.82
Doctor	1	16	110	127	15.56
Nurse	1	5	71	77	9.44
Other NHS			14	14	1.72
Outside NHS	3	36	57	96	11.72
Vacant		2	4	6	0.74
Total	14	191	611	816	100.00*

*to nearest 1%.

Source: Personal communication from the Department of Health 21.2.89.

the government intended, into health service management. Despite the direct intervention by health ministers to try to block some in-service appointments, some 80% of NHS general manager posts went to existing health service staff in 1985 (Table 5.1). The proportion had barely changed by 1987, nor was there any significant difference between the regional, district and unit general manager appointments (Table 5.2). Fixed-term contracts, low salaries relative to those available in the private sector and the total absence of fringe benefits were some suggested reasons – or it could have been an indication of the management ability of existing NHS staff (Alleway, 1985).

The general managers from the armed services saw themselves as in charge. The army model slipped in neatly for those from a military background but was at variance with decision making by committee, the plethora of meetings and deluge of paperwork (Sherman, 1985). Many DGMs who had been previous NHS administrators had much to learn to become more leader-like. Indeed by 1987, there had been a 5% turnover of general managers. The departures were largely explained by a misunderstanding over the nature and the culture of the job (Alleway, 1987).

Doctors and the outcome in the new management structure

For many doctors, the Griffiths' development seemed to herald the end of clinical freedom, even though the Griffiths MIT advocated the close involvement of clinicians in the management process. However, the immediate reaction of the medical profession to the Griffiths Report (1983) was mixed. The BMA expressed reservations and strongly recommended a trial run in one region. Doctors wished to see 'medical' general managers appointed but, on the whole, the doctors' stance was fairly positive (Taylor, 1984), more particularly amongst junior doctors (who, in the short term, had less to lose from the proposals).

However, increasingly doctors felt that the 'spirit' of Griffiths had been hijacked by health service administrators. Doctors were left behind in the general manager appointments, as few of them had management skills. Hospital and community doctors had secured only a small proportion of RGM and DGM posts by 1987 (Table 5.2), although a more significant proportion of UGM posts had been secured by doctors.

Clinicians faced a dilemma analogous with that of the technical expert in industry. To most clinicians/technicians management was not a 'real' job. Clinicians drawn into general management found themselves doing less work for which they believed they had been trained, while spending more and more time on administration. Even alternative careers, general manager's salaries and the lure of power were not sufficient attractions to most (Williams, 1987).

Some doctors might well have been reluctant to lose their former position. Historically, NHS priorities had been determined through a powerful combination of 'priorities by decibels', which worked to the advantage of prestigious specialities involved in heroic surgery and life-threatening conditions (Hunter, 1988). Neither the market nor the public sector had quite managed to tackle the problems stemming from the professional monopoly of all health care systems. The Griffiths' approach was to involve clinicians in management, principally through budgeting and resource management. More significantly, the Griffiths' reorganization set out to challenge 40 years of professional domination of the NHS (Petchey, 1986). Laurance (1988a) reported on individual doctors who were critical of the NHS being intimidated into silence by management.

Nurses and management

The position of nurses in the proposed management structure seemed to be under far greater threat: at least doctors, as a whole, held positions of prestige and power in the NHS. A major implication for nursing staff was that their unique position on management teams, given to them in 1974, looked to be in jeopardy if they did not secure representation and status within the new management arrangements (Taylor, 1984). The mounting level of anxiety among the nursing professionals over the Griffiths' implications was reflected in the massive Royal College of Nursing advertising campaign, launched in January 1986.

The forebodings of the nursing profession proved timely. Quite simply, nurses felt they had lost out on the Griffiths' deal. The fact that few nurses were appointed as general managers (2.8% in 1985: Table 5.1, although 11% of UGM posts had been filled by nurses in 1987) may have been welcomed by those who believed that nurse managers were of limited intellectual quality (Taylor, 1984) and lacking in managerial ability (Cox, 1986). As David Cox (1986) found in his research in South Birmingham, prejudices were strongly entrenched. It remained to be seen whether the culture of general management could overcome mutual scepticism.

Others saw the post-Salmon in-service management courses as the pitfall. The basic problem was that nurses had only limited training in management skills. The Salmon structure had proved double-edged as it encouraged nurses to concentrate on the clinical management of nursing alone and to develop a managerial system that appeared entirely self-contained, whereas the traditional view of general management was usually expressed in terms of wider functions such as planning, controlling, staffing, budgeting, organizing and directing. The top nurse at DHA level, the Chief Nursing Officer (CNO), was responsible solely for the organization and delivery of nursing services. Under the new management structure, DHAs saw no need for the advice to be channelled through CNOs, a third of whose posts were promptly axed. Professional nursing advice was rather more received at subunit level (Rowden, 1986).

A major study of the nursing management function (Glennerster et al., 1986) after the Griffiths Report (1983), described how initially many nurses feared that role conflict would arise from the separation of management control and professional advice, which was foreign to the hierarchical system of the Salmon nurse management structure. The study also suggested that a problem was arising for married women – over half of the nurse managers appointed were either men or single women with continuous employment records, although the new post-Griffiths' structure might enable younger nurses to make a career in management (Glennerster et al., 1986). Nevertheless, Glennerster's (1988) second report showed that many district nurse advisers, burdened by overwork, had accountability but no authority (and vice versa), that nurses had become demoralized and that their stress levels had been heightened by constant change in the NHS.

After researching nursing advice in seven varied health authorities in the aftermath of the Griffiths changes, Robinson and Strong (1987) indicated that the turmoil of the nursing profession could be assuaged by furthering the major asset of professional nursing advice – promoting quality of care – but this required the creation of a senior clinical nursing grade to monitor quality at clinical level. The basic argument presented was that, whatever the management arrangements, nursing's claim to power and influence and to sit at the management table ultimately rested on its knowledge of the quality of nursing care and the conditions for creating that care. Strong and Robinson (1988) reported that there were many first-class managers among nurses and that general management needed managers with extensive clinical experience. Indeed, in some districts, nurses were making a fundamental contribution to the new post-Griffiths' era.

The more stark reality was that, by 1989, there were still only six nurses who held DGM posts. The first to do so, Christine Hancock, the Royal College of Nursing's leader-in-waiting, described how she had to battle against discrimination to reach a top position in NHS management (Millar, 1989a).

Reorganization and management models

The reaction from several Regional Health Authorities was to express concern that the Griffiths' developments could amount to further NHS reorganization. Indeed, by 1985, the NHS management realignment had incurred the wide-scale abolition of jobs that had been created under the 1982 reorganization, as well as the creation of 2700 new DGMs and RGMs.

The reactions of DHAs to Griffiths varied. While making little pretence at any major rethink, some DHAs adopted a strategy of minimalism; others took the opportunity to develop a corporate approach to revise management structures and practices. The impact of change set in motion by the Griffiths Report (1983) did indeed trigger major restructuring, in which every NHS manager's job was affected and in which there was a significant movement of staff around the country. Griffiths proclaimed that this was not another reorganization – but, to those involved, the change felt very real (Cox, 1986).

A further significant outcome of the Griffiths' reorganization was the way in which the existing district management arrangements were made to accommodate the introduction of the general management function. In its implementation, the Districts were given considerable discretion, subject to DHSS approval. A wide variety of models evolved and at least five organizational types could be identified.

1 Peterborough DHA adopted a management development process in which the general manager was both specialist and team player (Tibbles, 1987).
2 Winchester DHA had general managers as the pivotal link, in which the management units were reduced to two: one covered acute services and the other embraced all remaining services. The Winchester model was unique in the shape of two district-wide bodies: one concerned mainly with managerial issues (the executive group) and the other with professional and policy issues (the strategic advisory group) (Nattrass et al., 1985).
3 A third model was taken up by a number of health authorities (Riverside, Wirral, Gloucester) with slight differences between them. Central to this model were two types of managers: the executive (or operational) DGMs and UGMs and the 'specialist' general managers, who had district-wide responsibilities for certain key functions such as personnel, planning or finance (Nattrass et al., 1985).
4 South Birmingham DHA implemented a simplified management structure in which three main health care areas (acute services, family services, mental handicap and mental health) were identified as viable and rationalized management units. Of interest here was the solution to the aggrieved clinicians, who felt penalized by the new management structure, through the appointment of a clinician as Director of Acute Services or 'Boss Doc' (Cox, 1986).
5 A fifth, more evolutionary, model was chosen by Newcastle DHA. In this the main consideration was to introduce general management without sacrificing many important and desirable features of the 1982 reorganization. The structure therefore incorporated an expanded district management team accountable to the DGM (Nattrass et al., 1985).

Within the variety of models implemented, three factors remained central: a desire to take account of the district's major strategic concerns and service policies, a wish to devolve managerial power and authority to unit level and the need to find a formula through which professional and general managers could work together to the mutual advantage of both (Best, 1985).

Overall, the implementation of the Griffiths Report (1983) had swept in a new era of management for the NHS. The changed structure and roles were aimed at gaining more control, through devolution, over the direction, planning, use of money and standards of performance in DHAs and at unit level, in order to integrate a corporate sense of priorities in health care.

General management: the impact of a national development programme, a new vocabulary and information technology

By the mid-1980s, wider changes were sweeping through the NHS. As the DHSS (1984b) explained, the introduction of general managers in health authorities was part of a national development programme, which included:

- Rayner-type scrutinies;
- annual accountability reviews;
- value-for-money audit programmes;
- tighter manpower planning;
- competitive tendering;
- setting up an NHS Training Authority;
- cash limits and cost improvement programmes;
- manpower targets.

The upshot was that that the NHS – managerially, financially and structurally – was having to absorb a level of change unparalleled in its history. On the one hand, efficiency (managerial and financial) had now been elevated from being one consideration in decision-making to the major policy objective. On the other hand, the battery of central activities, such as cash limits, manpower targeting and annual reviews, all reinforced the trend to centralization which had earlier been foreshadowed by narrowing local authority representation on health authorities and, later, by the creation of a central management board together with an influx of new general managers accountable to the centre.

The new wave of managerialism brought in a new vocabulary and organizational intent concerning resource priorities, targets and reviews. The terms included.

- *Cost effectiveness:* Resource allocation based on value for money by identifying the cheapest way of producing an agreed measure of health outcome such as the saving of life or additional life years (Maynard, 1987).
- *Management effectiveness:* Personal performance linked to the achievement of objectives.
- *Performance indicators (PIs):* Systems and management tools, based on comparative statistics used to analyse data, assess performance against objectives, measure efficiency and focus on possible underlying problems. Although PIs meant different things to different people, they were most commonly used in connection with bed use, medical and nursing staffing, clinical activity, finance and estate management (Payling et al., 1987; Jenkins, 1988). Some would argue that PIs provided a refined way of cost cutting.
- *Quality assurance:* A technique of comparing performance against expectations, implementing change where necessary, checking that action had the desired effect and taking remedial action if standards were not met (Shaw,

1987; Ellis, 1988). Many health authorities had appointed 'quality assurance' managers by 1988.

Closely linked to the new managerial modes was information technology. The Körner Steering Group (1982) had been set up to report on the information systems in the NHS. Their purpose was twofold: to enable collection and effective use of reliable and up-to-date data about supply, demand and services and to ensure the best possible patient care with the resources available. Indeed general management, as envisaged by Griffiths, was scarcely possible without major improvements in the NHS information services and systems or in the managers' capacity to use information to effect change.

Following the Körner Steering Group's recommendations, DHAs were asked to have the systems for collecting the Körner specified minimum data sets by April 1987 (1988 for community services). For many DHAs, the process of translating data into information for management and for making effective use of information to achieve patient benefits was a largely uncharted area (McClenahan et al., 1986). The challenge was for DHAs to use information effectively but to avoid the use of laborious paper systems as an end in itself.

The 1986 *Data Protection Act*, which was designed to protect the privacy of the individual and to regulate the processing of data by computer, also had to be taken into account in the use of the NHS information systems, as the Körner Steering Group advised in October 1984.

One major impact of both the Griffiths and Körner recommendations was that overt rationing and planning by managers, based on financial criteria and using information technology, were to replace the more covert rationing at the discretion of clinicians on medical grounds. As a result, Griffiths had confronted a conflict, inherent in the NHS since its inception, between bureaucratic and professional control: 40 years of professional domination had shifted towards managerial supremacy.

GENERAL MANAGEMENT AND THE NHS

Was it all worth it? Had the change in management structures achieved the results intended?

A survey of UGMs and their staff in the Trent and North West Thames RHAs suggested some success in achieving two of Griffiths' main recommendations: improved budgetary and costing arrangements and clearer responsive decision-making at local level. The achievement of greater devolution at unit level had contributed to the strength and status of units in the NHS but had failed to improve staff morale and motivation (Banyard, 1988). However, research on unit management groups at Birmingham University's Health Services Management Centre suggested that, within the new management arrangements, sustained change in attitude and culture were harder to achieve than organizational adjustments. There was a tendency to resume old habits once the dust of reorganization had settled (Williams et al., 1985).

Funded by the Economic and Social Research Council (ESRC), a Nuffield Institute/Open University survey of eight English DHAs and their regions specifically set out to establish whether the improvements intended by the Griffiths Report (1983) had been realized. The findings indicated that UGMs and nurses felt that decision-making had been speeded up; consultants, district-based planners and administrators were more sceptical. The improvements initiated by general management were therefore unevenly distributed, although most thought allocation of personal responsibility had become more precise. Conditions of severe financial constraint tended to reinforce top-down line management. Meanwhile, progress towards making services more consumer-oriented was less than spectacular (Harrison et al., 1989).

The ESRC-funded survey and a further Nuffield Institute study on the use of management budgets and resource management (Pollitt et al., 1988) found a few enthusiastic managers, but a greater number of cautious ones; a handful of keen consultants, but a large number of determinedly sceptical ones. The Griffiths Report (1983) had stressed the need to induce doctors to become more involved in costs and, more broadly, resource management (critical factors for effective management at local level). However, the Nuffield Institute showed that time was required to win over many clinicians to the principle of resource management and to allay their fears about losing clinical autonomy.

Strong and Robinson's (1988) research in seven various DHAs on Griffiths' new model management found that the initiative had introduced not merely an efficiency drive but a better way of providing health care under the guidance of a new sort of manager. Higher quality was being delivered to consumers from properly co-ordinated front-line workers.

More negatively, the price of administrative tidiness underestimated the costs to staff morale and patients, especially as the Griffiths' recommendations were based on, and directed at, the hospital services to the neglect of community-based health services (Carrier and Kendall, 1986). A Brunel University report warned that, while correct in principle, the Griffiths' general management revolution lacked effective implementation – a view shared by the Social Services Committee 1988a). In many districts, little of substance had changed; in some, change had even been harmful (Kingston and Rowbottom, 1989). However, while the introduction of the Griffiths' management model had favoured NHS administrators who had secured the greater proportion of management posts, the British Medical Association/Royal College of Nursing strategy of co-operating with implementation, in the hope of 'containing the fall-out', proved an almost complete failure (Petchey, 1986). What had certainly not changed was the sexist bias. There were barely half a dozen female managers at regional and district levels; the managers were essentially male. Nevertheless, general managers still faced incompatibilities between the political imperatives of the NHS and the principles of business management embedded in the 1983 Griffiths Report (Cousins, 1987: 171) and between the new managerial values and the caring values oriented to the health needs of the population.

6 POLITICS AND PRIORITIES: HEALTH CARE PROVISION BY 1988

The June general election of 1987 led to a crucial turning point in the provision of health care in Britain, although the impact on the NHS was not immediately apparent. Despite much 'New Right' rhetoric against the Welfare State, the first two Thatcher administrations (1979/83, 1983/87) did not seriously take on the public welfare sectors – with one single (but important) exception, that of council housing. The basic structures of social security, state education and the National Health Service were much the same in 1987 as they had been in 1979, which could not be said of former public activities such as the nationalized industries. The idea that the government should continue to provide health care, education and social security had proved remarkably resilient.

As the third Thatcher administration began in 1987, again with a significant majority, so the right-wing Conservative ideology and philosophy on welfare provision became strengthened and consolidated. As expressed in the 1987 *Conservative Party Manifesto* together with subsequent developments, the key principles on which the Welfare State now hinged included:

1 Privatization, exemplified by the encouragement of private pension plans (*Social Security Act* 1986), by pressure on the private sector to fund City Technology Colleges (*Education Reform Act* 1988) and to regenerate inner city areas.
2 Diminishing local government powers expressed by greater autonomy for parents of children in state schools who could vote to opt out of Local Education Authority control into central government direct-grant arrangements (*Education Reform Act* 1988); similarly, tenants could 'opt out' of local government housing and transfer to private and charitable sector management (*Housing Act* 1988).
3 Increasing centralization: polytechnics and 'opted-out' state schools were no longer directly responsible to local but to central government (*Education Reform Act* 1988).
4 Efficiency and cost effectiveness, set as supreme values against which health, welfare and education were to be measured.
5 Economic independence, reflected in rising home ownership aided by mortgage tax relief. Reliance on social security was regarded as 'dependence' on the 'nanny' state, a system to be administered selectively and stringently to the targeted poor.
6 Individual values and maximization of choice, promoted by lowering personal income tax at the expense of collective action in social welfare.

Social policy had become transformed. The Welfare State was at a point of radical transition. The politically successful policy of selling off council houses to tenants, under the 1980 Housing Act, heralded the outlook for the first half of the 1980s. By 1988, legislation in social security, housing and education underpinned the political values in social welfare for the 1990s. With this substantial social policy programme in hand, the government did not initially intend to alter the provision of health care in any significant way. The Griffiths management restructuring had, in any case, only recently been absorbed. Then, in the late autumn of 1987, the government was caught on the political hop over the financing of the NHS. An explosive public row erupted amongst health professionals and politicians over the inadequacy of resources to meet the needs of the NHS. To understand the background to this outburst, one must look at a series of issues that had increasingly put pressure on the NHS. Priorities became ever more influenced by the emergent values in welfare politics.

STAFFING THE NHS

One major issue that acted as a powder keg within the NHS, was the question of clinical staffing. Through thick and thin, medical and nursing professionals in the NHS had, on the whole, maintained high standards of recruitment, training and professional conduct. Until 1987 the standards of patient care, some failings and abuses apart, had remained good (Maxwell, 1988).

However, the failure to deal justly with many groups, such as junior medical and nursing staff, ward sisters and their equivalent, midwives, ancillary and other low-paid workers, was a major drawback (Maxwell, 1988; Widgery, 1988) which was aggravated by racism. Further, although women accounted for nearly 50% of doctors, discrimination led them to work largely in less prestigious specialities and to be less likely than men to reach higher grades (Allen, 1988). Altogether, bad working conditions and increased patient turnover had affected staff morale and decreased the chance to build up friendly and human relationships with patients (Widgery, 1988). The weaknesses of the NHS reflected the frustrations of working in a big politically led bureaucracy: inertia, neglect of capital investment and the sometimes shameful treatment of staff (Maxwell, 1988).

THE PLACE AND TRAINING OF CLINICIANS IN THE NHS

One direct outcome of the unrest was the pressure from junior doctors to reduce their alleged 120-hour working week. In 1989 a north London GP, Lord Rhea, through a House of Lords Bill, consequently sought legislation to reduce junior doctors' hours to a maximum of 72 hours a week by 1992.

A second bone of contention was the outcome of the Griffiths Report. In the clamour to introduce general management into the NHS, the effect of such a move on the career opportunities of staff was largely overlooked. For some, the introduction of general management was an opportunity for development – clinicians who had made the transition to general manager and who had negotiated safety nets to enable either their return to professional roles or their retention of clinical workloads (Linstead and McMahon, 1987). Clinical budgeting often brought loud objections from consultants, although clinicians could be won over to management budgeting at unit level if their legitimate concerns were respected (Wickings, 1983; Scrivens, 1988). More fundamentally, the Griffiths reorganization introduced a general management model which offered the possibility of controlling rampant medical dominance (Strong and Robinson, 1988). The previous classic medical model of an administrative system, within which doctors treated patients and controlled resources in the light of their professional judgement, had shifted in favour of managerial efficiency and cost effectiveness.

However, the nub of problems and pressures for doctors and consultants continued to be restrained resources and overspent budgets in acute services. Nevertheless, David Hunter (Harrison et al., 1989), health policy analyst at the King's Fund Institute, commented that 'mere influx of new money' would do nothing to alleviate the underlying problem of how doctors were trained and managed – or, rather, undermanaged. The politics of health was as much about the power and influence of particular professionals as it was about the policies of governments.

The training of doctors had remained unchanged for many years. Medical education had failed to keep pace with changing needs, with the new thrust of general management and with clinical budgeting. Trainee doctors received almost no practical training in dealing with patients; the prevention of illness and the promotion of health were also largely ignored. Students spent all but a few weeks in lecture theatres of high technology hospitals; often only four weeks of a five-year degree course were devoted to general practitioner work in the community even though half of all graduates became GPs (Collins, 1988). By August 1988, the World Federation for Medical Educations *Edinburgh Declaration* sought to change the obsolete training methods in Britain and abroad by placing greater emphasis on disease prevention, health promotion, health priorities, community resources and the management of patients (Douglas Home, 1988; World Federation for Medical Education, 1988).

Training for GPs had, however, developed: indeed, the requirement that all principals in general practice had, by 1982, to have undertaken a special three-year training scheme emphasized the recognition of the role of the GP and the increasing importance attached to primary health care.

GENERAL PRACTITIONERS AND PRIMARY HEALTH CARE

By the mid-1980s, priority considerations had shifted in favour of GPs playing a key role in community health. Under political focus was the whole development of primary health care by which the DHSS meant the work of dentists, opticians, pharmacists and GPs. The emphasis on consumer choice, financial incentives, privatization and cost accountability reflected the dominant political values in welfare provision. Initially, the DHSS (1986b) issued the consultation document *Primary Health Care: An Agenda for Discussion*. The direct outcome of the discussions was the 1987 White Paper *Promoting Better Health* (DHSS, 1987a) which led to the *Health and Medicines Act* 1988.

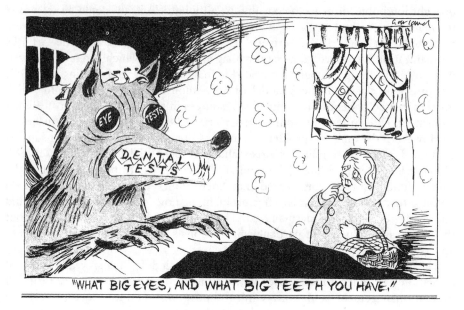

"WHAT BIG EYES, AND WHAT BIG TEETH YOU HAVE."

Source: The Independent, *1 November 1998.*
Reproduced by kind permission of The Independent *and Nicholas Garland.*

Three key features of primary health care arose from these developments. First, privatization was encouraged through a variety of measures.

1 Charges were introduced for eye tests and dental check-ups (despite opposition from the House of Lords).
2 GP private services were to be expanded.
3 The General Practice Finance Corporation, which provided for doctors' surgeries, was to be privatized.

The second main theme was the emphasis given to the prevention of ill health and the promotion of good health in which GPs, dental practitioners, health educators, health visitors and community nurses all had a part to play. GPs, who were required to retire at 70, were offered a series of financial incentives to help people to adopt healthier lifestyles and to make the GP services more responsive to consumer needs. Measures included incentives and allowances to provide:

- special target levels of vaccinations, immunizations and screening;
- comprehensive regular care for elderly people;
- minor surgery;
- health surveillance for children under five;
- health checks for first-time patients;
- support for doctors working in deprived areas;
- regular postgraduate training for GPs.

The third feature reflected the government's intention to make the provision of health care accountable to the public. The objectives of the primary health care plans were therefore to improve value for money, to give patients the widest choice in obtaining high-quality services and to make the services more responsive to the consumer.

Few believed that the existing primary health care system, centred on the GP, was entirely satisfactory but these plans seemed to duck real reform. Possibilities for co-ordinated and constructive change were missed; nor was it clear who was to take the lead in monitoring preventive services (Marks, 1988).

Although GPs were untouched directly by the Griffiths management reorganization, the proposed 5% increase on Family Practitioner Committee expenditure was unlikely to solve the funding problems. The demands of primary health care were therefore another pointer to the mounting financial difficulties in the NHS.

THE PLACE AND TRAINING OF NURSES, MIDWIVES AND HEALTH VISITORS

The nurses actually sparked the tinderbox of political trouble in the autumn of 1987, with various grievances. The problems started in the training programme.

Nurse training

Nurse education in Britain had been extensively reviewed by the statutory bodies for nursing, midwifery and health visiting set up in 1979. The United Kingdom Central Council for Nursing, Midwifery and Health Visiting (UKCC) found that nurse education was not fully oriented to service needs. The basic premise of nurse education was that students – some 85 000 of them in the UK – should be a major part of the hospital labour force. Apart from a minority of degree students on grants, student nurses therefore found themselves working for long hours on low pay. Furthermore, health visitors, district nurses and midwives all complained that their basic preparation was not a sound basis on which to build. Those who had been trained to educate were powerless to control the educational process (UKCC, 1986).

The UKCC proposed *Project 2000* as a means of reforming nurse training. *Project 2000* included:

1 Basic preparation for all, oriented to health as well as illness.
2 A new three-year programme of education and training, to comprise a common 18-month foundation programme followed by a further 18 months in a specialist branch programme. The outcome would be to reduce the level of service contribution by students to about 20% of their time.
3 The UKCC-registered nurse would, at the end of three years, be able to work with a specific client group in both institutional and non-institutional settings and would undertake much of the work of the previous two levels of nursing, enrolled and registered.
4 Specialist practitioners would undergo additional training in specific aspects of nursing (health visiting, occupational health nursing, school nursing, community psychiatric nursing, community mental handicap, district nursing).

5 A separate programme for midwives.

6 Helpers would support and be supervised by nurses, midwives and health visitors (UKCC, 1986).

Overall, the proposals were meant to offer a more flexible labour force and a practitioner ready to respond to changing health needs. By February 1987, the UKCC estimated that gross annual training costs were likely to be about £400 million (rising to £430 million in the transitional period) compared with £360 million in 1985, which represented an initial 25% increase on the training cost per student (UKCC, 1987). Therefore, by the autumn of 1987, one key question was whether the government was prepared to foot the bill.

By May 1988, in the wake of a political storm over nurses' pay, the then Secretary of State for Social Services, John Moore, had given qualified acceptance to the proposals (Moore, 1988). The general principles had therefore been accepted which were likely to lead to a smaller professional work force, backed up by a larger team of support workers, as the National Council for Vocational Qualifications and a training consortium for the care sector developed. However, detailed negotiations on costs, timing, staff numbers and midwifery training had still to be worked out before the UKCC proposals could be implemented.

Community nursing

Despite the fact that 90% of nurses continued to work in hospitals and institutional settings, prevention and health promotion in primary health care looked to be a key priority. Directly relevant was an extensive survey of community nursing undertaken by the Cumberlege review team. The Cumberlege Report (1986) called for nursing and primary care to be planned in 'neighbourhoods' of between 10 000 and 25 000 people, to be identified by District Health Authorities. The central recommendation was for a neighbourhood nursing service to be established, headed by a nurse manager, chosen for management skills and leadership qualities. Furthermore, while community nursing services should remain a DHA responsibility, all primary health care services (DHAs and FPCs) should be amalgamated under the control of one body because their separation was not in the best interests of the consumers, of professional teamwork in the community nor of joint planning with discharged hospital patients (Cumberlege Report, 1986).

The government immediately turned down the proposal for an FPC/DHA amalgamation, but to the idea of planning community nursing services on a neighbourhood basis the Government gave a cautious welcome. It was, however, left to the health authorities concerned to decide what was appropriate, although the approach was considered especially appropriate for inner cities (DHSS, 1987a). The outcome for community nursing therefore appeared to be gradual modification for the future, while the bolder ideas put forward by the 1986 Cumberlege Report were left in abeyance.

Nurses' pay

The key problem for nurses, which led directly to the political storm in 1987, was their preoccupation about pay and conditions of work. Nurses' pay had

Source: The Times, 2 February 1988.
Reproduced by kind permission of Mel Calman.

always been a problem. Nurses amounted to half of all the NHS staff – some half million in total. Their salaries bill accounted for £3 out of every £100 that the government had to spend on the NHS. Over the years, the nurses' struggles for a just reward had been set back by lack of unity, poor public image and the effects of inflation (Clay, 1987).

Following the 1982 dispute, an independent review body was installed whose deal, accepted by the nurses, remained in effect until March 1984. Based on a low starting point, further increases were eroded by time. By 1987, nurses were aggrieved over poor pay and status, long hours and lack of support. Furthermore, the next decade was likely to see difficulties in recruitment due to the decrease in 18-year-old school leavers and increased opportunities for those with basic qualifications to enter other professions. The situation was heading for a crisis. Even after the major political furore late in 1987, nurses remained deeply dissatisfied with their low levels of remuneration: the regrading exercise was politically mishandled and exacerbated their feelings of financial injustice, which led to disputes, disruptions, stoppages and 'working to grade'. By 1989, a new element – regional variations in pay – had entered the equation when the review body proposed to offer nurses and midwives supplements to move to areas of low recruitment (Davies, 1989a).

AN AGEING POPULATION

An ageing population had increasingly put pressure on NHS resources. By 1988, Great Britain had the highest proportion of people over 65 in the European Community: 15.3%. The proportion of over 65s was projected to increase to 19% by 2025 (Table 6.1).

Table 6.1   The elderly population of Great Britain, past, present and future.

		65+	%	75+	%	85+	%
Historical	1901	1734	4.7	507	1.4	57	0.15
trends	1931	3316	7.4	920	2.1	108	0.24
	1951	5332	10.9	1731	3.5	218	0.45
	1961	6046	11.8	2167	4.2	329	0.64
	1971	7140	13.2	2536	4.7	462	0.86
	1981	7985	15.0	3053	5.7	552	1.03
Projections	1985	8371	15.2	3544	6.4	671	1.22
(1985	1991	8847	15.8	3925	7.0	865	1.55
based)	2001	8995	15.7	4320	7.5	1146	2.00
	2011	9404	16.3	4374	7.6	1301	2.30
	2021	10562	18.2	4678	8.0	1300	2.23
	2025	11013	18.9	5177	8.9	1331	2.28

Source: Office of Population Censuses and Surveys (OPCS) (1981) 1901–1981; Census Data Population Projects by the Government Actuary 1985–2025, PP. 2, No. 5.
Crown copyright material is reproduced with the permission of the controller of Her Majesty's Stationery Office.

Future NHS financing was likely to put even more pressure on resources. Elderly people made seven to eight times greater demands on health and welfare services than the rest of the population. This trend was projected to accelerate as, between 1981 and 2001, the 75+ age group was anticipated to grow by 42% and the 85+ age group to more than double (Table 6.1). Furthermore, although in 1981 96.6% of people of pensionable age lived in private households (FPSC, 1988), local authorities had increasingly been unable to meet the rising demand for places in residential and nursing homes. Private residential care had therefore escalated dramatically between 1979 and 1986 (Table 6.2), augmented by those on supplementary benefit who could claim for all or part of private care fees. About 45% of those in private or voluntary homes were funded through social security payments (FPSC, 1988), but those places were increasingly in jeopardy due to the reduced level of benefits (Peaker, 1988).

The pressure of an ageing population on NHS resources was therefore inextricably linked with joint financing and policies between health services, community care and social security, which required close co-ordination. However, Challis et al. (1988) showed that joint approaches to social policy

Table 6.2   Residential places for elderly and younger disabled persons in England 1979 and 1986.

	1979	1986	% Change
Local authority	113564	115609	+1.8
Voluntary	33898	36000	+6.2
Private	31999	92605	+189.4

Source: FPSC (Family Policy Studies Centre) (1988).
Reproduced by kind permission of the Family Policy Studies Centre.

were difficult to achieve, although essential for managing the ever increasing complexity of society.

In reviewing residential care, the Wagner Report (1988) argued that, aided by community care allowances, people had to be given real choices. The experience of residential care should be positive in relation to real alternatives, although the priority should be to help people to live independently in their own homes where possible. In this context, the district nurse played a vital role in meeting the nursing needs of patients in the community (Allan and Jolley, 1982).

Both the Wagner Report (1988) and the Griffiths Report (1988), which provided an official review on the use of public funds to support community care, came down firmly on the side of local authorities assuming a lead role. The Griffiths Report (1988) proposed that social services departments should become managers, not simply providers, of care for elderly, mentally ill and handicapped people, across the state, private and voluntary sectors. A Minister for Community Care should be appointed to implement effective joint planning mechanisms between health, housing and social security.

The government's reaction to these far-reaching proposals, which had a mixed reception, was muted. The notion of extending the role of local authorities – financially or otherwise – was contrary to the government's political outlook. However, despite initial government opposition, by June 1989 the outcome looked as if local authorities were to be given a key role in the running of community care. The question of an ageing population remained complex and the pressure on NHS resources continued – relieved, however, by an estimated saving of £15–24 billion annually on family care provided by 6 million unpaid informal carers in Britain (Green, 1988; see Table 4.1).

PREVENTIVE HEALTH CARE: PRIORITIES AND INEQUALITIES

HIV and AIDS

In contrast to an ageing population, which could be projected, the acquired immune deficiency syndrome (AIDS) arrived unexpectedly. Official recognition was eventually given on 21 November 1986, when the Secretary of State for Social Services, Norman Fowler, outlined the first £20 million anti-AIDS package (Hansard, 1986). By then it had become clear that AIDS was a major health problem affecting almost all countries.

Although medical technology had made advances in the knowledge of the agent responsible, the human immunodeficiency virus (HIV), it was clear that both cure, and even effective treatment, were still years away. As the number of sufferers inexorably mounted, AIDS presented a major challenge to preventive health care in Britain and new pressure on NHS resources. By the start of 1989, more than 1000 people had died of AIDS in England and Wales, the number of reported cases had reached almost 2000, while there were more than 9600 HIV-antibody-positives (Gunn, 1989; Hansard, 1989a). Table 6.3 sets out sex differences and groups at risk amongst the total cases and deaths in the UK reported by June 1988.

Table 6.3   AIDS – total cases and deaths reported in the UK, by sex and by patient characteristic/presumed risk group, June 1988*.

	Cases		Deaths	
	Males	**Females**	**Males**	**Females**
Homosexual/bisexual	1315	0	738	0
Intravenous drug abuser	20	7	14	3
Homosexual and intravenous drug abuser	27	0	12	0
Haemophiliac	107	1	67	1
Recipient of blood – abroad	10	9	7	5
– UK	9	3	7	3
Heterosexual – possibly infected abroad	36	14	11	6
– UK[†]	4	6	3	4
Child of at risk/infected parent	6	10	2	6
Other/undetermined	12	2	6	2
Total	**1546**	**52**	**867**	**30**

*Data shown are cases and deaths reported to the Communicable Disease Surveillance Centre and Communicable Disease (Scotland) Unit up to the end of June 1988.
[†]No evidence of being infected abroad.

Source: CSO (1989).
Crown copyright material reproduced with the permission of the controller of Her Majesty's Stationery Office.

World-wide the number of HIV-positive people was estimated at between five and ten million, with about 350 000 cases of AIDS (Gunn, 1989). The figures in Britain were, however, likely to increase significantly, according to a government working party chaired by Sir David Cox, Warden of Nuffield College, Oxford. Health authorities and the government were warned to plan for at least another 13 000 cases of AIDS by 1992, although the figure could fall anywhere between 10 000 and 30 000. By the end of 1992, deaths from the disease were expected to be at least 7500 and possibly as high as 17 000, based on estimates that between 20 000 and 50 000 people were infected with HIV in England and Wales by 1987 (Cox, 1988).

In 1987, the DHSS launched a nation-wide campaign of action: a prevention policy of virus containment. The government's strategy on AIDS included:

1 Public education in order to increase public awareness of AIDS, to counter popular press misconceptions and to motivate modification of at-risk behaviour – especially among homosexual men and drug addicts.
2 Public health measures, infection control and surveillance.
3 Research, especially into vaccines.
4 Developing care and treatment services.
5 International co-operation through intergovernmental agencies (Hansard, 1989a).

Criticism that the government's programme was too little, too late and insufficiently targeted was balanced by praise from pressure groups that Ministers had headed off demands for a harder line from the moral right.

The impact of the strategy was difficult to assess. Qualitative research in Scotland found that, although the mass media had succeeded in giving people basic facts about AIDS in a programme which included a prominent government television and leaflet campaign and a co-ordinated AIDS week, there was still confusion, uncertainty and anxiety (Hastings and Scott, 1987). A survey of 16–25 year olds in the West Midlands revealed that, while youngsters had a high level of knowledge about the dangers of AIDS, only 18% had changed their sex lives through fear of AIDS; a subsequent survey of UK teenagers found that more than a quarter did not think that AIDS concerned them (IPPF, 1988). According to the Minister of Health, David Mellor, although evidence showed that the homosexual community had heeded health warnings and changed their behaviour, the AIDS epidemic was in danger of spreading rapidly to hetero-sexuals because drug users were refusing to stop sharing needles (Hansard, 1989a).

Alongside key issues concerning the ethics of screening for AIDS and sex education for AIDS in schools in line with the moral parameters set by the 1986 *Education Act*, the major implication of AIDS for the NHS was the consequent pressure on expenditure. In the light of mounting health care needs, the DHSS funded an advisory service for UK health authorities to provide free and confidential telephone advice on national AIDS helplines; DHSS policy groups were formed; health educators were drawn into major training programmes; and the Health Education Council was dissolved when, in April 1987, the Health Education Authority took charge of the government's AIDS campaign. Substantial sums of money went into research programmes in which a hierarchy in the allocation of medical research money soon became established. Prestigious research centres benefited at the expense of other research (Small, 1988). The National AIDS Trust was launched in 1987 by Robert Maxwell to raise £50 million within two years. The drug companies were also beginning to move in for a financial scramble for profits in the largest new pharmaceutical market in history (Campbell, 1988).

Meanwhile voluntary bodies, with special expertise and experience, were put under mounting pressure for advisory services and help. Particularly involved were the Terrence Higgins Trust, Body Positive, Crusaid, the London Lesbian and Gay Switchboard, as well as the Family Planning Association. New groups were also rapidly being launched, including Lambeth AIDS Action, 'Buddy' schemes, self-help schemes and hospice care (which opened up at the Mildmay Mission Hospital, Hackney in May 1988, followed in November 1988 by the residential and support centre at the London Lighthouse). The contribution of the voluntary and self-help movement (largely underfunded) was therefore of great importance (Small, 1988).

Despite considerable input from the voluntary sector, costs were escalating. NHS health care expenditure was approaching an average of £30 000 per person – in other words, about £30 million a year was being spent by the NHS on treating AIDS and HIV infection (Campbell, 1989). Parliament's Social Services Committee was critical of the government's failure to provide adequate hospital and community resources. The absence of any strategy was preventing health authorities from planning (Laurance, 1988b). The Minister of Health promised that the £62 million earmarked to fight AIDS for 1989 would rise to £130 million in 1990 (Hansard, 1989a). The resource demands from preventive health measures for AIDS/HIV infection were therefore a significant factor in the increasing pressures on NHS expenditure.

Continuing inequalities in health

By the end of the 1980s, AIDS had been given a relatively high level of priority for NHS resources. Other aspects of preventive health provision received less political and financial attention.

One striking example was the lower level of priority accorded to the varying aspects of inequalities. Significant social class differences in health and access to health provision remained. Factors fully documented in the Black Report (1980) and subsequent studies (BMA, 1987; Cox et al., 1987; Smith, 1987; Whitehead, 1987) had persisted throughout the decade. By 1988, the divide between north and south, rich and poor, was again emphasized by a major study on *The Nation's Health*, Smith and Jacobson (1988), which investigated the inequalities in the health of the country's population. Strong evidence indicated that deprivation associated with unemployment was damaging to health. A strategy for national health promotion and prevention policies was put forward (Smith and Jacobson, 1988). However, the negative response from politicians reflected the low level of priority accorded to many aspects of this report.

PRIORITIES IN WOMEN'S PREVENTIVE HEALTH CARE

Family planning

The priority and financial recognition given to the needs of women's health in the NHS was variable. From the start of free family planning on the NHS in 1974, the pressure on resources had, by the mid-1980s, curtailed clinic provision. Increasingly, DHAs (funded at district level) were cutting sessions, closing clinics and pressing services over to the seemingly more favourable centrally funded option of GPs. Largely prescribing the pill, GPs saw more patients – some 2.5 million annually (1986 figures). Nevertheless, 1.4 million women preferred to go to clinics as they offered a greater choice of methods (cap, IUD, sheath, natural methods, sterilization as well as the pill), specialist knowledge, anonymity, a non-disease-oriented setting and the greater chance of seeing a woman doctor (Snowden, 1985). Constrained resources had therefore led to diminishing choice for women in methods and facilities which reflected the lower priority given by NHS regions to family planning services and to Well Woman Clinics (Leathard, 1987) than to other aspects of preventive health care.

The politics of abortion

Access to abortion facilities was largely determined by the NHS resources available, the views and control exercised by local doctors and consultants and pressure group politics (Allen, 1981). Increasingly, the private and charitable sector responded to demand. By 1987, the OPCS Monitor AB 88/3 showed that the percentage of abortions performed in the NHS had fallen to 44%; NHS agency arrangements accounted for a further 5%.

Abortion was dominated by politics. The issue continued to be fiercely fought out between the 'right to life' lobby (drawn from such groups as the Moral Right, the Society for the Protection of the Unborn Child, Life, the Catholic Church and those opposed to a 'woman's right to choose') and the pro-choice lobby (variously supported by women's groups, pro-abortionists, family planners and health professionals). Anti-abortion bills were continuously presented in Parliament by private members, despite the Lane Committee's (1974) official review which gave unanimous support for the 1967 *Abortion Act* and its provisions.

In 1979/80, Labour MP John Corrie's *Abortion (Amendment) Bill* – which sought to curtail the grounds for abortion through a qualified 20-week time limit – was one of the most keenly fought in Parliament. The bill galvanized the pro-choice lobby into co-ordinated activity and, as a result, was finally defeated (Marsh and Chambers, 1981).

Twenty-one years after the 1967 legislation, Liberal MP David Alton's 1988 private member's bill to lower the legal abortion time limit from 28 to 18 weeks reached the furthest stage in the legislative process – the report stage and third reading – but eventually ran out of time. Supporters refused to admit defeat and pledged to return to the fight, regardless of public opinion which showed clear support for a woman's right to choose an abortion in the first few months of pregnancy (Jowell et al., 1986: 155; Gillie, 1988a). Conservative MP Ann Widdecombe sought, early in 1989, to force extra parliamentary time for the Alton bill, which represented the fifteenth attempt to amend or destroy the original 1967 *Abortion Act*. Priorities for abortion provision were therefore influenced as much by political as financial pressures.

The new reproductive technologies

New demands arose as new techniques in human reproductive technologies developed. As the social, ethical, legal and medical issues became ever more complex, the government set up the Warnock Committee to examine the implications of human fertilization and embryology. In 1984, the Committee recommended that a statutory authority should be set up to license test tube babies, embryo research up to 14 days, together with other forms of infertility treatment, but the Committee was opposed to commercial surrogacy (Warnock Report, 1984).

Legislation was swiftly passed to outlaw commercial surrogacy under the *Surrogacy Arrangements Act* in 1985. Following the exposure of legal loopholes, further legislation was introduced in 1986 which made surrogacy wholly unlawful. Meanwhile, unsuccessfully, the anti-abortion lobby was again active in seeking to ban all research on human embryos, through the Powell and Hargreaves private members' *Unborn Children (Protection) Bills* in 1985 and 1986.

The implications of the new reproductive technologies, for the estimated one in ten infertile couples, opened up wider choices for women in one sense – to overcome infertility – but posed new health risks, pressures and problems. Then again, women themselves were divided in their views on the developments (Corea et al., 1985; Feldman, 1987; Corea, 1988). Financial pressures on the NHS were somewhat restricted because only one of the 22 *in vitro* fertilization units offering treatment in Britain was funded by the NHS.

Impatient for government action, the Medical Research Council and the Royal College of Obstetricians and Gynaecologists in 1985 set up a Voluntary Licensing Authority for human fertilization and embryology to impose their own limits and to monitor developments. Following consultation, a 1987 DHSS White Paper proposed a framework for legislation, embodying the Warnock principles, which the government accepted. However, the controversial issue of research on human embryos was to be left entirely open for Parliament to decide (DHSS, 1987b).

Given the inadequate provision made by the NHS for infertility treatment (Warnock Report, 1984; Pfeffer and Quick, 1988), NHS priorities for this treatment were obviously not very high.

Screening and preventive health

Screening for breast and cervical cancer commanded a higher level of NHS recognition. Breast cancer killed more women in the UK (about 15 000) annually than any other cancer. Although breast screening centres had been set up in each of the 14 Regional Health Authorities (RHAs) by 1988, it was estimated that it would take five years to cover the target population of four million women aged 50–64. A government-commissioned study anticipated that up to 2000 lives could be saved annually (Forrest Report, 1987).

Cervical cancer was claiming 2000 lives a year. Demands for a routine comprehensive screening programme came from the Women's National Commission (1985), the British Medical Association (BMA) (1986) and the Commons Public Accounts Committee (1986). By 1988, call and recall systems had been computerized in England and Wales. All women aged 20–64 were to be invited for a cervical smear test at least every five years, but the slow rate of take-up gave rise for concern. Fear, lack of information and impersonal computer invitations were the main reasons for women not coming forward. Labour MP Harriet Harman's 1988 survey claimed that, despite the £10 million nation-wide screening programme, women were still not protected from the risk of death from cervical cancer (Harman, 1988). According to the Chief Medical Officer's annual report for 1988, women were dying unnecessarily of cervical cancer in six RHAs. Lung cancer was also killing more women each year (Smith and Jacobson, 1988), as women had taken up smoking in greater numbers than in the 1950s and 1960s. Amongst the possible causal factors, such as parents or close friends who smoked, or smoking seen as a means of calming nerves or becoming slimmer, Hilary Graham (1988) suggested that single parents found in smoking a way of coping with a stressful life of deprivation and constant child-caring demands.

In all, preventive health care for women had received a lower priority for NHS resources than other health needs. Although the government had made certain attempts by the late 1980s to direct facilities to the prevention of avoidable deaths amongst women, there was still a long way to go. Pressure therefore continued for further action.

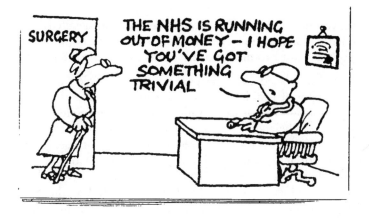

Source: The Guardian, 20 February 1988.
Reproduced by kind permission of The Guardian and Hector Breeze.

CRISIS IN THE NHS

As the government sought to juggle priorities in health care provision, the NHS began to look like a terminal case. The crisis in the NHS was compounded by four crucial factors: an ageing population, advancing technology, the pressure from staffing costs and rising consumer expectations. The NHS proved increasingly unable to cope with the financial requirements generated. The government's response was to try to force the system to confront economic reality by restraining the growth of real resources below the rate warranted, while using relative underfunding to secure greater efficiency (Social Services Committee, 1988b).

However, the crisis seemed to be founded on a paradox. On the one hand, the government had repeatedly claimed that more than ever was being spent on the NHS (DHSS, 1983b). Indeed between 1978 and 1987, not only had the NHS received a substantial growth in income, but the NHS was also treating more patients in fewer beds (Laurance, 1987b). On the other hand, the NHS budget was severely strained. Resource restraint, efficiency savings and the adverse effect of RAWP on some health regions had all led to cuts, shortages and rationing, as demand had outstripped supply.

ECONOMIC PROBLEMS IN THE NHS

Lessons perceived by health analysts, economists and other bodies pointed to certain fundamental flaws in the system which included:

- serious neglect of capital investment and maintenance (Maxwell, 1988);
- almost total lack of competition nor any incentives to greater efficiency (Peet, 1988);
- paucity of consumer choice (RCN, 1988);
- absence of costing data or any effective in-built cost-containment mechanism, apart from the external political imposition of resource restraint (Whitney, 1988);
- performance indicators revealed slack in the system: detailed studies of costs and outcomes indicated inefficiencies (Social Services Committee, 1988a);
- the service was failing to meet modern needs (Whitney, 1988).

Dissatisfaction was voiced over the persistent gap between demand for health care and the supply of health services. The gap reflected a problem inherent in any system that made health care available to everyone solely on the basis of need, regardless of their ability to pay (Gardner, 1988). Furthermore, because health care was generally provided free at the point of use, patients had no incentive to economize. Unbridled clinical freedom had pre-empted scarce resources, which reduced their availability for patients, while there had been little incentive to practice prevention (Owen, 1988). For the Social Services Committee (1988b) the key issues were underfunding and the need to develop an improved measurement of NHS effectiveness.

The fundamental question therefore remained: how to get better value for money and at the same time make the NHS more responsive to patients' needs and demands?

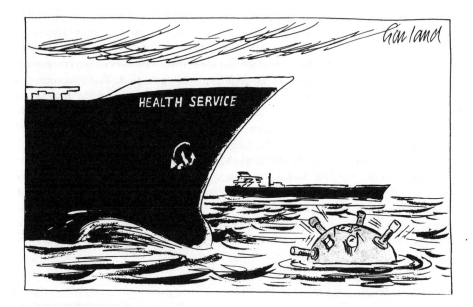

Source: The Independent, 9 October 1987.
Reproduced by kind permission of The Independent and Nicholas Garland.

THE CRISIS GATHERS MOMENTUM

The public mind was immediately alerted by banner headlines about the lack of facilities for hole in the heart operations (in particular the David Barber case; Grice, 1987), by the mounting concern with hospital waiting lists and by the impeded access to provision due to cuts (especially to DHA clinic services). A poll showed that public opinion still held an overwhelmingly (67%) favourable view of the NHS, although the rating had dropped during 1987 from 76%. However, results suggested that individuals were influenced by media reports rather than by first-hand experience (Davies, 1988).

The poll findings underlined a further background feature in the impending crisis: an inherent tendency for the NHS (as in any nationalized service) to denigrate its achievement in order to attract more government funding. Unlike the private sector seeking to attract customers, the NHS had therefore been continually belittled rather than defended and promoted (Gardner, 1988).

THE POLITICAL STORM BREAKS: DECEMBER 1987

The public controversy about NHS financing took many, including the government, by surprise when it burst into the headlines late in 1987. The controversy was not of the government's choice: education and housing reform were seen as the priorities in the Conservatives' third term of office. Two key factors led up to the eye of the storm.

First, early in December 1987, protests by the nursing profession over pay and conditions were mounting. John Moore, the then Social Services Secretary, and Tony Newton, the then Health Minister, sought to prepare concessions against the background of fierce Opposition criticism of the government's handling of the NHS.

Secondly, by 7 December 1987, the three heads of the Royal Medical Colleges made a statement of unprecedented and blistering criticism on the crisis in the NHS (Wright, 1987). The government had no immediate answer to the problems of the NHS. Under pressure from the Opposition, which had at last found an issue on which the apparently armour-plated government seemed vulnerable, the Prime Minister announced a government review of the NHS.

Overall, far from celebrating its 40th birthday in July 1998, the NHS faced a mounting crisis and a greater challenge to the fundamental basis of the National Health Service than at any time in its history.

7 FUTURE OPTIONS FOR THE NHS: LESSONS FROM HOME AND ABROAD

The announcement of the government's NHS review heralded a spate of publications that sought to advise on future options. One approach was to draw on lessons from health care systems abroad; another was to provide a range of internal solutions for the NHS.

There have been three basic models by which international health systems have been resourced: national taxation, social insurance and private insurance. However, the financing of health care has always been complex. Even within these three models, various distinctions could be made between 'direct' (fee-for-service) and 'indirect' (payment by government) revenues. Further, in all International comparisons, what might perform well in one country would not necessarily be successful in another. Countries differ significantly in geography, demography and in their constitutional and administrative systems. Accordingly, a variety of health care systems have emerged. Nevertheless, lessons from abroad, more particularly from developed countries, might provide a perspective on the NHS in Britain as to whether the financial problems were universal or whether there were more effective ways forward.

THE NATIONAL TAXATION MODEL

The NHS system is essentially a national taxation model: universal in coverage, largely free at the point of use, run by the state where government intervention has been direct; private health insurance has played only a marginal role. Although inefficient in its use of resources and somewhat ignorant about outcomes, NHS funding has proved cheap-to-collect and able-to-control cash limits. Have other countries employed a national taxation model more effectively?

The Nordic countries: Denmark, Norway and Sweden

Despite certain differences, the Nordic countries have relatively uniform health systems. The basic arrangements in Denmark indicate the pattern overall.

Denmark
Health care provision is almost completely funded out of general taxation to cover all forms of sickness. National health insurance includes the whole population: 95% belong to a basic scheme, the other 5% belong to a more liberal scheme which allows greater choice of treatment. Hospital doctors are employed by the 14 counties and the local government of Copenhagen, while General Practitioners are private contractors controlled by the health scheme. In all three Nordic countries, in contrast to Britain, local government plays a significant part in the administration of health care. Hospital and medical treatment is generally free in Denmark, but patients pay the pharmacy for their medicines,

Table 7.1 Public and private health expenditure as a percentage of gross domestic product, 1984.

	Total	Private	Public
Sweden	9.4	0.8	8.6
France	9.1	2.6	6.5
The Netherlands	8.6	1.8	6.8
West Germany	8.1	1.7	6.4
Ireland	8.0	1.1	6.9
Italy	7.2	1.1	6.1
Denmark	6.3	1.0	5.3
Norway	6.3	0.7	5.6
Belgium	6.2	0.5	5.7
Great Britain	5.9	0.6	5.3
Spain	5.8	1.5	4.3

Source: OECD (1987).
Reproduced by kind permission of the Organisation for Economic Co-operation and Development.

for which they are reimbursed, although patients pay 40% of the cost of all prescriptions.

At first sight, in comparison to Britain, Danish health care looks impressive: more modern hospitals, high standards and free hospital care. Spending as a percentage of the gross domestic product (GDP) was 6.3% compared with 5.9% in Great Britain (1984 figures: Table 7.1). However, Denmark's problems largely mirrored those of the British NHS: waiting lists, rising consumerism, planning difficulties due to the decentralized system (Timmins, 1988), rising costs (despite counter-measures), interference with the doctors' freedom, prescription charges which have provided difficulties for poorer patients unable to receive financial help from the social security system. Delays in the availability of treatment in Denmark had led to a two-fold rise in private health insurance in the previous ten years and the building of new private hospitals (OHE, 1988).

Norway's national health plan

Of interest in Norway was the national health plan. On regaining power in 1985, the Labour government established a national health plan to provide an overview of health staffing and incomes and to set goals for health advancement within the framework of national, economic and human resources. The plan called for the weakest sectors of society (elderly, mentally ill and physically disabled people) to receive top priority in funding.

The Norwegian government therefore attempted to confront the issue of an ageing population as well as the problem of nursing shortage but had also to contend with confrontation from the doctors. Norwegian doctors campaigned for salary increases, against the government's view that health care resources should be directed to lower-paid staff and primary care. The strength of Norway's state-funded system was the planning and strategy potential which was employed in the determination of priorities. As a result, the Norwegian government said 'no' to state funds for some forms of provision – such as high-technology medicine with little or unknown therapeutic value – while low priority was accorded to test-tube reproduction, sports surgery and artificial insemination. A drawback in the system was the disruption and confrontation with those who disagreed with the overall plans.

Sweden

The comprehensive nature of the Swedish health system, together with the extent of state control over the finance and delivery of health care, provided a system which closely resembled that of the British NHS. The entire Swedish population was covered by a national health insurance scheme: 90% of the cost was covered by various forms of taxation. Spending was therefore financed from a combination of general taxes and social insurance (Ham and Calltorp, 1992). However, instead of pointing the way forward for the NHS, there was the drawback that the Swedes paid higher health charges across a wider range of provision: some 10% of health care costs were raised by patients' out-of-pocket payments. However, Sweden attached high priority to providing health services in the public sector: spending was therefore above the average for developed countries (see Figure 7.1). As in Norway, nearly all hospitals and health service facilities were run by local authorities at a high standard, but the corollary of high investment in institutional services has been lower spending on primary and community care (Ham and Calltorp, 1992).

The British NHS had less administrative complexity, in that Swedish hospital patients made certain direct payments which were then deducted from their cash sickness benefit. The County Councils charged patients for their first 15 visits to the doctor each year. Critics also claimed that the system's resources had been used inefficiently (Ham and Calltorp, 1992) but, as in Britain, the public were

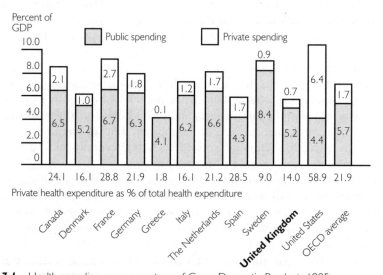

Figure 7.1   Health spending as a percentage of Gross Domestic Product, 1985.
Source: Timmins (1988).

generally satisfied with their health care delivery (OHE, 1988). However, the rise in Swedish standards of living put pressure on demands for higher standards of medical care. Although private medicine was provided by only about 5% of doctors and some private nursing homes, there had been a gradual increase in private medical care.

Overall, the national taxation models abroad had both positive and negative features, although none offered a 'pure' practice, all examples contained an element of private practice. However, countries that had largely adopted the national taxation model had encountered similar problems to those in Britain, particularly rising costs, without necessarily offering appropriate solutions to the financial crisis in the NHS by the end of the 1980s.

Canada

Canada provided an example of a country that had much in common with the British health system, although geographically and culturally closer to the USA than to the Nordic countries. Canada had slowly been moving closer to a system based on the NHS model and away from the market system. Concerned by rising costs, from 1968 the Canadian government had developed a publicly funded universal health system.

The key elements of the arrangements meant that the health needs of all Canadians were funded by global budgets financed by general taxation or by compulsory insurance premiums. Physicians (except those working in teaching hospitals) were reimbursed on a fee-for-service basis from health insurance plans. Run by boards of trustees, acute care hospitals were generally owned by municipalities, voluntary societies or universities. In the actual delivery of care there was little public intervention, which was largely confined to the determination of reimbursement at provincial government level.

The positive features suggested that the Canadian system was perceived as being egalitarian: there was only one point of access (which was free to all), people could choose their own doctors and hospitals and most used the public system (Millar, 1988). Universal public insurance had also brought firmer cost control. The standard of patient care was regarded as excellent. The Canadian system also recognized and treated the patient, with rights and choices, as a 'customer' with whom the system was consistently popular (Owen, 1988). The private management of hospitals as well as public and private sector collaboration, although much discussed, had rarely been tried in Canada as privatization per se did not necessarily, in their view, guarantee good management (Millar 1988). Nevertheless, private sector capital was under consideration to fund health care developments, given the problems in Canada of raising taxes. Meanwhile, a quarter of Canada's health spending remained private: chiefly dental work, drugs and some long-term care (Timmins, 1988).

Problems of the day included escalating costs. Although the Canadian government was a monopoly buyer of physicians' services and provinces were able to set the fees, increased use meant that costs were rising remorselessly

(Millar, 1988). Some doctors and hospitals argued that the system was under-funded, which resulted in outdated equipment, growing waiting lists and overcrowded hospitals (Owen, 1988). Even so, Canada's health spending absorbed a significant proportion of national expenditure: 8.6% of the GDP in 1985 (Figure 7.1) – high by international standards. Indeed, Taylor (1989) reported that a comparative survey of Britain, the USA and Canada by Louis Harris and Associates, New York and Harvard School of Public Health, showed that by almost any measure (except cost) the Canadian health care system performed much better than either the British or American systems.

THE SOCIAL INSURANCE MODEL

The social insurance model has universal coverage, generally within the framework of a state-run social security system, financed by compulsory employer and individual contributions through non-profit insurance funds.

West Germany

The first system of social insurance began in Germany under Bismark in the 1880s. Under the post-war West German health system up to 1989 (when Germany's national health insurance system was extended to cover East Germany) insurance was compulsory. Free medical care was provided although, as in Britain, cost-sharing arrangements existed for prescription drugs and dentures. The system was regulated and supervised by the government. Those who earned the British equivalent of £18 000 could opt out and join a private scheme. About 9% of West Germans had private health insurance. However, some 90% of the population was covered by about 1200 public insurance schemes run by independent bodies with their own board of management composed of local employers (30%) and unions (50%). The insurance funds paid the cost of medical treatment in whole or in part, either directly or by reimbursing patients.

The hospital system was planned by state governments. About half the hospitals were publicly owned and run by local councils; a third were non-profit-making organizations; the rest were run for profit. Doctors in the community, including specialists, were private practitioners. Hospital doctors were employed by the hospitals. Outpatient doctors were either paid directly by privately insured patients (who claimed reimbursement) or paid fees for service by public insurance organizations. Doctors bargained directly with the insurance funds over pay. Most medical specialists operated outside the hospitals in clinics (OHE, 1988).

The comparative interest in the West German health system was that, unlike the NHS which was grappling with shortages and waiting lists, West Germany faced a situation of over-supply (Owen, 1988). For example, each clinic felt that investment in the latest high technology equipment was necessary in order to compete with their medical neighbours (Gardner, 1988). In comparison with other European countries, (alongside a shortage of nurses) a high average density of doctors had resulted in serious problems of medical unemployment (Moran, 1992). There was, however, close financial integration of the private and public sector; consumer choice was available between hospital and clinic treatment and amenities; while virtually every citizen was guaranteed access to a high standard of health care largely free at the point of treatment.

The fundamental flaws, from the NHS perspective, in the West German system were wastage and slack in hospital bed use, rising costs and inefficiency in the insurance scheme due to the payment of fees for items of service which encouraged supply of treatment as well as problems of acceptability, equity and accountability (Moran, 1992). In contrast to Britain, West Germany had more limited powers to control the costs of health care. Their health insurance costs were rising sharply due to more comprehensive and advanced medical care and to longer life expectancy. Drastic proposals to reduce health care costs had been discussed in West Germany, but were supported by only 30% of the population (OHE, 1988).

France

Many other countries have adopted a system similar to that in West Germany. In France, 95% of the population is covered by a national health insurance scheme financed as part of the social security system. Compulsory contributions are made by employers, employees and individual contributors in proportion to their earnings. The rates vary for different classes of employees and for the self-employed. The occupational basis of the sickness funds leaves a small minority, mostly those with no income, without insurance protection. As a safety net, local authorities provide cover and may reimburse health care providers (Chambaud, 1993). The government also contributes to the cost of health care from the proceeds of motor insurance premiums and taxes on pharmaceutical advertising, alcohol and tobacco. In 1991, a controversial health service tax, the Generalized Social Contribution, was introduced by the Socialist government, under Michel Rocard, to raise further revenue of 1.1% of gross income (Nundy, 1993). In addition to the social security fund, over 30 million people have supplementary insurance through a non-profit network (Chambaud, 1993). Overall, the financing of French health care is complex.

Regional governments are responsible for the administration and funding of health care subject to central regulations. About 70% of hospital beds are publicly owned, mainly by local government hospitals. Some 20% of hospitals are profit making; the rest are run by voluntary organizations. Doctors are either paid by the state hospitals or, more generally, receive a fee per item of service from the patient, partly reimbursed by the insurance fund.

Patients (except those in receipt of social assistance and treatment for one of 30 defined illnesses) usually pay for the full cost of any treatment (except treatment as inpatients). The social security system then reimburses up to 75% of doctors' and dentists' fees and 80% of hospital treatment, minus a small hotel charge (Gardner, 1988) – which explains why so many French people take out supplementary private insurance: in order to cover the part of their costs the social security scheme does not include. However, as in Germany, patients are free to choose where they are treated.

The advantages of the French system included the genuine co-operation between the public and private sector, an impressive range of modern facilities, easy accessibility to medical care and the choice afforded to the consumer between specialists or doctors. Furthermore, the system was popular with the French public (OHE, 1988).

From the NHS perspective, the snags were large: the French social security scheme has faced continual financial problems because the scope for medical treatment continually expands. Extensive consumer choice for diagnosis and treatment has led to costly use of scarce skills (Owen, 1988). The array of exemptions and reimbursement scales have been extremely complicated, in contrast to the simplicity of the straightforward NHS health care delivery system. Under the French multi-provider arrangements, planning is difficult; demand is unrestrained, administrative costs are high. This health care system has been one of the most expensive in Europe (Table 7.1; Figure 7.1).

Overall, despite certain positive features, the social insurance model had therefore not revealed any significantly effective ways of overcoming the problems that besieged the NHS in Britain.

THE PRIVATE INSURANCE MODEL

The United States of America

The third model, based on private insurance, is not run by the state; coverage is not universal but is financed by individual contributions, employer contributions or a combination of both. Right-wing economists in Britain (Orros, 1988) were greatly attracted to the American system. Per capita health spending was running at the equivalent of £1000 sterling each year, nearly three times the British figure (Owen, 1988), yet American public spending on health formed a smaller proportion of total spending than in any other developed country (Figure 7.1). However, the American system was spending a higher proportion of its GDP on health overall (11–12%) when the private sector was included. As a result, the USA health care system was costing twice as much as the NHS by 1988.

On the positive side, for many Americans the private insurance system (which covered three-quarters of the population) provided:

- very high-quality health care (for those who could afford the best insurance coverage) in cleaner, newer, better equipped hospitals and medical centres than in Britain and most other countries (Owen, 1988);
- substantial freedom of choice and innovation (Gardner, 1988).

On the negative side, from the viewpoint of the British NHS

- one-tenth of the population had no insurance cover at all;
- many suffered because they were inadequately protected against illness;
- private insurance inevitably led to a marked emphasis on the more easily quantifiable hospitalization rather than on preventive medicine;
- the largest share of insurance coverage (55%) was through the major commercial insurance companies, which retained large profits but showed

little concern for the content or quality of the care rendered to policy holders (Roemer, 1986);

- experience rating was practised by nearly all insurance companies so that high-risk populations, with the greatest health needs, paid the highest premiums (Roemer, 1986: 135).

Furthermore, the American health insurance system has been largely based on a fee-for-service model where the insurer pays the provider for each procedure. Consequently, the system provides no incentive for doctors to use resources economically. Medical costs have therefore escalated, although alternative systems have emerged.

Health Maintenance Organizations (HMOs), which covered 30 million of the 230 million North Americans by 1988, have developed as a favoured means of controlling health care costs. The main feature is that, for a prepaid annual fee, the organization either provides all the care needed by the patient or manages care by contracting out with doctors and hospitals to provide health care for a year for a fixed payment. There has been some evidence that HMOs have reduced health care costs, but some organizations have experienced bankruptcies, mergers and financial loss (Timmins, 1988; Gardner, 1988).

Although the role of government in American health care has continuously been more limited than in Britain, federal, state and local government spending still constitutes over 40% of the total of which about three-quarters finances the two major government programmes: *Medicare* and *Medicaid*. The remaining 60% of American health care spending is divided equally between payments from private insurance companies and direct payments by the patients.

Medicare is a federal government programme for people aged over 65, which provides limited coverage, so many elderly people take out 'top-up insurance'. *Medicaid*, jointly funded by federal and state governments, provides health care for the poor, but eligibility is incomplete and coverage usually excludes dental services and prescribed drugs. The federal, state and local governments also run 40% of hospitals which tend to fulfil a charitable 'last resort' function but are decreasing in importance (Gardner, 1988).

Most GPs work in the private sector. Over 60% of hospital (and nursing home) beds are privately owned, but only 15% are in profit-making organizations (Gardner, 1988). Although systematic planning of health resources has been increasing, it is still principally on a decentralized basis.

As a result, the American health care system has become a fragmented jumble of unco-ordinated services which offer different patterns of care to different groups. Nevertheless, regulation is, paradoxically, highly developed. To some extent because of the pluralistic and somewhat easy-going form of health service administration, problems and abuses have developed which government regulation has been imposed to prevent. Medical audits, 'peer reviews' and evaluation of health care services have become highly developed. Meanwhile, as provision has been increasingly financed by government or by large groups of people, so questions have become more insistent (Roemer, 1986: 27).

Even though social and political forces were driving the American health care system towards greater co-ordination and central controls, there remained significant diversities in the patterns of financing and delivery of health services between states, or even within different sections of one state.

In drawing lessons for Britain, the health care system in the USA was haunted by a dilemma. The extraordinary contribution to the expansion of the scientific and technological basis of medical practice encouraged public demand for universal access to everything that medicine could make available, which in turn lead to a costly consumer outlook. Where the federal, state and local government have been involved in funding their own health care schemes (such as *Medicare* and *Medicaid*) the same problems the NHS encountered have had to be faced: cost containment and underfunding (Cousins, 1987: 154). By 1988, it was, however, the achievements of the Health Maintenance Organizations that left the British radical right 'positively dewy-eyed' (Timmins, 1988: 77).

LESSONS TO BE LEARNT FROM ABROAD

In his evidence to the Social Services Committee (1988b) on resourcing the NHS, Professor Alan Maynard from York University summarized the lessons to be learnt from abroad.

1 All countries have had to face difficult choices. Resources were scarce; rationing was unavoidable.
2 It was essential for the NHS to measure health care costs and benefits systematically (based on quality-adjusted life years (QALY) or the enhancement in the patient's length and quality of life) in order to determine the cost effectiveness of health care therapies.
3 While the NHS, like all other health care systems (public and private) was inefficient in the use of resources, the major advantage was that the NHS funding source (taxation) was cheap to collect and, with one source of funding, expenditure could be controlled by cash limits.

HEALTH EXPENDITURE COMPARED

Great Britain was one of the lowest spenders on health amongst the developed countries and certainly below the average in 1984 and 1985 (Table 7.1, Figure 7.1). France, Sweden, Canada and the USA were amongst the highest. However, in France, and particularly in the USA, the margin between public finance and total expenditure was largely covered by health expenditure from private funds. Although the French health system boasted an impressive range of modern facilities, much of its high-level finance was inefficiently spent or uneconomically invested. The NHS appeared to be more cost effective than most other health care systems (Owen, 1988). Nevertheless, the difficulty of defining and measuring health outcomes remained (OECD, 1987).

More problematically, although simply spending more on health care had solved some problems, it had created others (such as insatiable demand). Nor was it certain that greater spending on health care necessarily generated better health for the country as a whole because other factors, such as the environment, life-styles, social investment and efficient expenditure, were also relevant (Abel-Smith, 1976).

All health care systems in developed countries faced similar problems, such as the increasing costs incurred by high-technology medicine, an ageing population and rising consumer expectations. However, evidence from all over the world strongly implied that greater consumer choice, responsiveness and efficiency could be achieved only at a considerable price. The clearest evidence for this could be found in the USA where market forces played a larger role in health care than in any other OECD country (Best, 1988). Nevertheless, contrary to the Reagan adminis-tration's commitment to free market principles and reductions in government regulation, a centralist system of price controls for *Medicare* had been introduced, health care cost containment had become a priority and private corporations were also seeking measures to limit the costs of health care (Cousins, 1987: 155).

As Professor Teeling-Smith's briefing on 11 West European countries (including Great Britain) concluded, no country had perfectly solved the difficult problem of providing optimum medical services at an acceptable cost (OHE, 1988).

ADVICE FROM FOREIGN HEALTH ECONOMISTS

To outsiders, the NHS did not appear grossly inefficient. There was admiration for the low administrative costs, tight cost control, high degree of equity, treatment regardless of ability to pay, a strong network providing effective primary care and the family doctor system which acted as a gatekeeper to the expensive hospital services. Asked for the weakness of the NHS, foreign health economists pointed to lack of consumer choice, monolithic supply through effectively government-owned hospitals which led to resistance to innovation, misuse of nurses, the size of the waiting lists and underfunding. The one clear-cut message from abroad, reported Nicholas Timmins (1988), was that there were no easy answers.

Consequently, as the government's review of the NHS continued throughout 1988, few instant remedies for the financial problems in the NHS could be readily found.

FUTURE OPTIONS FOR THE NHS

The Private Sector

If health care systems abroad provided no immediate solution, could private medicine point the financial way forward for the NHS? The private sector had indeed expanded between 1979 and 1986 by when there were some 193 private hospitals. Outpatient treatment had risen steadily, private beds had increased by 50% and, although the sharpest increase in the number of people covered by private medical insurance had taken place between 1979 and 1983, membership increased by nearly 8% from 1984 to 1987, from 5.0 million to 5.3 million. By the end of 1987, over 9% of the population of the United Kingdom was covered

(CSO, 1989: 131). However, going private remained an overwhelming upper and middle-class activity: people from families classified as unskilled manual workers accounted for only 1%; skilled and semi-skilled were recorded as no more than 2% each (Laing, 1987). Furthermore, the bulk of private medicine involved a narrow range of around 30 surgical activities, such as hernia operations, abortions and vasectomies. Generally, the private sector had therefore not provided emergency care or care for long-term chronic patients. To the extent that the NHS sought to offer universal comprehensive medical care, free at the point of use, the selective operation of the private sector could not necessarily solve the financial difficulties faced by the NHS.

At the height of the NHS crisis in 1988, *British Social Attitudes* (Jowell et al., 1988) indicated that the general public still strongly supported the basic principles of the NHS, but remained hostile to private treatment (pay beds) in NHS hospitals. Nevertheless, the majority of the public supported the view that doctors and dentists should have the right to take on private patients, while only 20% were opposed to private hospital treatment.

However, the general performance of the NHS was causing concern. Those expressing dissatisfaction were increasing in number (from 25% in 1983 to 39% in 1987), amongst whom the higher-income groups were both more dissatisfied with the NHS but more likely to be covered by private medical insurance. Overall, amongst those identifying with all the main political parties, health was named as the main priority for extra public spending (Jowell et al., 1988: 96).

Significant changes in the private sector had taken place since 1979; the discernible trends included:

- the expansion of for-profit medicine;
- the growth of American-owned hospitals (rising from 2% of all private beds outside the NHS in 1979 to 22.5% in 1986) which had provided newer, larger and more sophisticated private hospitals than average together with a wide range of patient services;
- a transition from private medicine as a cottage industry to a business enterprise with an emphasis on incentives and efficiency;
- the growth of employer-financed care with a small but significant shift away from financing and provision by the state (through pay beds) when, by 1985, 75% of private sector bills were settled by insurance companies (Higgins, 1988).

The private health care market in Britain had, however, shown ways in which the NHS might improve public sector services to the user, particularly in hospitals, as well as meeting the demands of patients concerning waiting lists, admission arrangements, privacy and medical communication. Nevertheless, for many, the supreme value by which a private health care system would have to be judged concerned moral criteria about justice, fairness and equity rather than its cost effectiveness or its effects on NHS waiting lists. Joan Higgins (1988) concluded, in her analysis *The Business of Medicine*, that the growth of for-profit medicine in Britain had weakened the commitment to equal access to health services for all, irrespective of age, gender, race, class or ability to pay.

Whatever lessons the private sector had for the NHS, the economic reality was that Britain's major private health insurers were making a healthy return but at the expense of private hospitals which were only just making a profit. More than half of London's 29 private hospitals were making losses (Health Care Information Services, 1988). Both private (more particularly the not-for-profit) and NHS hospitals increasingly faced similar problems: mounting expenditure in the face of advances in medical technology and costly labour-intensive staffing which required strict financial control. While the private sector could therefore offer no effective solution to the financial problems in the NHS, health economists and analysts produced a wide range of internal proposals for the National Health Service which tended to form into two groups: funding and management options.

FUNDING OPTIONS FOR THE NHS

The range of funding possibilities, discussed in the late 1980s, are now summarized in Table 7.2, together with the perceived advantages and disadvantages.

All the various proposals to fund health care in Britain had therefore as many disadvantages as advantages. If all financial options were to be rejected, the final option was, in Professor Brian Abel-Smith's (1988) view, to give the hospitals and nurses the money they needed to do a proper job which might prove politically successful at the next general election.

The future financing of the NHS was therefore a complex issue. As there were no magic answers from the funding options, what possibilities were there to make the health services more efficient? Amongst the second main group of proposals, the emphasis was placed on efficiency through improved management and greater competition.

MANAGEMENT OPTIONS

Internal markets

Much interest and discussion were aroused by the advocacy of creating internal markets and managed health care in order to introduce competition within the NHS. Exponents (NAHA, 1988b; National Consumer Council, 1988; Peet, 1988; Robinson, 1988) argued that competition for goods and services in general brought more choice for consumers as well as incentives for greater efficiency. Professor Alain Enthoven (1985), who put forward the idea of internal markets in the mid-1980s, criticized the British system on the grounds that few positive incentives were offered to do a better job for the patients, nor were District Health Authorities properly compensated for treating patients from other districts, between which waiting lists varied widely. Under an internal market, NHS hospitals and districts would buy and sell services from each other on a cost-effective basis.

The basic idea underlying an internal market arrangement was that the health districts' responsibilities for financing and providing health care services for their resident population should be separated. Districts would continue to finance

Table 7.2   Funding options for the NHS.

Method	Advantages	Disadvantages
National Health Insurance (NHI): Raising money from compulsory NHI contributions	a) NHI would bring home to payees what the service was costing b) People would therefore make more rational choices about levels of spending	a) NHI was not a true insurance system b) Individual payment rates would bear no relation to the amount of health care received (Gardner, 1988) c) Raising money from compulsory NHI reduced the financial incentive for unemployed people to take on whatever low paid jobs there were d) If employers were to pay instead, either wages would be reduced or goods would be less competitive abroad (Abel-Smith, 1988) e) Unless compulsory, the 'healthy wealthy' would tend to opt out, as they would be able to purchase insurance more easily; high-risk groups would then face high premiums if they were expected to cover costs (Robinson et al., 1988)
Private Health Insurance (PHI)	a) Potential scope for PHI in line with that of the major European countries was recommended by the Institute of Health Services Management (Orros, 1988) b) Availability of consumer choice c) There was a place for the private sector to contribute to health care improvement through a relatively small-scale supplement to the NHS, according to the King's Fund (Robinson et al., 1988).	a) International evidence showed that where private insurance was the main method of health finance, adverse selection would mean that high risk groups would find it difficult to obtain cover at affordable premiums (Robinson et al., 1988). b) Analysis had shown that the high cost of private medical care had placed a limit on its growth (Laing, 1987) c) PHI led those involved to pay for health twice over, since the NHS was largely financed from taxation
Health Vouchers, Health Credits: People would be given, or opt for, a credit or voucher to cover all or part of the cost of their health care – but excluded long-stay provision for elderly, handicapped and mentally ill people (Green, 1988; Whitney, 1988)	a) Vouchers were seen as a means to provide people with more choice and to attract more funds into health care b) Extra resources for health care could relieve some of the pressure on the NHS	a) There would be no guarantee that people would be able to obtain satisfactory coverage for their voucher or credit (Gardner, 1988) b) There was no way in which the value of vouchers could be geared to individual risk c) The poor and chronic sick would be likely to be denied health care because they would not necessarily find an insurer willing to take them (Abel-Smith, 1988)

(continued)

Table 7.2 Continued

Method	Advantages	Disadvantages
Tax Relief: A variant on deductible cost: health insurance had only been tax deductible for employees earning less than £8500 p.a. who were included in a scheme by their employers	a) If extended, the private sector contribution could increase significantly which might then relieve some of the burden on the NHS b) A lighter deadweight alternative could be effected through a tax relief system available to elderly people only (Gardner, 1988)	If extended, the 'deadweight' cost would be around £200 million per annum with no immediate savings for the NHS
Hypothecated Tax: An earmarked tax specifically to raise funds for the NHS	a) Increased spending of £3 to £5.5 billion, through a tax to increase revenue only for the NHS was favoured by David Owen (1988) b) The aim would be to raise NHS annual spending from 6% to 7.5% of the GDP c) The NHS Royal Commission had already acknowledged the funding advantages (Merrison Report, 1979), even through a tax on health harming goods such as alcohol and tobacco	Although the NHS might have a source of revenue outside the immediate control of ministers and insulated from government public spending policy, this was precisely why such a tax would meet strong Treasury opposition
Lotteries: A means to raise money for the NHS	a) In February 1988, a private lottery was launched to raise £40 million annually b) After the legal problems were cleared, the NHS lottery was relaunched in October 1988 by the National Hospital Trust, who expected to raise £17 million within a year	a) By April 1988, the Gaming Board (which registered and oversaw big lotteries) had misgivings. The Home Office was asked to look into the legality of a privately run lottery to raise cash for the NHS (Brindle and Johnson, 1988) b) The Royal Commission on the NHS had already dismissed lotteries as inadequate to fund the NHS while likely to favour glamourous causes (Merrison Report, 1979)
Income Generation: The government estimated some 1000 projects were intended to yield a target of £20 million in 1988	The 1988 *Health and Medicines Act* provided new powers and a statutory framework for income generation to take on a more significant role	Despite the opening of shops, the franchising of bookstalls, florists and hairdressers in hospital reception areas, the promotion of catering facilities and corporate hospitality packages, concerns remained that the government would reduce the health authorities' financial allocation proportionate to income (Ham and Robinson, 1988)

services but could choose to buy some services from other districts, if financially advantageous, or even sub-contract to the private sector (Robinson, 1988).

The benefits of an internal market, argued Ham and Robinson (1988), would include:

- increased efficiency between DHAs (just as competition was claimed to have achieved in the private market);
- lower costs from economies of scale which might arise through the specialization of services;
- reductions in slack or spare capacity.

However, there were potential snags to internal markets:

- the power of decision-making was likely to be taken even further away from the consumer;
- anomalies within RAWP (the Resource Allocation Working Party) would be highlighted: therefore a more sensitive mechanism for allocating resources in districts would be needed (Owen, 1988);
- potential confusion over the notification to GPs as to which local hospital they would be sending particular patients;
- problems of access to health care together with travelling long distances for treatment which could exacerbate inequalities;
- updating hospital lists would be a constant task;
- the severance of long-established relationships with consultants would be unwelcome to GPs.

Furthermore, it was not entirely certain that the specialization incurred by internal markets would bring economies of scale and savings, except possibly by shortening the length of stay in hospital. The expectations of greater efficiency were also highly speculative (Abel-Smith, 1988; Robinson et al., 1988). Meanwhile, the Canadian experience of internal markets had made little progress because of the difficulties in designing systems (Millar, 1988).

Health maintenance organizations

Several commentators (Green, 1986; Butler and Pirie, 1988; Whitney, 1988) put forward a variety of more radical proposals, which were designed to adapt the American experience of HMOs to the NHS.

As one example, the Centre for Policy Studies proposed that DHAs (District Health Authorities) should be replaced by competing Managed Health Care Organizations (MHCOs) which would combine the financing function of both DHAs and FPCs (Family Practitioner Committees). The MHCOs would be purchasers and managers of health care, not the providers, who would contract with doctors and hospitals for the provision of services. A Health Care Finance Administration would finance the MHCOs on a variable capitation basis, taking into account age, sex and morbidity rates. Hospitals would come under the control of their local communities while MHCOs would be free to contract with them or with private hospitals for the provision of individual services. Patients would be free to choose between different MHCOs which would be smaller than existing DHAs, but patients would not be able to choose who treated them nor where they were treated. Consumers would also be free to use their own funds to buy extra services, notably hotel facilities such as single rooms (Willetts and Goldsmith, 1988b). MHCOs would be one means of introducing an internal market into the NHS.

Overall, the case for managed health care was based on the need for competition in both the financing and the delivery of health care, while results should include improved efficiency, innovation and greater choice. The NHS would, however, be preserved free for all. Nevertheless, any variant of managed health care contained disadvantages in the NHS setting. The imposition of an American HMO-type system on virtually all British doctors would not be welcomed. In Abel-Smith's (1988) view, the fatal flaw of the managed health care model was how the NHS budget would be distributed among organizations managing care: there was no basis for making a completely fair distribution. Then again, as NAHA (1988b) pointed out, after major reorganizations in 1974 and 1982, followed by the Griffiths management reorganization from 1984 onwards, further change in the NHS – which was always costly – would be unwelcome.

Resource management initiative

Another method which sought greater efficiency in the delivery system was the emphasis on resource management initiatives. The intention here was to manage budgets more efficiently. The initiatives sought primarily to provide information about the use of resources to enable clinicians, managers and others to identify the costs involved in providing services; to translate district priorities and agreed budgets into action; and to evaluate the outcome in terms of efficiency and effectiveness.

One problem in encouraging greater efficiency was that improvements in clinical performance often led to increased total expenditure. Treating more patients by cutting lengths of stay lowered unit costs but increased total costs (Robinson et al., 1988).

Ham and Hunter's (1988) extensive analysis of the management of clinical activity in the NHS warned ministers against proceeding too quickly. Resource management had so far been mainly confined to a handful of carefully selected demonstration sites where doctors were, in principle, supportive. Support would need to be won elsewhere. Formidable problems had to be overcome before health services could be provided more effectively and efficiently. To succeed, the resource management initiative had to change not only the management culture in the NHS but also the clinical culture.

NHS reorganization

Others argued that the NHS could be made more efficient through structural reorganization (Whitney, 1988). The Royal College of Nursing (RCN, 1988) called for the abolition of the Regional Health Authorities and greater DHA devolution, because the NHS was top heavy with frequently blurred lines of accountability. The RCN's emphasis was placed on a consumer revolution in which patients could choose how they wished to be treated and by whom, aided by a National Health Inspectorate to monitor care at hospitals, GP surgeries and nursing homes in the public, private and voluntary sectors. The RCN (1988) and David Owen (1988), amongst others, called for the amalgamation of FPCs and DHAs, to enable a unified delivery of health care in both hospital and community settings, based on an NHS which remained comprehensive, free at the point of delivery and funded mainly by taxation.

WHAT WERE THE VIEWS OF THE GENERAL PUBLIC?

No-one asked the users of the NHS what they might wish as their future option, apart from opinion poll surveys. A Marplan poll on the NHS, commissioned by the National Association for Health Authorities and the *Health Service Journal* in April 1988, showed the following.

1 Nearly 40% of people were prepared to travel anywhere in the country for treatment to avoid waiting; most were prepared to travel up to 25 miles to a neighbouring district. The distance content of internal markets therefore had a measure of public support.
2 Lotteries were popular, more so in the south than in the north. Charges to patients remained as unpopular as ever. Voluntary donations and income generation schemes attracted only lukewarm support.
3 The public mind boggled at the complexities of an additional separate health tax. Such a move therefore appeared to be a dangerously unpopular avenue for the government to pursue, while one in ten people questioned were too flummoxed to endorse any additional source of money (other than general taxation) for the NHS.
4 All social classes and age groups were united in their conviction that the NHS should have more money.
5 Once again, although the 1988 *British Social Attitudes* report showed only 41% to be satisfied and 20% to be neither satisfied nor dissatisfied (Jowell et al., 1988), the Marplan Poll found that 87% of individuals and their families who had actually used the NHS were fairly or very satisfied with their treatment (Davies, 1988).

Overall, despite the criticisms, problems and ongoing financial crisis, the NHS received a massive vote of confidence from the one group of people who mattered: the general public.

EVALUATING THE NHS

According to the government's perspective, the NHS review was intended to ensure a future for the beleaguered NHS rather than termination, as some had envisaged. Although various options for the future had been published by 1988, a thorough audit of inputs and outcomes, or indeed any rigorous evaluation, of the NHS was lacking. Charles Webster's (1988) major historical analysis *The Health*

Services since the War was based on the problems of health care before 1957. As Martin Powell (1997) has pointed out, apart from the work of the Guillebaud Committee (1956) which concentrated mainly on costs, the Royal Commission on the NHS (Merrison Report, 1979), which looked at the performance of the service and an article by Klein (1982), there was little evaluated evidence on the NHS at this stage. As the House of Commons Social Services Committee (1988a: xi) commented:

> *The last major weakness of the NHS is that it is not possible to tell whether or not it works ... As a result, the correct level of funding for the NHS cannot be determined and the public and politicians cannot decide whether they are getting value for the resources pumped into the National Health Service.*

THE DEMISE OF THE DHSS

There was little time for evaluations on which to base appropriate changes in the NHS. Political events suddenly moved fast. In a surprise political shuffle in July 1988, the Department of Health and Social Security was split in two. The Social Services Secretary, John Moore, who had been in charge of the government's review of the NHS, was by-passed for the plum political job of the day: the Prime Minister decided that Kenneth Clarke, former Chancellor of the Duchy of Lancaster and Commons Cabinet Minister at the Department of Trade and Industry, should be put into the front-line job of Secretary of State for Health. John Moore was appointed Secretary of State for Social Security. Anthony Newton, who was Minister of Health, was promoted to Kenneth Clarke's former position, while David Mellor was moved from the Foreign Office and appointed Minister of Health. Edwina Currie remained as Under-Secretary of Health until December 1988 when, amid her accustomed blaze of publicity, she resigned over her controversial comments concerning the extent of *Salmonella* infection in the national egg production. The flamboyant media-minded junior Health Minister was replaced by Roger Freeman, former Parliamentary Under-Secretary for the Armed Forces.

The Prime Minister justified her decision to split the DHSS on the grounds that the Department was more than any one person could handle. Kenneth Clarke's unflappability, communication abilities and affable approach were seen by Mrs Thatcher as essential skills for the task of selling the reforms of the NHS to a doubting public.

Throughout the autumn of 1988, leaks of the NHS review began to appear. The appointment of Duncan Nichol, former general manager of Mersey Region, as chief executive of the NHS Management Board heralded, it was suggested, a new era of managerial independence. Everyone was waiting to see which of the funding and management options were to be chosen, whether radical new initiatives were to be proposed or whether the outcome was to be evolutionary. At last the date for the publication of the NHS review was announced: Tuesday 31 January 1989.

8 THE NHS REVIEW 1989

The White Paper *Working for Patients* (DoH 1989a) represented the most far-reaching reform of the NHS from the start in 1948. According to the Prime Minister's foreword, the NHS would continue to be financed mainly out of general taxation, available to all, regardless of income. The main aims were to extend patient choice, to delegate responsibility to where the services were provided and to secure the best value for money. The proposals, to be applied to the whole of the UK, were intended to put patients' needs first.

The White Paper's two main objectives were to give patients better health care and greater choice of the services available, as well as greater satisfaction and rewards for those working in the NHS who successfully responded to local needs and preferences. Once again, the programme was essentially evolutionary: there were no revolutionary proposals, for example, to move the system over to either a private insurance or social insurance model. Further, the sweeping reforms, which set out to make the NHS cost-effective and competitive, continued the government's policy of trying to improve the managerial efficiency of the NHS. The main proposals of the White Paper are summarized below.

1 *Self-governing status.* From 1990 hospitals and community trusts could apply for self-governing status, independent of health authority control but remaining part of the NHS, providing specified management criteria were satisfied. Run by boards of directors, the new hospital trusts would be free to settle the pay of their staff but would raise their income from selling their services, from contracts won, to DHAs, GP fundholders and private patients.
2 *The hospital sector.*
   - All hospitals would be expected to have better appointment systems, more rapid notification of results and would be encouraged to sell 'amenity' services – single rooms, choice of meals, television and phones – to NHS patients.
   - Consultants' distinction awards were to be reformed. Some 100 new consultant posts would be created to reduce waiting lists. Job descriptions would more clearly reflect consultants' commitment to the NHS.
3 *Audit.*
   - Private hospitals would be required to audit their work before health authorities signed contracts with the private sector.
   - Medical audit – a systematic analysis of the quality of medical care – was to be improved in all hospitals through a local medical audit advisory committee, chaired by a senior clinician. Medical audit in primary care was to be in place within three years, to be supervised by a medical audit advisory group accountable to the Family Health Services Authority (FHSA) (the reconstituted Family Practitioner Committee from 1990).

- An NHS audit, to assist in the aim of achieving better value for money, would be undertaken by the Audit Commission.

4 *General Practitioners.*

- GP fundholding (initially denoted as budget holding) would be available for larger GP practices that satisfied certain criteria, who could apply to control their own budgets, which they would receive direct from the Regional Health Authority. The money would be used to buy hospital care for patients, compete with other practices for patients, run their own businesses and plough back savings into their own practice.
- Non-fundholding practices would receive 'indicative' prescribing budgets, monitored by the FHSA.
- Patients would be able to change doctors more easily.
- GP capitation fees, which accounted for 46% of a GP's income, were to be raised to 60%, as an incentive to satisfy patient choice, by increasing the income attributable to the number of patients on GPs' lists.
- From 1991, GP indicative drug budgets would lower the £1.9 billion drugs bill through a prescription-monitoring procedure which would not, in any way, prevent people from obtaining the medicines they needed.

5 *Management changes.* Through a 'purchaser-provider split' within 'an internal market', the main role of DHAs would be to assess the health needs of the population in order to purchase services to meet those needs. No longer would RHAs nor DHAs have to provide all the services themselves. DHAs would be able to trade with each other, with self-governing trusts, hospitals in other districts, the private sector and the voluntary sector. Core services, such as emergency services, would still have to be provided locally, but patients might have to travel for specialist operations or even routine surgery.

- Resource management was to be speeded up: all major acute hospitals could join the programme by March 1992.
- Money was to follow the patient through a weighted capitation system of funding which was to replace RAWP, phased over five years. DHAs were to receive allocations for their resident populations, but were to pay each other directly for services provided across boundaries.

6 *Privatized initiatives.* The private sector and co-operative ventures with the NHS (competitive tendering, use of facilities, joint construction programmes) were to be further encouraged. From April 1990, tax relief on private health insurance would be extended to people over 60.

7 *Structural changes.*

- Family Practitioner Committees (FPCs) would be reduced from 30 members to 11, half lay and half professional, to include a doctor, dentist, nurse and pharmacist. The chair was to be appointed by the Secretary of State. New chief executives would be appointed and management teams strengthened.
- RHAs and DHAs would be slimmed down from their previous 16–19 members to five executive members (to include the general manager and finance director) and up to five non-executive members, appointed for their

individual skills by the Secretary of State/RHA. Local authorities would no longer have the right to appoint members to DHAs, but teaching districts would continue to include someone drawn from the local medical school.
- At central level a new policy board, chaired by the Secretary of State, was intended to oversee the strategic direction of the NHS, while the NHS Management Executive, chaired by the Chief Executive, was to carry it out.

8 *Timing.* The government intended to implement the whole programme by 1991, in three phases, to begin in 1989.

In the wake of the crisis in the NHS, there was no doubt that reforms were needed. Some of the proposals reinforced changes that had already begun (resource management; medical audit) and were welcomed. Changes in the method of resource allocation also seemed to address RAWP funding problems such as inadequate compensation for workload or for recognition of good performance (Ranade, 1994). However, the introduction of an internal market, in which the demand for health care was to be separated from supply to encourage competition between the providers, was more controversial.

Although the British public had remained steadfastly loyal to the concept of the NHS, there was a widespread sense that resources could be used more efficiently, while an increasingly affluent society had the right to a better service. However, the complexity of changes contained in the White Paper (DoH, 1989a) set the NHS onto an uncharted course. Taken together with the subsequent eight *NHS Review Working Papers* (DoH, 1989b), some details were clarified but many questions remained outstanding. Sorting out what *would* happen from what *should* happen would be a daunting task (Timmins, 1989a).

THE NHS STRUCTURE

While other areas of the NHS were being changed radically, management at the centre altered little. Despite pressure from the Institute of Health Services Management and the National Association of Health Authorities for reform, the NHS Management Board was simply transmuted into the NHS Management Executive, chaired by a Chief Executive, to deal with operational matters. A new NHS Policy Board, chaired by the Secretary of State, was to determine the strategy, objectives and finances – as did the former Supervisory Board. The separation of the political role of setting objectives and the managerial one of implementing policy therefore continued as before.

Regardless of calls for their abolition, the 14 Regional Health Authorities (RHAs) in England were left in place. The boundaries of the 190 District Health Authorities (DHAs) similarly remained unchanged, which continued to bear no relation to any other political, social or administrative unit – such as those of local authorities.

Community Health Councils (CHCs) were to continue as channels for consumer views to health authorities and FPCs. However, FPCs were intended to be accountable to RHAs, as were the DHAs. The intention was to bring responsibility for primary health care and hospital services together at a strategic level in order to plan and monitor comprehensive policy initiatives effectively. Previous suggestions to bring DHA/FPC services under common management at local level were rejected, although such a feature was being examined for Wales. The NHS structure to emerge overall for England (Figure 8.1) was therefore similar to former arrangements.

Wales

Some of the RHA functions in England were the responsibility of the nine DHAs in Wales. Other responsibilities were carried out by the Welsh Health Common Services Authority or were the special remit of the Welsh Health Promotion Authority. The NHS in Wales was to continue to work under the strategic direction of the Health Policy Board, chaired by the Secretary of State, as the arrangements had proved their worth under the NHS management inquiry of 1983. However, DHA membership was to be reconstituted with the creation of new style boards. It was also suggested that the 22 CHCs should be realigned, to match one CHC for each DHA area.

Scotland

The responsibility for health service policy continued with the Scottish Home and Health Department, strengthened by the appointment of an NHS Chief Executive for Scotland. The Scottish Health Services Policy Board was to be replaced by a new Advisory Council. At local level, health boards were to be smaller; membership would include general managers and more business interests.

Northern Ireland

All boards were asked to review their management structure in order to submit proposals for reform.

CENTRALIZATION AND DEMOCRACY

One major implication of the structure proposed (Figure 8.1) was the firm control from the centre over health authority and FPC membership. All FPC nominees, RHA chairs, RHA non-executive members and DHA chairs had to be submitted to ministers for prior (some would contend 'political') approval.

However, while the whole tenor of the White Paper (DoH, 1989a) was to give the NHS back to the people, the removal of local authority representatives from DHAs ran seemingly counter to the notion of increasing local choice and participation. Furthermore, CHCs feared that self-governing hospitals would scrap all consultation with them and local people and would deal solely with health authorities.

Nevertheless, democracy in the NHS had never been a strong element (Widgery, 1988: 42) even before the NHS review. The White Paper (DoH, 1989a: 64) suggested that health authorities were neither truly representative nor management bodies. In choosing the management option, the democratically

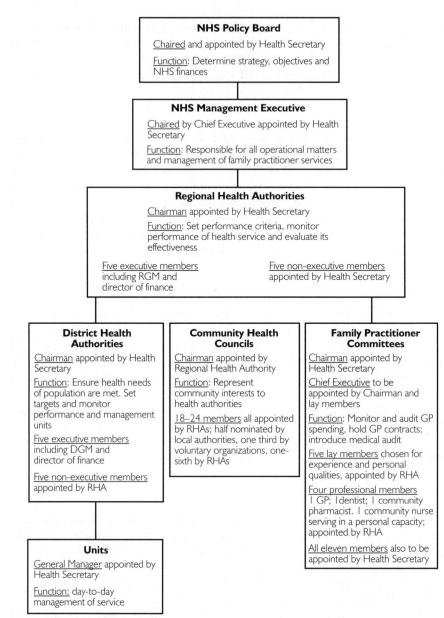

Figure 8.1   New structure proposed for the NHS under the White Paper *Working for Patients*.

Source: (DoH, 1989a).
Reproduced by kind permission of the Department of Health.

elected local authority links were finally severed, while the NHS was rendered less accountable.

INTERNAL MARKETS

The crux of the White Paper's (DoH, 1989a) proposals was the separation of demand (purchasing based on assessed needs) from supply (provision). The model for reform followed the Griffiths (1988) recommendations for community care which, by 1989, remained unimplemented.

The organization of provision therefore represented a major change. The responsibilities of budget holders (hospital managers and GPs) were to be more clearly identified; encouragement was to be given to search out the cheapest forms of health care provision, public or private.

Amongst the management options considered, internal markets had been chosen with all the speculated advantages and very considerable disadvantages of 'managed health care' (see Chapter 7). Where internal markets were to be taken forward, arrangements for patient services' contracts were likely to become increasingly central to NHS management. Lessons from abroad and from the commercial sector had clearly shown that patient services needed to take into account not only money cost but also the quality and reliability of the service provided. However, there was little precedent for assessing the quality and reliability of services within the NHS (Best, 1989).

A modest internal market, in which health authorities bought and sold from each other at negotiated prices, had already started to emerge. Patients from Lincolnshire had been treated in West Lambeth; patients from Gloucestershire had travelled to Riverside in London; NHS Districts had also bought in operations from private hospitals with over capacity. However, any expansion of internal markets was likely to lead, in the view of Brotherton and Jenkins (1989), to chaos, hardship, more paperwork and loss of consumer choice as no DHA would be able to provide the full range of services, so patients would have to travel further for treatment. Meanwhile, the *Independent* (13 February 1989) reported that the East Anglian RHA was to pioneer parts of an internal NHS market of the kind the government planned for the entire NHS in the 1990s (Timmins, 1989b).

THE PRIVATE SECTOR

Central to the notion of managed care and the internal market was the place and development of the private sector. The government now sought to expand on previous initiatives; competitive tendering could extend beyond non-clinical support services as far as the wholesale buying-in of treatment for patients. Joint ventures between the public and private sectors could include sharing the construction of hospital facilities and the leasing of NHS land, buildings and other facilities.

However, the time bomb set to blow the NHS apart, according to Frank Field

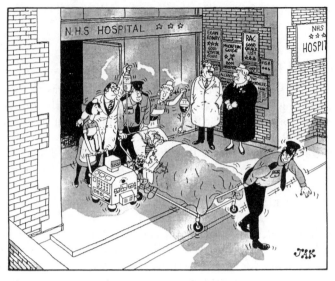

"Make a note to get black silk sheets, matron. That's the third patient we've lost to a
Five Star hospital in a week!"

*Source: The Evening Standard, 2 February 1989.
Reproduced by kind permission of The Evening Standard and Jak*

(1989), Labour MP for Birkenhead and Chairman of the Commons Social
Services Committee, was the proposed tax relief on private insurance premiums,
from April 1990, for those aged 60 and over, whether paid by them or their
families. Despite Treasury resistance, based on the argument that such a subsidy
would be unlikely to increase the numbers opting for private cover, the tax
subsidy was included in the White Paper (DoH, 1989a) at Mrs Thatcher's insistence. The proposition, feared Frank Field, was couched in such terms that the
scheme could be extended to the entire population, ultimately creating a two-
tier system that would erode the basis of a free NHS. Overall, the NHS was not
so much being privatized as commercialized, in Social Democratic party leader
David Owen's view, and even the concept of an internal market, supported by
Dr Owen in order to provide a more efficient patient-oriented health service,
was being corrupted. What was being proposed was an 'open market'. For those
with poor health records and low incomes, there was little comfort (Owen,
1989).

THE HOSPITAL SERVICES

Overall, the government was seeking to diminish the separation between the
public and private sectors and to devolve responsibility across the whole NHS.
The next logical step, according to Health Secretary Kenneth Clarke (1989), was
to allow individual hospitals to become self-governing while remaining within

the NHS. Opting out of DHA control, contended others, was likely to lead to a 'Cinderella' system alongside sparkling 'health condominiums' to which the best doctors and managers would gravitate. Containing the excess of the larger hospitals had always been important in the NHS in order to encourage them to link in well with the rest of the system, but the self-governing concept flew in the face of the principle of NHS unity (*Health Service Journal*, 1989).

Strong reservations about the government's plans for hospitals to become self-governing emerged from the six key hospitals (Guy's in London and the Freeman in Newcastle amongst them) which had been running an experimental scheme to give doctors their own budgets and price treatments – essential requirements for self-governing status. Although doctors were enthusiastic about the 'resource management initiative', most remained pessimistic about becoming self-governing. Doctors were concerned that the need to run their hospitals at a profit would undermine their capacity to provide a full range of services (Laurance, 1989a).

Other concerns over self-governing hospitals included the harking back to the pre-1974 days of the hospital Boards of Governors with their elitist tendencies, a possible threat to future research and medical training, lack of accountability (Millar, 1989b) and the temptation to dispense with unprofitable services

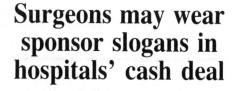

Surgeons may wear sponsor slogans in hospitals' cash deal

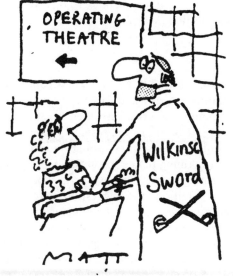

Source: The Daily Telegraph, 10 February 1989.
Reproduced by kind permission of The Daily Telegraph plc.

(*Lancet*, 1989). Freed of pay controls, self-governing hospitals could be a potential destabilizing element in a cash-limited NHS (Timmins, 1989c).

The *NHS Review Working Papers* (DoH, 1989b) made it clear that any hospital, as well as community units, would be free to opt out of Health Authority control by seeking self-governing status. Critics commented that costs would spiral. In contrast, Dr David Green (1989), Director of the Institute of Economic Affairs' health unit, argued that the proposal to establish self-governing hospitals was a step in the right direction. For David Willetts (1989), Director of the Centre for Policy Studies, the 'charm' of the self-governing hospitals was that change was optional.

Meanwhile, the implications for the non-opting-out hospitals involved, first, the outcome of the proposed weighted capitation system of funding RHAs, which was to replace RAWP (Regional Allocation Working Party), which would in turn directly affect DHA and hospital finances. Some regions feared that the principle of the RAWP policy (which favoured some RHAs but not others) had been abandoned. In 1992–93, all RHAs would receive their main allocations on the basis of their population, adjusted for age, morbidity and the relative costs of providing services (DoH, 1989b: *Working Paper 2*).

Secondly, the resource management initiative, which provided doctors with detailed information about the costs of their work, was to be rapidly expanded. However, ministers had not waited for the evaluation of six resource management initiatives, due later in 1989, although the outcome was crucial to the intended extension of resource management in acute hospitals, in self-governing hospitals and for GP budget holders (Macpherson, 1989).

Thirdly, the use of information technology (IT) was also to be significantly expanded. Collecting and using information had long been a weakness in the NHS. The government proposed to spend £40–43 million on IT, but many thought much more was needed (Macpherson, 1989).

GENERAL PRACTICE

Strong opposition was voiced by GPs to the White Paper's (DoH, 1989a) plans to change GP remuneration radically and to sanction those who prescribed drugs excessively. There were, however, other anxieties.

The British Medical Association expressed immediate concern that GP budgets for drugs and for buying care would reduce, not increase, patient choice. The indicative prescribing budget proposals were perceived as an attempt to set limits to spending, which, the BMA warned, would lead to putting money before medical need. In addition, the suggestion that GP fundholders should hold contracts with hospitals for non-urgent operations was seen by the BMA as likely to restrict, not to improve, choice, as the patient would have to go to the contracted hospital. The BMA was equally concerned about the ethical implications of holding back GP fundholders' money to buy special hospital 'bargains' (DoH 1989a: 52), which might defer treatment to take advantage of 'offers'.

GPs had an uneasy feeling that the government appeared to be shifting the blame for under-resourcing of the NHS onto GPs, by removing the responsibility for rationing scarce NHS resources from the centre to family doctors.

Constraints included the apparent loss of GP freedom of referral. The *NHS Review Working Paper 2* (DoH, 1989b) established that GPs who did not hold budgets for hospital care would be told with which hospitals the DHA had contracts in order to encourage GPs to refer patients to those hospitals whose care, in the DHA's view, offered the best value for money. However, patients would not be allowed, according to the NHS review on GP practice budgets (*Working Paper 3*: DoH, 1989b), to top up a family doctor's budgets by paying extra for quicker hospital treatment.

Hospital gynaecologist Wendy Savage and GP David Widgery (1989) were especially critical of the proposal to raise the capitation element in GP's income from the average of 46% to 60%. The implications would reverse the steady (and welcome) fall over the past few years in the average GP's list which allowed more time to be spent with each patient. A number of GPs regarded the whole package as one which presented largely unworkable plans for hard-pressed surgeries (Cohen, 1989; Davies, 1989b).

The concern of GPs was reflected in various straw polls. On 4 February 1989, the *Independent* published a poll of 60 GPs whose names had been taken from *The Medical Directory*. By more than two to one, family doctors believed patients would lose rather than gain from the proposed market-like NHS. The March 1989 issue of *Medeconomics* published the first major survey of GP reactions to the government's (DoH, 1989a) proposals for the NHS. More than three-quarters of the 2231 GPs who replied felt their independent contractor status and clinical freedom would be restricted; nor did they believe that any real improvement in the management of primary care would be achieved.

GP FUNDHOLDERS

The Secretary of State for Health assured MPs that doctors, who opted to run their own practices along more commercial lines, would not be put in a position where proper medical care could not provided for elderly or chronically sick patients (Hansard, 1989b). Indeed, the GP budget holder idea was the most radical proposal for primary care in the White Paper (DoH, 1989a): some larger practices were to be given budgets with which to buy services on behalf of patients. However, *Practice Budgets* (DoH, 1989b: *Working Paper 3*) went beyond the White Paper (DoH, 1989a) in suggesting that practices smaller than the 11 000 list minimum originally put forward could group together if they wished to opt for a practice budget. The crucial details about which hospital treatment would be included in practice budgets as well as how their costs would be calculated, were left to the NHS Management Executive to develop. However, if GPs decided not to opt for their own budgets, one of the chief instruments of the proposed internal market would remain unused.

Both negative and positive implications arose from the notion of GP fundholders, whose budgets would be directly financed by the relevant RHA. There was concern that many GPs lacked the skills required of efficient budget holders: considerable investment in both training and computer hardware would be necessary. Labour's shadow health spokesman, Robin Cook (1989), pointed to the likely outcome of replicating the experience of managed care in American Maintenance Organizations in which the fatal flaw of market medicine was the concentration on the fit and healthy who needed health care the least. Health economist Alan Maynard (1989a) raised other questions: whether GP fundholders could offer the choice of good quality care for their patients at stable prices, whether GPs would create new firms with consultants to provide good quality as well as cheap day surgery and whether GP budgets would be adequate to meet patients' needs. Experiments and research were necessary to test the viability of the GP provider market (Maynard and Holland, 1988).

On the positive side, some family doctors welcomed the chance to manage their own budgets, as long as they were given enough money (Ballantyne, 1989). GPs could employ physiotherapists and other specialist health workers: GPs could also act as travel agents, guiding their patients through the system while spending money on their behalf, as the money flowed with the patient (Willetts, 1989). The government argued that, through competition with other practices and improved services, GPs would have an incentive to put the patient first (DoH, 1989a: 48).

The crucial question remained unanswered – just how many GPs were going to opt to become fundholders? The BMA launched a determined campaign against many of the key government proposals, including self-governing hospitals, the internal market and GPs as fundholders. By 9 March 1989, the family doctors' local medical committees in Leeds, Birmingham and Sheffield had voted overwhelmingly against the government's plans for the future of the NHS. Winning over GPs was to be the Health Secretary's chief task.

MEDICAL AUDIT IN THE NHS

In contrast to the concern amongst GPs about the impact of the government's plans for family doctors, the proposed reform of medical audit was generally well received by the medical profession and public alike (*Lancet*, 1989; Macpherson, 1989). Even the most critical of the government's proposals (Savage and Widgery, 1989) welcomed the idea of medical audit, in which doctors would compare the quality of the clinical decisions taken and the treatment given with those of other doctors. However, while the move towards ensuring quality was applauded, medical audit might highlight deficiencies in the NHS, which only further resources could improve (Timmins, 1989a).

THE NURSING PROFESSION

Significantly, nurses were allotted no major heading of their own in the White Paper (DoH, 1989a). The Royal College of Nursing (RCN) criticized the proposals for hospitals to opt out of DHA control, as such hospitals were likely to concentrate on profitable forms of treatment which would undermine the NHS as a comprehensive health care system. RCN general secretary, Trevor Clay, welcomed the fact that the NHS would still be funded from taxation, but was concerned that self-governing hospitals could become targets for privatization. However, plans to reshape the NHS amounted to another management reorganization which the nurses distrusted after the 1988 regrading dispute (Pallot, 1989).

The most serious consequences were likely to be for community nurses and midwives. The care of mental handicap, mental illness and elderly people had not been addressed at all. The risk was that these groups would be dumped with all the difficult and long-term care issues in a no-man's land between the new GP group practices and hospital trusts.

Questions remained for nurses in primary health care. Would the new small business-type GPs really participate as equals within primary health care teams? Powerful checks would be needed to guarantee the development of primary health care policies (Clay, 1989).

On a more positive note, a *Nursing Times* (8 February 1989) editorial pointed out that midwives should look with glee on the two lines on page 15 of the White Paper (DoH, 1989a) that stated that their skills should be used fully. Further, on page 15, the extension of the role of nurses, to cover specific duties normally undertaken by junior doctors, might be welcomed as recognition of the nurses' contribution.

As a general manager in the late 1980s, Ray Rowden (1989) explored some wider implications for the nursing profession. In view of the likelihood of patients travelling longer distances for surgery, there was the need for a total overhaul of liaison between care agencies together with greater planning on patient discharge. Further, nurses would have to ensure that their profession had both an effective and valued voice at local level, especially where, under the new arrangements, there was no automatic representation of nurses in health authorities. On the other hand, nurses might have a major contribution to make to the NHS trusts, if trusts were to be expanded to embrace entrepreneurial ideas. The nursing profession would also need to be mindful of nurses' educational needs in the NHS of the future.

Above all, information technology was going to be the key to the success or failure of the new proposals. Some £43 million was to be spent in the community and the hospitals, which could be good news for ward-based staff, as the government proposed to extend the resource management initiative in which nurses and doctors would have a more accurate picture of costs and activity through better information (Rowden, 1989). Overall for nurses, as for the NHS as a whole, implementing the government's proposals was about managing change.

PATIENTS AS CONSUMERS

The White Paper (DoH, 1989a) was entitled *Working for Patients* or, as the *Daily Express* (1 February 1989) headlined: 'Health Revolution will give value for money: POWER TO THE PATIENT'. *Would* the rationing of resources give power to the patient? The White Paper's (DoH, 1989a) proposals were likely to transfer the rationing function from the hospitals to GPs. How would the transfer, asked correspondent Peter Jenkins in the *Independent* of 31 January 1989, make things any better or more acceptable to the patient? Did the doctors really know best?

Regarding hospitals which opted out of DHA control, the *Health Service Journal* (21 January 1989) contended that opting out was designed to service not patients but providers of health care.

Similarly, the flaw in the government's logic, argued Julia Neuberger (1989), then chair of the Patients Association, was that the purchasers of the hospital services would be the GPs and DHAs not patients – as the NHS was largely free at the point of use. It was hard to make the mechanism of the market work unless the purchaser was the consumer.

On the question of patients' choice, which the government sought to further, Klein and Day (1989) pointed out that competition between internal markets could not be equated with consumer choice. Cash limits on GP practices were also likely to discourage chronically sick, disabled and elderly patients. The complexity of the needs of these vulnerable groups made them a more expensive group to care for; choice was therefore only likely to be more readily available to the broadly healthy. Such an outcome then raised the question: 'would a true internal market ensure adequate services for the unlucrative, unglamorous, troublesome services (geriatric wards, for example)?'

The traditional voice of the patient at local level, the Community Health Councils, was not being strengthened either. How effectively CHCs would continue to act as a channel for consumer views was not entirely clear, as CHCs were to have no automatic right of representation on the new slimmed-down DHAs nor FPCs (Neuberger, 1989).

PARADOXES AND OMISSIONS

The White Paper (DoH, 1989a) contained several financial paradoxes. First, what started out as a review of finance emerged as a review of management and organization. The crisis in the NHS was therefore sold, in Savage and Widgery's (1989) view, as a result of the underlying structure but not of prolonged under-funding.

Second, as Robin Cook, Labour health spokesman, pointed out, a review which had grown out of a cash crisis in the NHS had resulted in further cash limits on the NHS through tighter cost controls all round (Jenkins, 1989a).

Third, despite intentions to control expenditure, spending on the NHS was to increase by £1.3 billion in 1990 and a further £2 billion in 1991–92, to reach a total of £21.7 billion. Based on an estimate of 5% inflation, the increase was to take account of the government's reform package. In the short term, extra spending on the NHS looked inevitable in order to implement the government's more controversial ideas: self-governing hospitals and GP fundholders. What remained to be seen was whether the government was prepared to tackle the financial pressures that change would inevitably generate.

The White Paper (DoH, 1989a) was, however, full of white spaces. Prevention was never mentioned, except briefly in the section on Wales although patients, even before treatment, would wish access to prevention. Details were lacking on community care and priority services. Facilities for women did not feature in the 'core services' that self-governing hospitals would have to provide: thus questions were raised more generally about the place of maternity provision. Abortion did not even appear in the section about the number of private operations performed, although it was the most commonly performed private operation (Savage and Widgery, 1989). The style of the White Paper (DoH, 1989a) was not necessarily to itemize particular groups and their needs, but where they were omitted they were significantly absent. The needs of neither women nor ethnic minorities were mentioned.

The original eight documents contained in *The NHS Review Working Papers* (DoH, 1989b) were intended to fill in the details of the White Paper (DoH, 1989a). However, omissions and uncertainties remained. Overall, the primary paradox was that the Health Secretary (Kenneth Clarke) was firmly on record as supporting the traditional principles of the NHS, yet his proposals implied a fundamental break-up of the existing unified system in the NHS.

WIDER REACTIONS AND RESPONSES

The unions greeted the NHS review as the start of a two-tier NHS. Rodney Bickerstaffe, general secretary of the National Union of Public Employees, said the review was a cynical charter to dismember the NHS; members would be mobilized to challenge the plans. Hector Mackenzie, General Secretary of the Confederation of Health Service Employees, commented that patients would be on the receiving end of a commercialized system where competition could lead to needless overtreatment of those requiring profitable care but, as in the USA, chronic undertreatment of those most in need. Ada Madocks, staff side secretary of the NHS Whitley Council, which represented NHS employees, stated that the review was a big step towards privatization.

Various health organizations had mixed reactions. The Association of Community Health Councils considered that the outcome would be the reduction of patients' choice. The National Association of Health Authorities (NAHA) welcomed the commitment to a high-quality health service, free at the point of delivery, but wished to see guarantees that comprehensive care would be available to all areas. The Institute of Health Services Management (IHSM) similarly wished to be assured that local community needs would not be neglected, although the IHSM welcomed more flexibility for managers.

Within the NHS, health authority chairs were understood to be privately delighted by the proposals. Many believed that smaller health authorities, modelled on management boards, would make their work easier. Health service managers gave the White Paper (DoH, 1989a) a qualified response although some were concerned that community needs might be neglected.

In Parliament, right-wing Conservative MPs greeted the White Paper (DoH, 1989a) enthusiastically. The shadow health secretary, Robin Cook, described the government's NHS review plans as the first step (Cook, 1989) and the subsequent eight *NHS Review Working Papers* (DoH, 1989b) as a further eight steps, towards full-scale privatization of the NHS. SDP leader, David Owen feared the NHS was to be commercialized and atomized by fragmenting care to create a series of autonomous financial circles, despite the more sensible provisions for GP health maintenance (i.e. fundholding; Owen, 1989).

For the general public, the White Paper (DoH, 1989a) was too big and too diffuse to focus on any particular issue. The proposals were daunting and confusing to absorb. However, public unease over the government's plans for the NHS was first seen in a mid-February Gallup Poll conducted for the *Daily Telegraph* (1989) ('Voters concern over NHS cuts Tory lead to 1.5%'), which showed that the majority of the public did not believe the NHS was safe in the Conservatives' hands, suspected that the Government intended to privatize the NHS and thought the NHS would be in worse shape in 10 years' time. The poll recorded that 71% of voters disapproved of Mr Clarke's plans, 14% backed them and 15% did not know what to think.

In a Guardian ICM poll the following day, the overall Tory lead was cut to 3%, after a spell of unusual turbulence for the government over trouble with water privatization, higher interest rates and contaminated food. The findings confirmed the importance of the National Health Service in the eyes of the majority of voters. Health care concerned the whole nation and was placed as first choice for additional spending by voters of all parties, all social classes and both sexes (McKie, 1989).

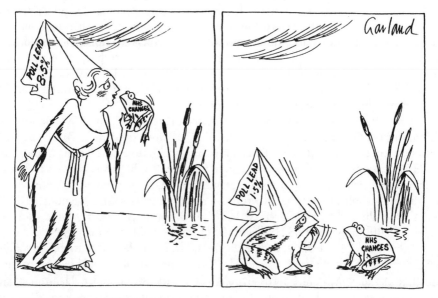

The Independent, *17 February 1989.*
Reproduced by kind permission of The Independent *and Nicholas Garland.*

CONCLUSIONS ON THE NHS REVIEW WHITE PAPER

First, on the positive side, the proposals set a new style for the NHS which promised a more flexible organization – as with wages and salaries – capable of adapting to new circumstances. Klein and Day (1989) pursued this point by suggesting that a more open learning organization could enable the NHS to accept and adapt to change which, in turn, would be more appropriate to coping with the uncertainties of the future.

Secondly, in contrast, there remained a very big query against the need for radical revision of the NHS structure. The NHS had been reorganized three times in ten years (1974, 1982 and 1984); the effects of the last two upheavals were still being felt. What was needed, argued Savage and Widgery (1989), was a period of stability in the NHS during which time the systems needed to monitor expenditure could be installed.

Thirdly, many shared the view of consultant physician Robert Elkeles (1989), who argued that health care was not a business, in which profit was the driving force, but a service.

Fourthly, the changes created by the government's proposals would certainly be a 'bonanza' for management consultants and computer wizards. To run the business of internal markets, the health authorities and hospitals had to acquire expertise to draw up contracts and price systems (Timmins, 1989a). In this competitive arena much was being asked of family doctors, as dissatisfied patients would be able to vote with their feet.

Mr Clarke's White Paper (DoH, 1989a) effectively gave notice to two powerful groups. For 40 years, the Treasury had controlled aggregate spending in the NHS, while the doctors had largely controlled the professional resources. Now the turn of managers and market forces had seemingly come.

Finally the government's proposals appeared to have set out three main objectives (Klein and Day, 1989).

1 To ensure central control over the policies and priorities through a tightened NHS management structure.
2 To raise efficiency through competition.
3 To increase consumer choice.

Professor Alan Maynard (1989b) suggested the following markers by which to question and judge the reforms:

● Would there be greater incentives to minimize costs?
● Would health be enhanced by lower cost?
● Would there be increased equity in order to reduce inequalities in health?
● Would consumer choice be increased in terms of their deciding who would treat them, and when?

Then suddenly and quietly, into the middle of all the hubbub of the questions and anxieties, the polls and campaigns, the Health Ministers on roadshows to promote *Working for Patients* (DoH, 1989a), the Office of Health Economics

(OHE, 1989) published *People as Patients and Patients as People*. This report claimed that hospital waiting lists had been bolstered by people waiting for types of treatment that would have been impossible 40 years ago. Overall, the low-cost NHS had, indeed, been outstandingly successful in achieving the original objectives envisaged.

REVOLUTION OR EVOLUTION?

While the outcome of *Working for Patients* (DoH, 1989a) was likely to be a radical transformation of the NHS, evolution still remained the key factor in health care provision in Britain.

The NHS, from 1948, introduced certain fundamentally new features: universal access to a comprehensive health care system free at the point of use, nationalization of hospitals and a personalized family doctor service. However, two aspects had changed little.

First, community care, GP services and hospital provision remained administratively separate. The divisions were a legacy from the pre-war arrangements which the NHS inherited but never reconciled. Except for a brief period between the 1974 and 1982 reorganizations, even co-terminosity of health and local authority boundaries never became an article of policy. Centralized administration rode rough-shod over municipal boundaries, thrust local interests to the sidelines of policy and separated treatment of sickness from care in the community. Efficiency, as well as a wish to placate the doctors, dictated that local authorities should withdraw from personal to environmental health care (Tonkin, 1988). The NHS White Paper (DoH, 1988) did nothing to alter these basic patterns (Figure 8.1). The DHAs, FPCs and local authorities remained separately administered – all with separate boundaries, although DHAs and FPCs were both accountable to their RHAs. Furthermore, membership apart, the 14 RHAs not only remained intact but moved into the 1990s unaltered for 40 years, in size and function.

The second feature to evolve without change across the post-war decades was the heavy resource and policy emphasis on the acute sector. As Bosanquet (1989) commented, the NHS White Paper (DoH, 1989a) might lead to radicalism in marketing but to conservatism in perpetuating patterns of acute hospital treatment.

A third aspect was that the White Paper (DoH, 1989a) fitted well into the evolutionary mould. The Prime Minister's foreword gave an assurance that the NHS would continue to be available to all, regardless of income, to be financed mainly out of taxation. However, the proposals did mark a new emphasis on resource management, consumerism, marketing and management.

From the various options set before the government in the late 1980s, revolutionary change had been largely put aside. Although certain major new elements were proposed (self-governing status for hospitals, GP fundholding, the internal market, albeit influenced by US managed care), the NHS review (DoH, 1989a) essentially set out an evolutionary pathway for the future.

The big question for the 1990s was whether the proposals would work. Were the professions prepared to implement the changes put forward? Without support from the health care professions, the notion of an internal market could not function.

By Easter 1989, although doctors faced dilemmas, the political battle lines had been drawn. All echelons of the medical profession were ranged against the Health Secretary's plans for reforming the NHS. Amongst the main anxieties expressed by doctors and nurses were the risks to patient care from a 'cut-price' NHS, the government's disregard of the main NHS problem (gross underfunding) and the concern that GPs would be sending batches of patients from one district to another in search of cheaper operations (Timmins, 1989d). The government therefore had a stand-up fight ahead.

In a forecast of future probabilities one of the shrewdest political commentators, Peter Jenkins (1989b) of the *Independent*, suggested that, while the Health Secretary might succeed in forcing through the NHS reforms in the face of medical opposition, the political war was unlikely to be won. Mrs Thatcher's great assets as a leader were accepted by the general public in the realm of enterprise and wealth creation but the welfare ideal still ruled over considerations of commerce. In her third term of office, Mrs Thatcher might have stepped over the welfare line. The general public held a deep-rooted and pervasive suspicion that the NHS was an area where the government could not be trusted. People were quite capable of holding two sets of values simultaneously which applied a work ethic to work and a welfare ethic to welfare. Privatizing gas and telecommunications was one thing; venturing into the heartland of the Welfare State was another.

HEALTH CARE PROVISION IN A WIDER SOCIAL POLICY CONTEXT

To set the proposed NHS reforms into a wider context, a broader dimension of health care provision could be seen by the end of the 1980s, through the pattern of public spending on social services as a whole. Paradoxically, despite the government's determination to curb public expenditure throughout the 1980s, resources had been increasingly made available to the major social services (Table 8.1). Increasingly, housing, however, was the one element that had been notably cut back. Although cuts had been imposed variously on social security, education, health and the personal social services throughout the 1980s, the actual resources allocated showed a gradual rise, although each service differed significantly.

By far the largest social services element was absorbed by social security (where financial commitments were legally earmarked for pensions, unemployment benefit and single parent families amongst other increasing pressures). On the other hand, expenditure on the health services had kept on a relative par with education. However, in both cases, the increased financial outturn disguised the drastic measures that had had to be taken by health authorities and education services, especially in the tertiary sector, in the face of

Table 8.1 Public spending in the UK (£ billion) in real terms by function 1981–1989.

Function	1981–82 outturn	1987–88 estimated outturn	1988–89 plans
Social security	37.7	45.9	45.9
Health and personal services	20.2	23.3	23.6
Education and science	18.5	20.1	20.1
Housing	5.4	3.5	3.8
Total of public expenditure on the major social services	81.8	92.8	93.4
Planning total for public expendiure overall	133.0	141.3	143.9

Source: CSO (Central Statistics Office) *(1989; 112).*
Crown copyright material is reproduced with the permission of the Controller of Her Majesty's Stationery Office.

severe cuts and resource restraint. Efficiency savings was one method of bridging the gap; rationing (waiting lists), raising private funds and low-paid staff were others. Even the planned public expenditure in 1989, for the combined state provision of health and personal social services, did not exceed the £24 billion that informal caring was estimated to be saving the Treasury (Green, 1988).

So the question for health care in the 1990s was how far, within the tightly controlled resource limits, could the proposals in the NHS White Paper (DoH, 1989a) be effectively implemented? Indeed, what was the outcome to be overall?

9 THE NHS REFORMS 1990–1997

The National Health Service and Community Care Act was passed in 1990. The NHS reforms, outlined in *Working for Patients* (DoH, 1989a), were thus implemented from 1 April 1991, by which time Mrs Thatcher had been replaced as Prime Minister (in November 1990) by John Major. William Waldegrave was appointed Secretary of State for Health until the general election of April 1992, whereupon Virginia Bottomley took over, to serve under John Major's Conservative administration until 1995, when replaced by Stephen Dorrell (see Appendix 1 for a record of Prime Ministers and their Health Ministers 1945–1999). The recommendations from the Griffiths Report (1988) on community care were largely implemented under the 1990 legislation. The implications will be discussed in Chapter 12.

This chapter sets out to consider the key elements in the NHS reforms (the internal market, contracting health care, the place of purchasers and providers) followed by a review of developments in primary health care. Chapter 10 will look at some wider aspects of the reforms across the 1990s.

THE BACKGROUND CONTEXT

The reforms in 1990 introduced the most fundamental change since the start of the NHS (Butler, 1992; Le Grand and Bartlett, 1993). The crucial difference was the shift from a command and control economy to a managed market approach. Previously, the hospital and community services and the separately administered family practitioner services were effectively under the vertical control of the Department of Health (DoH). Under a managed market, the horizontal relationships between purchasers and providers became of greater significance at local level, although the roles of the NHS Management Executive (NHSME – renamed the NHS Executive (NHSE) from 1994) and the DoH remained (Allsop, 1995).

Above all, providers had to compete annually for funded contracts which were intended to maintain their financial viability. Nevertheless, the basic NHS principles of comprehensiveness, universality, equity and a service funded out of taxation remained unaltered. *Working for Patients* (DoH, 1989a) had added greater choice for patients as a further principle, but the need to contain public expenditure, to learn lessons from private sector management, to uphold greater efficiency and value for money continued as before under public health care management. The process was essentially evolutionary in drawing on both the old and the new, perceived by Webster (1998) as 'continuous revolution'.

THE INTERNAL MARKET

At the outset

The internal market formed the basis of the 1990 NHS reforms. The format was much influenced by Professor Alain Enthoven's (1985) diagnosis of the NHS's problems wherein the resource allocation system to meet health needs at district level was separated from the planning process at both district and regional level.

Amongst the various proposals put forward to reform the NHS at the time (see Table 7.2), Enthoven's (1985) advocacy of managed health care, based on integrated health care plans geared to consumer choice, drew on the experience of competing Health Maintenance Organizations (HMOs) in the USA. Crail (1999a) reported that Enthoven's (1985) ideas for an internal market provided Kenneth Clarke with a solution when Margaret Thatcher sprang the 1989 review at short notice.

As devised by the 1990 NHS reforms, the essential elements of the internal market for the NHS introduced a split between the purchase of health care and contracted provision. Managed competition between providers was intended to regulate the advantages of markets without their inequities. As the Department of Health's (1993a) overall map shows (Figure 9.1), the purchasers at local level were the DHAs, FHSAs (reconstituted from the former FPCs) and GP fundholders. The providers covered the hospital and community health services, which had largely qualified to receive NHS trust status by 1994 (but until that point were managed by district managed units), together with the separately managed GP and primary care services.

Potential benefits

The potential benefits of the internal market, at the start, included the following.

- Purchasers could buy from providers who offered good value.
- Purchasers could identify who was providing what services, together with their cost and quality (Ranade, 1994).
- Importantly, health authorities were to base the purchase of services on the assessed health needs of their population, which could, in turn, lead to restructuring services in order to produce greater health benefit (for example, through prioritizing prevention and health promotion). The reforms therefore gave much greater scope for managers to meet health needs in the community.
- The internal market became the only real option to further the aims of decentralization (Bosanquet, 1993).

Drawbacks

The likely drawbacks of the internal market quickly revealed the complexities involved.

1 For a start there were the anomalies. While the supply side of the market was opened up to competition, on the demand side consumer choice was limited to GP regulation through the services purchased by GP fundholders or to the

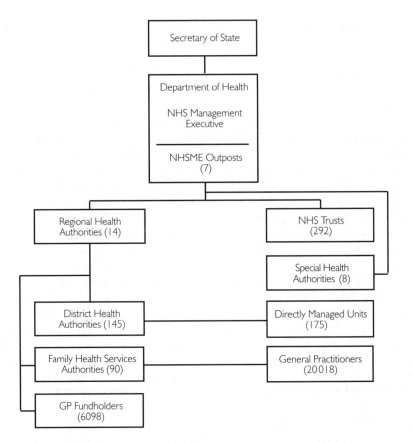

Figure 9.1 Structure of the NHS, March 1993.
Source: DoH (1993a).
Reproduced by kind permission of the Department of Health.

purchasing decisions made by the DHAs and FHSAs, who thereby acted as agents of patients. In contrast, members of the public who chose to enter the market as private patients had wider choice.

2 GP fundholders anomalously acted as both purchasers and providers of care.

3 The initial notion of one internal market provided a simplistic view of the reality: a collection of different types of market existed. In theory, the internal market was to be driven by purchasers (not providers as previously) who would determine the local population's needs and services. In practice, the providers had the expertise and information about services to give the providers a monopoly in some markets (ambulance, accident and emergency) although in other markets (elective surgery, pathology) competition did exist (Klein, 1995: 205).

4 Providers soon began to discharge hospital patients to the community early to cut costs, unless prevented by regulation (Paton, 1992: 80). Not only was such regulation more cumbersome than under previous public planning but,

more especially where the care of elderly people was involved, the community services quickly felt the financial strain as a result.

5 The problems of the internal market reflected the tensions between a commercial market and a government body (the DoH) which required financial controls and accountability. As a result, the NHS trusts were given less freedom than anticipated in *Working for Patients* (DoH, 1989a) to borrow from the public and private sectors to finance capital investment. Furthermore, the power of professional groups to win concessions and the political need to guarantee equality of access, led the government to limit the arena of competition. However, as Ranade (1994) has pointed out, the more heavily regulated the market, the less scope there was for the benefits of competition to emerge. Indeed, Paton (1998: 46) has questioned whether a market system was appropriate at all in the provision of public services; whether such a mechanism was directly transferable or could even cope with issues of equity and ever increasing demand. According to Baggott (1994: 265), markets have had a poor record in relation to health care.

6 Further political tensions continued between those who favoured the former integrated NHS model in contrast to those who pressed for radical reform, based on a market model which encouraged consumer choice and a greater role for private financing (Paton, 1998: 142). In this light the purchaser/provider split was seen as a compromise which overlooked the lessons from Health Maintenance Organizations in the USA that had led to Enthoven's (1985) recommendations for competing but integrated health plans in which benefit could be gained from the integration of purchasing and provision of health care.

7 A more immediate problem was the question of costs, both administrative and regulatory, which could offset any efficiency gains generated. The internal market was unlikely to perform adequately without extra funding (Baggott, 1994). At the introduction of the internal market, substantial costs were incurred through the link up with information systems and computer technology. By 1997, with the approach of a general election, the Labour party claimed that the internal market had added £1.5 billion to management costs (Webster, 1998: 203).

Early on, Le Grand and Bartlett (1993) showed that the internal market was not a market at all in the true sense of the word: the NHS reforms in 1990 had introduced more of a 'quasi-market'. Along the lines of other welfare developments in the fields of transport, education and housing in Britain, as well as in the social housing programmes in Europe, quasi-markets were considered markets because they replaced monopolistic state providers with competitive independent ones. However, welfare quasi-markets differed from conventional markets in three ways.

1 As non-profit organizations competing for public contracts, sometimes in competition with for-profit organizations.

2 Where consumer purchaser power was either centralized in a single

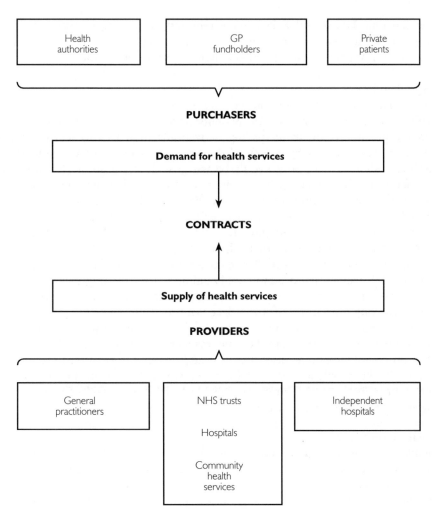

Figure 9.2 A simplified map of the NHS internal market by 1996.

purchasing agency or allocated to users in the form of vouchers rather than cash.

3 Where consumers were represented in the market by agents rather than operating by themselves (Le Grand and Bartlett, 1993: 10).

Contracting health care

At the centre of the internal market was the place of contracts. During the first two years of the 'quasi-market', contracts between purchasers and providers varied considerably, largely as a result of differing local circumstances (Paton, 1998: 76). Figure 9.2 sets out a simplified map of operations by the mid-1990s, by which time DHAs and FHSAs were required, under the *Health Authorities Act 1995*, to amalgamate into one local purchasing body. The amalgamation took place in April 1996 when 100 health authorities were formed as a result.

Hospital contracts

Competitive contractual action on the map was largely concentrated in the NHS hospital sector. As before, private patients negotiated their own requirements from the private sector, as fee-paying or insurance-based customers (of whom there were 6.46 million by 1997). However, Laing's (1997) review of private health care showed that, after five flat years, growth in private health insurance remained sluggish, influenced by the need to charge higher premiums. In order to ensure that competition between the NHS and independent sector would be fair and equitable, the differential treatment of capital in the public and private sectors needed to be rectified (Butler, 1992: 38). Even so, the system did not really involve a greater contractual role for the private sector (Bosanquet, 1993) although, by 1997, NHS trusts had increasingly turned to private earnings. In 1996–7 NHS trusts earned almost £249 million from treating private patients (an increase of 14% over the previous year) but, for the NHS as a whole, the figure was a tiny proportion of the budget (Munro, 1997/98).

While competition for contracts between the NHS and private hospitals was thus limited, other drawbacks became evident in contracting NHS hospital provision on a competitive basis. The cost and quality information were initially lacking. As the problems persisted (Ranade, 1997: 89), in practice purchasers were limited in the use of prices as reliable 'value-for-money' comparisons or indicators of comparative efficiency.

Primary health care

Competition for contracts was largely irrelevant. GPs had either become fundholders or received general practice budgeted contracts from their corresponding health authority. Nor could GPs' extra-contractual referrals be really described as competitive, even though an integral part of the NHS market, when referrals were made for non-budgeted care to be delivered outside contracts.

Types of contracts

Behind the idea of contracts was the view that competition between the providers would press down costs. Given the complexities and contractual variations between the GP services, the force of the exercise tended to be focussed on the acute sector. As a result, a sharper edge was increasingly applied to the type of contracts designed for hospital treatment.

- *The block contract (or simple contract):* the purchaser paid the provider a fixed sum for access to a defined range of services or facilities. Under a *sophisticated block contract* targets or thresholds with 'floors' and 'ceilings' were included as well as agreed mechanisms if targets were exceeded.
- *Cost and volume:* outputs were specified in terms of patient treatment. Purchasers did not necessarily purchase fixed volumes but sometimes

developed contracts with a fixed price paid up to a certain volume of treatment or a price per case up to a volume ceiling.

● *Cost per case:* based on a given contract price for individual cases, a hospital agreed to provide a range of specified treatments.

Paton's (1998) analysis showed that the simple block and sophisticated block contracts accounted for most transactions. Almost one-quarter of all providers indicated that all of their health authority income was held in simple block contracts; a further 36.5% indicated that all their health authority income was held in sophisticated block formats. The remaining NHS trusts obtained their income from a variety of different types of contract.

During the development of contracting throughout the 1990s, various issues have arisen.

● The *contract workload* in terms of negotiations, documentation and administration has increased significantly, which has resulted in an additional category of expenditure that did not occur before the 1990 NHS reforms (Paton, 1998: 86).

● *Quality assessment*, in a way never considered before, the NHS internal market saw the introduction of service contracts between purchasers and providers which heralded a new approach to negotiate quality standards and targets. Questions of quality, monitoring, audit and evaluation have had to be addressed; these will be reviewed further in Chapter 10.

● *Extra-contractual referrals (ECRs)* have been problematic, especially for GPs, where specific interventions might not be included in their overall budgeted contract. Individual demands for *in vitro* fertilization (IVF) have been a case in point. General practices would then have to make a special submission to the respective health authority. Patients referred under ECRs were treated quickly or not, according to waiting lists, waiting times or rationing procedures (Paton, 1998: 61). In contrast, GP fundholders could decide to fund the item themselves from their own budget. By 1997, infertility treatment had become a lottery in which IVF costs varied widely across the country; many health authorities no longer funded the treatment (Revill, 1997). However, although only 4% of all health authority budgets were allocated ECRs, for whatever intervention, ECRs have incurred disproportionate costs and bureaucracy to administer and service which, according to Paton (1998), represented the 'illegitimate' or unplanned aspects of treatment by the criteria of the reformed NHS.

● *The annual chase of yearly contracts* has also driven up costs significantly. Block contracts had initially started out on a three-year basis, but increasingly all forms of contracts moved to an annual basis. By 1995, the Director of the National Association of Health Authorities and Trusts, Philip Hunt, called for contracts to be agreed on a rolling, indefinite basis, with prices amended annually – in anticipation of a Labour government (Brindle, 1996a).

● *Legality:* Hughes (1990) then Dingwall and Hughes (1990) had, from the start, pointed out that only in contracts between the purchaser and the private

sector could the commitments be legally enforceable. All other forms of contracts between NHS purchasers and NHS providers could only be managerially negotiated and regulated where liability might be incurred. The issue of legal liability raised some interesting questions, such as whether comprehensive health care could be enforced in the courts (Hughes, 1991) or whether NHS health authorities could be held liable for what happened in NHS provider units (Old, 1993).

- *Contracts for the community health services:* while most attention had been given to the contracting process in the acute hospital sector, another important – but neglected – sector of health care was the community health services. Both the specification and implementation of contracts had been particularly difficult. Contrary to the competitive formula envisaged in the NHS internal market, Flynn et al. (1995) showed conclusively, from qualitative evidence drawn from case studies, that community health services were intrinsically problematic in the quasi-market. The nature of the services and the system of delivery militated against provider competition. Community health services had more in common with 'clans' and 'networks' than markets and hierarchies; collaborative rather than adversarial relationships were therefore more appropriate between purchasers and providers.

THE PURCHASERS/COMMISSIONERS OF HEALTH CARE

In looking at the place of purchasers, then providers, within the internal market, a striking contrast emerged: increasing collaboration among the purchasers, while competition between the providers, more particularly, in the NHS acute sector became over taken by 'contestability'.

The collaborative momentum

The economic imperative to control public expenditure led to the NHS and *Community Care Act 1990*: competition between providers was to be the mechanism with which to curb costs. Through the creation of a purchaser/provider split, collaborative developments became a driving force to rationalize health purchasing agencies within the internal market (Leathard, 1998). Significantly, no longer would the demand-led process dominate, assessed need would be budgeted through contracts. While rationalization and economy of scale were the key motivators amongst the purchasers, joint working between DHAs was also prompted by deficiency in contractual purchasing skills.

The patterns of collaboration and rationalization from 1991 to 1997

RHAs, whose main function was to allocate NHS resources, were reduced by the Department of Health from 14 to eight by April 1994. Under the Health Authorities Act of 1995, the RHAs' functions were then taken over by eight regional offices of the NHS Executive (Webster, 1998: 201).

DHAs started to work together informally which escalated to 'mergermania' as Harrison's (1992) continuum of purchasing indicated (Figure 9.3).

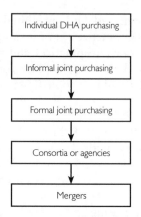

Figure 9.3 A continuum of purchasing.
Source: (Harrison, 1992).
Reproduced by kind permission of the Kings fund.

Ham and Heginbotham's (1991) study, *Purchasing Together*, revealed that some DHAs were too small to form viable purchasing organizations. Reasons for joint purchasing also included the availability of greater financial leverage, the potential to increase competition among providers, ease of formation of 'healthy alliances' with FHSAs and local authorities, and assistance of integrated purchasing across primary care, secondary care and community care.

Family Health Authorities (FHSAs) (responsible for services provided by GPs, pharmacists, dentists and opticians) and DHAs collaborated:

- informally then formally;
- FHSAs and DHAs were then required to integrate by law in April 1996 under the 1995 Health Authorities Act.

Under the 1990 legislation, GP fundholders could apply for the status to run their fundholding practices, employ their own staff and to raise funds over and above the NHS monies budgeted according to the assessed needs of the fundholding population. The budgets covered only hospital diagnosis and investigations, out-patient services and a range of elective, surgical procedures. GP fundholding in the managed market was, initially, somewhat experimental. Only practices with over 11 000 patients were allowed to become fundholders in 1991. To increase the range of practices eligible, the government reduced the maximum number of patients to 9000, then 7000 and finally to 5000 in 1996 (Webster, 1998: 199). The 'first wave' of fundholding involved 291 practices (roughly 7% of GPs) which represented some 7% of the population. By 1996, about half of the population of England and Wales were covered by fundholding practices (Audit Commission, 1996a). However, GPs soon perceived the resource potential of rationalization and collaboration.

- Multifunds became established, which led GP fundholders to work together on purchasing. This development was followed, more ambitiously, by

- Total fundholding, which merged and integrated purchasing across health authorities and fundholding practices. For example, total fundholding in Berkshire integrated six consortium practices and the DHAs which managed funds for 85 900 people (Smith, 1994). The West Yorkshire 'total fund' covered a combined population of 2.1 million people (Hunter and O'Toole, 1995).

Some purchasing/commissioning issues

As the Audit Commission (1993a: 8; 1993b: 65–9) pointed out, the practice of health care was changing rapidly, with an increasing emphasis on primary care and patient involvement for which really effective commissioning involved joint working. The terminology was also evolving as purchasers increasingly became known as commissioners.

By 1997, the patterns of purchasing and commissioning had become complex. Mays and Dixon (1996) described the developments in UK health care, as 'purchaser plurality', for which a typology was mapped out (Figure 9.4).

Mays and Dixon (1996: 52) concluded that each model of purchasing had a different combination of merits and drawbacks. Owing to the complexity and diversity amongst commissioners, no single 'best way' to purchase health care could be signalled (Mays and Dixon, 1996: 72). However, any extension of the role of GPs as purchasers could sensibly proceed only with careful monitoring and regulation.

As purchaser plurality in the NHS developed, changes were not so readily matched in the degree of patient involvement and choice which continued to be limited. As Le Grand and Bartlett (1993) pointed out, only in services purchased by GP fundholders was competition at all relevant as patients had, in theory, a choice of GP but no choice of a DHA or FHSA, which were effectively local monopolies. Therefore, even in practice, patients could find selecting or changing a GP fundholder problematic or even geographically unobtainable.

Paton's (1998: 110) analysis concluded that health care purchasers were essentially a means for the government to conduct centralized planning through decentralized provision. All the main political parties seemed to agree that, whatever else happened, purchasing in the future in the NHS would rely heavily on the skills and judgement of GPs.

THE PROVIDERS OF HEALTH CARE

From the 1990 reforms onwards, the structure of the NHS had been continuously modified. Figure 9.5 has captured the national picture by early 1997 but which was soon to change again.

Special health authorities

A further complication in the pattern of the internal market continued with the special health authorities whose provision covered a range of specialist treatments – from renal dialysis to infant cardiac surgery – not found in every hospital. The services featured small patient numbers, high cost of treatment and

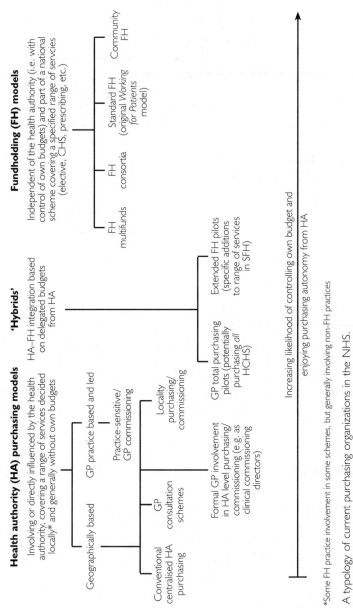

Figure 9.4 A typology of current purchasing organizations in the NHS.

Source: Mays and Dixon (1996: 15).
Reproduced by kind permission of the King's Fund.

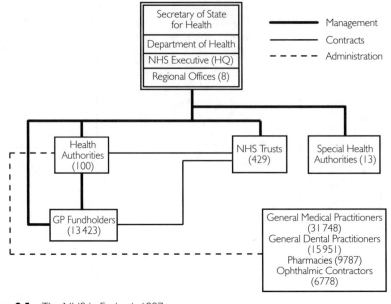

Figure 9.5   The NHS in England, 1997.
Source: DoH (1997).
Reproduced by kind permisisn of the Department of Health.

rapid changes in technology, which presented difficulties for health authorities to commission but which accounted for some £1.4 billion of NHS expenditure. Patients gained access to these 'tertiary centres' either through a hospital consultant or a GP extra-contractual referral. As the Audit Commission's (1997a) review showed, health authorities needed to develop strong alliances with other health authorities and with the clinicians and managers who provided the specialized services, to make the most of scarce resources and maximize the benefits for the users.

NHS trusts

The two main features to emerge from the development of NHS trusts between 1991 and 1997 were as follows.

1 By the mid-1990s, despite the political pressure to engage in competition between NHS trusts, NHS hospitals increasingly began to appreciate the financial value of rationalization. 'Contestability' became the term used to indicate a pathway towards a modified market and hospital mergers.
2 The initial emphasis of the NHS reforms on the acute sector, as the government sought to address funding problems in the hospital services, was overtaken by the increasing importance attached to primary health care.

The development of NHS trusts was conducted through a series of 'waves' as hospital and community units qualified to become self-governing. Assets had to be costed and financial viability had to be demonstrated as a non-profit agency.

From *Working for Patients* (DoH, 1989a; see also Chapter 8), one key principle was for the money to follow the patient to create an incentive for hospitals to provide high-quality specialist services. NHS trusts could rationalize or alter their services to reflect judgements about market movements as, indeed, the main role of the trusts was to provide the services which purchasers wanted. By August 1992, 156 'first-wave' trusts (35% of all hospital and community units) were accepted; in 1993, 129 followed. By April 1994, some 450 NHS trusts, which provided 90% of all hospital and community health services, had emerged. By the last wave in 1995, effectively all units had been absorbed into various patterns: some FHSAs combined with community units; others were split between acute, community and family health services.

By 1997, amongst the significant issues that had arisen in the development of NHS trusts, were the following elements.

Information systems
Information systems needed much improvement from the start of the NHS trusts (Rivett, 1998: 422). The government promised to cover investment in information systems (amongst other factors), the cost of services, the processes through which services were produced, the benefits brought to NHS users, help for GP fundholders to calculate their budgets, to assess the prices of hospital services and to monitor the costs of drug prescriptions.

In early research on the 156 first wave trusts by 1991–2, most had met their financial objectives – but these results were not altogether surprising as the self-selected group of first wave hospitals were significantly more efficient than their non-trust counterparts (Bartlett and Le Grand, 1993: 71). However, in reviewing initial first wave trust annual reports, Hodges (1993) found a wide variation in the quality and quantity of information available, although of 57 trusts who provided accounting information, 55 showed an average return on assets of 8.8%. As Butler (1992: 39) pointed out at the time, the market needed to be protected against the charge of placing profitability before quality of care. In 1994 alone, the cost of installation of NHS information technology totalled some £780 million (Lamb, 1994). By the mid-1990s, an NHS-wide computer network was becoming a reality, although difficulties over implementation and the need to ensure confidentiality remained problematical (Cross, 1995).

The pace of change and management tensions
NHS managers had to adapt to an unprecedented pace of change (Allsop, 1995). According to Rivett (1998: 432), never had the acute hospitals been so efficient nor under such strain. The 1990 NHS reforms had generated competitive pressures. Clinicians knew that their budget might suffer if their hospital service and waiting times fell below the standards elsewhere.

Doctors were drawn into management as heads of clinical directorates to make decisions about what could be provided within the financial targets of annual business plans. Increasingly, clinical directorates had to make rationing decisions about levels of activity and new developments (Allsop, 1995;180).

Tensions arose between clinicians, who were concerned with the quality of patient care and professional standards, and administrators, who were pre-occupied with cost efficiency and effectiveness. While the clinical management roles could be summarized under the headings of functional management, strategic management and human resources management, difficulties remained over the principles of governance, hierarchical control, service co-ordination, clinical autonomy and self-regulation (Lorbiecki, 1995). Further contentions occurred when management changes introduced chief executives from outside the NHS to run the trusts and boards of directors, some of whom did not always share the long-held NHS tradition of public service. While the more technocratic chief executives promoted efficiency and responsiveness, the turnover was both substantial and expensive as chief executives and consultants battled for power (Rivett, 1998: 422).

As the numbers of health service managers needed to run the contractually based internal market increased from 300 in 1985 to 23 000 by 1994 (Appleby, 1995), so Members of Parliament and the popular press maintained that any extra resources should be spent on patient care not on managers' salaries. Concerns over management costs were slightly curtailed when the Health Secretary (Stephen Dorrell) announced at the 1995 Conservative party conference that cost targets for managers were to cut numbers by 5%. Nurses, who had sought to further their careers through the nursing management developments, suddenly found themselves caught out between traditional nursing posts and the new possibilities in the management structure.

By February 1996, some health authorities (on the purchasing side) also planned to cut up to 23% of management staff (Butler, 1996a).

The regulation of market forces in the hospital sector
In order to protect the quality of patient care and equity of access, NHS trusts could not be allowed to fail. The market forces therefore had to be regulated: limits were placed on the ability to borrow capital nor could trusts be allowed to incur a financial collapse (Allsop, 1995).

Managed closures
The Tomlinson Report (1992) on the impact of the internal market on London's health services revealed the need to rationalize the existing pattern of services, which was unsustainable. Set up by William Waldegrave, when Secretary of State for Health, the Tomlinson enquiry embarked on a strategic planning and consultation exercise in London. Influenced by a King's Fund (1992) Commission on London's health services, the Tomlinson Report (1992) recommended that London's acute services should be rationalized and primary health care improved. The Department of Health accepted the main thrust of the recommendations. The government therefore provided £170 million over six years for a 'London Initiative Zone' to facilitate the development of primary health care where health care needs were uppermost as well as to strengthen educational and managerial effort. The London Implementation Group was set up; six

specialty groups were formed to examine clinical requirements and undertake a research review of London's postgraduate hospitals.

The upshot led to the rationalization of London's medical schools which involved tough negotiations. The then Health Secretary, Virginia Bottomley, was continuously involved in difficult decisions which her predecessors had sought to avoid but for which her successors would be indebted (Rivett, 1998: 441). As a result, four main centres were to absorb the existing London medical schools. Each centre would be related to a multi-faculty college: Imperial College; King's College; Queen Mary and Westfield College; and University College. In south-east London, protracted discussions took place over the future of Guy's and St Thomas's: the latter was to become the main centre for acute inpatient and emergency care. Meanwhile, St George's maintained an independent position within the University of London. However, to remain on one's own was likely to be somewhat financially hazardous. Within four years, St George's had teamed up with Kingston University to form an innovative Joint Faculty of Healthcare Sciences.

The effect of market forces was most clearly seen, therefore, in London as referrals from out-of-London districts dropped in the light of higher costs, which led to the Tomlinson Report's (1992) recommendations that some of the most prestigious teaching hospitals should close or merge. Similar problems developed on a smaller scale in some other cities, such as Newcastle and Birmingham. Further, as Le Grand's (1993: 254) early evaluation of the 1990 NHS reforms showed, competition depended in part on the willingness of patients to use alternative, perhaps more distant, providers and on the willingness of GPs to refer their patients to such providers.

The place of community health trusts

The provision of community health services (CGS) for children, elderly people and those with mental illness or learning difficulties (formerly termed mental handicap) were increasingly based in the community and managed by community health trusts. A wide range of professionals worked in the community health services – mostly in community nursing – including district nurses, health visitors, community midwives, community psychiatric nurses, nurses for people with learning difficulties, school nurses and community specialist nurses (such as stoma, diabetes and continence nurses). Midwives have tended to be hospital-based so community midwives might work for a hospital rather than a community trust. About one-third of total NHS revenue expenditure was spent in the community: about one-quarter of the total was used to finance CHS; the remaining three-quarters was allocated to the GP, dental, optical and pharmaceutical services (Audit Commission, 1992a).

There has therefore been a considerable variation in the composition, mix, management and organization of community health services between different (former) DHAs. According to the Audit Commission (1992a), community health services were inherently complex and varied, with diverse management systems. As a result, any evaluation of the effectiveness of the services, outcomes of treatment and quality assessment has been notoriously difficult (Flynn et al., 1995).

Nevertheless one striking factor was to emerge: because the services were delivered in the home or within a neighbourhood, community health trusts increasingly sought to extend services by developing local teams to provide the relevant services in co-operation with voluntary bodies and to develop good relationships with GPs and the local population (Rivett, 1992: 422). Overall, the place of the internal market was inappropriate for community health trusts as providers.

Hospital mergers

From the perspective of the acute sector, the end of the internal market seemed increasingly 'nigh'. The need to curb costs, face cuts, rationalize services, address poor financial stability and compete for contracts had increasingly led hospitals into merger discussions. By 1993, NHS trust leaders were calling for greater colla-boration between trusts to enhance services. Mergers were about to soar (Chadda, 1993). More dramatically, by 1996, two lead hospitals in Leeds (St James' Hospitals Trust and the United Leeds Teaching Hospitals Trust) were set to merge to form the UK's biggest trust due to an anticipated multi-million pound shortfall, although they were subsequently bailed out by the NHS Executive (Hunter and Shamash, 1996). The two trusts commented that their unproductive rivalries had ill-served the NHS. By 1996, NHS trusts were merging to secure rationalization, to reduce duplication and to ensure survival, as in Wales (Chadda, 1996a). Threatened by a financial squeeze, the Hampshire market town of Andover was even considering a merger between a community health care trust and fundholding practices to create a purchaser hybrid. Ham described how purchasers and providers were displaying more mature recognition of the need to work as partners as well as to improve the health of patients through 'contest-ability': a middle way between old-style NHS planning and outright competition (Millar, 1996; Chapter 12 looks at merger outcomes more widely in conjunction with care in the community). Meanwhile, the question for the future was: how long could the internal market hold out as mapped by the NHS reforms in 1990?

THE NHS INTERNAL MARKET: SOME OUTCOMES

By 1997, certain problems had arisen. First, the government decided not to set up any systematic evaluation of the reforms in general, nor of the working of the internal market in particular. Further, the government embarked on wholesale implementation rather than, as experts advised, controlled trials (Webster, 1998: 204).

Secondly, variety and change have been constant. Different patterns of service had been based on local circumstances. While such developments did reflect the policy intent to encourage decentralization and local initiative, standard patterns could not be readily assessed. The NHS structure had also been continuously modified (see Figure 9.5 for further changes) by early 1997.

Thirdly, terms altered: purchasers subsequently became known as commis-sioners; amalgamated DHAs and FHSAs became health authorities; GP fundholders were initially entitled 'budgetholders'; 'self-governing hospitals' were later referred to as NHS trusts. So was the NHS internal market all worth it? The 'official' historian of the NHS, Charles Webster (1998), has commented that, while the market reforms did not go unmonitored, early research findings tended to follow a pattern. The results suggested that the market changes showed some beneficial results, but other outcomes were adverse. The overall conclusions were 'lukewarm'.

On the positive side, it could be argued that, at the very least, health authorities had built up data on the health needs of their local population on which to base an assessment of requirements for provision. Progress had been made in the collection of data on service use, in the acquisition of methods for assessing needs and in the recognition that questions of quality, audit and health outcomes had to be evaluated. Further, giving budgets to GP practices, or groups of practices, had produced innovation as well as benefits to patients, according to a review of evidence from Le Grand et al. (1998).

Amongst the more negative outcomes was the questionable viability of an internal market across the NHS. While referred to as a 'quasi-market' or 'managed market', the concept of an internal market in health care had become an illusion (Paton 1998: 46), more especially where issues of equity and mounting demand, unmatched by the resources available, all had to be addressed, but which were incompatible with a 'market' process. Furthermore, the internal market had actually led to adverse outcomes, which included high management and contracting costs, incurred by the purchaser/provider split (more especially in establishing GP fundholding). Next, the internal market was intended as a means of increasing productivity which would thereby decrease rationing health care; in effect, rationing escalated (due to rising demands unmatched by the resources made available) as indicated by Figure 11.2.

From the perspective of patient choice, intended to be upheld under the 1990 NHS reforms, the internal market could not be compared with a private market, manifestly based on consumer choice. Private health care could offer choice for those with financial means, albeit with some restrictions on access to certain forms of treatment. In contrast, within the NHS internal market patient choice remained at a minimal level in reality, governed by contractual arrangements between purchasers and providers, although GP fundholders did have some leeway to act on behalf of their patients for specific needs. The outcome, in the light of Paton's (1998: 46) analysis, was to have created management by contract which represented a partial alternative to hierarchy and bureaucracy.

A further suspicion lingered over the place of perverse incentives to NHS patients: discriminatory 'adverse selection' by which less money was made proportionately available to meet the needs of high cost, less marketable, low political visibility patients (for example, elderly people; Paton, 1995). The charge tended to be levelled especially at GP fundholding. However, by 1997, the case was not proven (Le Grand et al., 1998), while Paton's (1998: 154) later research showed that the best purchasers could do, within the financial limitations, was to meet demand as far as possible.

By 1998, the King's Fund had published a comprehensive review of the evidence of the main elements of the 1990 NHS reforms. What was the impact of the internal market on efficiency, equity, choice and responsiveness, quality and accountability? asked Le Grand et al. (1998). Although it was acknowledged that assessing the overall effect of the internal market was almost certainly impracticable, from the evidence most analysts would agree on the following.

1 The purchaser–provider split, together with the development of contracts between purchasers and providers, were desirable innovations which should be retained in any future development of health care provision despite the fact that, for some commentators, the extent of regulation weakened the incentives in the system.
2 If the policy aims were to promote quality, choice and responsiveness, it was important to develop purchasing with some degree of GP involvement in the commissioning process. Further, the best way to sustain productive GP involvement was for the relevant agency to have a measure of budgetary control.
3 The conclusions regarding equity and efficiency were not so clear. Devolution of power to smaller purchasing units had led to variations. The most important prerequisite for equity appeared to be for each purchasing agent to have equal resources relative to the composition of the population. However, efficiency problems had arisen with devolved purchasing. The Audit Commission's (1997a) investigation into the purchasing of specialized services had identified scarcity of expertise in the NHS as a whole. Smaller purchasing units could create difficulties for provider planning and stability; the provision and maintenance of expensive facilities might require guarantees of future income streams which raised a more general question of the appropriate size of purchasing units.
4 Although budgetary control appeared to be desirable for achieving changes in a particular direction, it was insufficient on its own. As the Audit Commission (1996a) had shown, it was only the innovative and well organized practices within fundholding that had transformed patient care.
5 On the most fundamental question 'should there be competition at all?' the review of the evidence offered little help. Competition had been patchy. No conclusion could therefore be drawn as to whether the impact of competition had been detrimental or beneficial.

Paton's (1998) findings on the place of competition, mirrored the King's Fund analysis (Le Grand et al., 1998). In his study on *Competition and Planning in the NHS* Paton (1998) found that 57.3% of NHS trusts felt that health authorities did not encourage competition. Paton (1998: 98) has suggested that the explanation could reflect confusion in national policy. On the one hand, there had been acceptance of co-operative relationships; on the other, at different points in time, there were demands from the top for renewed or continual competition. As market structures had been shown to be inadequate to enable competition and were further undermined by mergers and rationalization of services amongst the providers, Paton's (1998) study showed how the conflict between competition and increasing collaboration achieved neither the benefits of a market nor the gains of planning.

Contestability

As the internal market in the NHS never really became established as a competitive market between providers, terms varied between a 'managed market' and 'managed competition', to reflect a form of regulated health care provision which was intended to secure the benefits of competition as distinct from the drawbacks. 'Contestability' then gained favour as the term to denote a middle way between old-style NHS planning and the competitive potential of market forces, which became in actuality a health care market characterized by *ad hoc* arrangements with competitive possibilities, wherein competition between providers in many cases did not exist. Then again, as Le Grand's analysis found, even when potential competition existed the extent to which health authority purchasers or GP fundholders actually used the threat of competition was far from clear (Le Grand et al., 1998: 12). Further, health authorities had an interest in supporting, rather than threatening, local providers based on a more collaborative basis.

By 1997, a political consensus had concurred on the worth of retaining the split between purchasers and providers in the NHS. The value of the split was seen as a means to promote change in local services and to secure costed benefits from health needs assessments. Alongside the purchaser/provider split, developments in primary health care began to move apace – but what were the main outcomes of GP fundholding and non-fundholding?

GENERAL PRACTICE AND PRIMARY HEALTH CARE PROVISION

Two fundamental issues continued to underpin the provision of general practice. The tension between professional autonomy and managerial accountability in primary health care services has been one factor. A second feature has reflected the dichotomy between the encouragement of local autonomy and diversity alongside the safeguarding of quality standards and equity. Such matters have involved all GPs, whether non-fundholding or fundholding. Further, some elements of the 1990 GP contract encouraged competition between GPs as a means of improving the quality of primary care services and increasing choice for patients (Glendinning, 1998). The new targeted payments led to an increase in new activities in general practice. Such developments as health promotion, chronic disease management and minor surgery have taken place. The practice nursing staff have undertaken many of these services for which additional allowances could be claimed (Paxton et al, 1996). Practice-based nurses have also become involved in counselling and advice activities (Figure 9.6) and with family planning provision.

Non-fundholders as providers

In contrast to fundholder, much less has been researched on non-fundholding activities and outcomes. By the mid-1990s Nick Goodwin (1996), a research

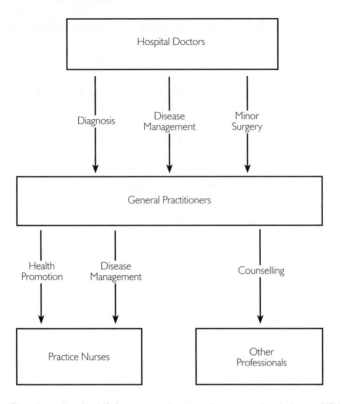

Figure 9.6   Changing roles. (A shift from secondary to primary care has led to a shift in roles.)
Source: Audit Commission (1993b: 70).
Reproduced by kind permission of the Audit Commission.

officer from the King's Fund Policy Institute, contended that many non-fundholding practices had, in fact, achieved efficiency improvements equal to, if not better than, fundholding. Further, the literature had shown that some non-fundholders have been able to perform as well as, if not better than, fundholders as well as being more dynamic.

Once again, even with non-fundholding practices, developments have increasingly taken place to involve GPs with the purchasing and commissioning of health care on a collaborative basis (see Figure 9.4). Of particular interest has been the Nottingham Non-Fundholders Group which was set up in 1992 to represent the views of non-fundholding GPs. Fundholding never really took off in Nottingham; little more than a quarter of the population was ever covered by fundholding practices. The lack of enthusiasm for fundholding may have been explained by the very success of the Nottingham Non-Fundholders Group, guided by principles of equity and co-operation, in working together with the health authority on placing the secondary care contracts in Nottingham. Representing the views of 67% of Nottingham GPs, the group offered the main source of advice to the health authority on health care commissioning matters (Earwicker, 1998).

Fundholders as providers

GP fundholding has been one of the more controversial aspects of the 1990 NHS reforms. However, the underlying rationale was entirely consistent with government policy of encouraging the process of decentralization in the health services. In April 1991, there were 720 GPs in 306 fundholding practices with over 11 000 patients. By 1994, nearly three-quarters of all eligible GP practices with 7000 patients or more were fundholders, serving 37% of the population in England (Appleby, 1994a). By 1997, 59% of the population in England and Wales was covered by fundholding practices. However, as Rivett (1998: 425) has pointed out, the expansion was driven by GP demand which required courage, hard work and professional unpopularity.

Implementing GP fundholding: the balance sheet

Research undertaken with ten first-wave practices in three regions in the south-east of England, supplemented by a sample of second and third-wave practices (Glennerster et al., 1993, 1994), was largely supportive of the GP fundholding scheme.

The case for GP fundholding:

- GPs were better contractors than DHAs as GPs were closer to their patients and more responsive to their needs.
- GP fundholders had the motivation to improve service standards because they suffered from delay and patient dissatisfaction.
- GPs could make marginal decisions while not being involved with big public confrontations, faced by DHAs, if the provider was changed.
- GP fundholders had greater independence than DHAs, which enabled GPs to make the market work quickly and efficiently in order to obtain gains for patients which were highly appreciated.
- GP fundholders had stronger incentives than their non-fundholding colleagues to secure more efficient methods of treatment.
- GPs could use their budget flexibly between outpatient referrals and GP services, between community services and GP practice services, or between staff such as a practice manager, medical partners or assistants, practice nurses or nurses, receptionists, physiotherapists, health visitors, computer experts, district nurses, a social worker, a dietician, an ophthalmologist (one practice even had an operating theatre). All of these strands enabled the people concerned to ask where and how services were best located and organized within the budget constraints.

The case against GP fundholding:

- GP fundholding had rather higher costs than district-wide purchasing: one of the regions studied calculated that total administrative costs came to 5% of the fundholding allocation. Fragmenting contracting by individual practices was wasteful of time and money (Glennerster et al., 1994).

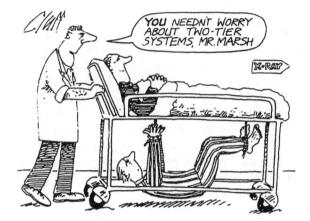

Source: The Times *Magazine, 18 December 1993.*

- DHAs lost their capacity to plan overall services for their populations.
- The gains made by first-wave fundholders might not be repeated by subsequent GP fundholders at a later stage of acceptance.
- The creation of a two-tier service was the complaint levelled against fundholding from the start: that the practices were allocated more money to buy services than the resources allocated to non-fundholders via district allocations. Glennerster et al. (1994) were, however, unconvinced by the equity case against fundholding, although some claims had validity. Even in 1996, evidence was surfacing over inequities – for example, when East London and the City Health Authority had a shortfall of around £14 million. One of the two main local NHS acute trusts, Newham Healthcare, had to suspend health authority-funded elective operations; only patients registered with fundholders then received non-urgent treatment (Butler, 1996b).
- Cream skimming (turning away expensive patients) had also raised early fears. Such concerns were somewhat dispelled when it was shown that GPs did not stand to lose personally if a patient was very costly, although other patients in the practice could receive less treatment. However, the £5000 limit on practice liabilities and the non-emergency nature of the categories covered had put fundholding on a more secure footing than the American HMOs (Glennerster et al., 1994: 174). Le Grand et al.'s (1998: 58) review of the evidence concluded that despite the claimed allegations and theoretical incentives, the general view from the literature was that fundholders had not undertaken cream-skimming.
- Whether patients in fundholding practices were any healthier remained unanswerable.

The Audit Commission (1995) found that, at the stage when 41% of patients in England and Wales were registered with a fundholding practice, one third of all such practices had marked regional variations. Thirty-three per cent were found in the south and west; 51% in the West Midlands. More significantly, fundholding practices were most common in the shires and suburbs and less so in the cities.

The Audit Commission (1996a) followed up with an 18-month study to provide the first comprehensive assessment of fundholding. By now, 53% of patients were covered by GP fundholding. Entrepreneurial doctors had achieved much; there was little doubt that the successful fundholders had often obtained better services for their patients. On the other hand, some doctors had neither the skills nor the motivation to make the scheme work. However, fundholding practices had stood out from equally large non-fundholding practices as having more of the features normally associated with high standards and better quality. Nevertheless, most fundholding practices did not appear to be especially good at management, networking nor achieving benefits for their patients. Whereas (more rarely), the best practices had thought carefully about what they could achieve, were well managed and had achieved much for their patients. The Audit Commission (1996a: 95) recommended that measures were needed to improve management, training and opportunities for development.

Tinsley and Luck (1998) concluded that the principal theoretical advantage of fundholding was that it had proved market sensitive. Furthermore, GP fundholders, unlike health authorities, had been both able and willing to shake up providers. Nevertheless, while in the general application fundholding had shown considerable potential, at the same time serious weaknesses had been revealed.

A primary care-led NHS

One of the first references to a new 'buzz' term came from the NHS Executive (1995) in their publication *Developing NHS Purchasing and GP Fundholding*, significantly subtitled *Towards a Primary Care-Led NHS*. The renewed policy emphasis on primary care implied that there would be a substitution of some hospital care with primary care although, as Paton (1998; 52) later pointed out, there was no evidence that increased primary provision would reduce demand for secondary care. Nor was it clear whether a 'primary care-led NHS' was real primary care or merely secondary care outside hospitals in the hope that the former might be a cheaper option.

Health care provision in the primary care sector included GPs' responsibility for diagnosis, general personal treatment, referral to a specialist, health promotion and prevention. This last role was also shared with district community nurses (Paton, 1998: 53). If other primary care services were included – such as dentists, pharmacists and opticians – primary care has provided most people, most of the time, with the treatment and care they have needed (Holland, 1996). Primary care has two major roles: as a provider and as an integrator of services. From a GP background, Patrick Pietroni (1996) has clarified the often confused difference between *primary health care*, which was rooted in models of evidence-based medical outcomes, drawn from quantitative data, while *primary care* has referred to a social/anthropological understanding of human experiences in health and disease, drawn from the collection and analysis of relational and qualitative data. The NHS Executive (1995) discussed a 'primary care-led NHS' in simpler, policy terms which involved the extension of GP fundholding, a clear role for the new health authorities, a growing partnership between both and for NHS decisions about health care to be more responsive to the needs and preferences of patients and local people.

The commitment to a primary care-led NHS would, in Bosanquet's (1995) view, need a firm strategy to provide investment and to focus on the patient, while assisting local initiatives. In this context new technology offered an opportunity for more information but less bureaucracy. Harrison and Neve (1996) similarly recommended the development of a local primary care strategy from a broad-based consultation process, to identify principles and aims, clarity about resource allocation and to enable partnership, collaboration and the integration of functions across commissioning, provision, monitoring and evaluation.

By whichever pathway, primary care would be placed under increasing pressure. The need to share responsibility for patient care between different organizations involved co-operation, collaboration and the strengthening of networks as the basis for inter-organizational relationships, rather than competition. Pietroni's (1996: 12) conclusion, based on considerable experience with collaborative care, was for a 'Community-oriented Primary Care-led National Health and Social Service'.

The concept of a primary care-led NHS led to a number of White Papers in 1996. The sequence started in June with *Primary Care: The Future* (DoH, 1996a), which concluded that the independent contractor status of general practice was a positive feature that had allowed innovation, diversity and variation. However, inconsistencies and inequalities remained in the range and quality of primary care services; this was a disadvantage of diversity. The report identified a set of principles that should govern primary care services, such as the need for continuity of care, comprehensive services, and co-ordinated provision to enable professionals to work together to meet patients' needs and address the health needs of individuals and local communities while remaining the gatekeeper to secondary care. The report identified five 'touchstones' of primary care: quality, accessibility, fairness, responsiveness and efficiency. Of interest in general practice was the significant rise (69%) in the proportion of women GPs between 1984 and 1994 (DoH, 1996a: 18). Overall, greater flexibility in primary care was called for so that more appropriate organizational structures and financial movement could be developed in response to local problems and shortcomings.

In November, the Secretary of State for Health (1996: 40) presented *The National Health Service: A Service with Ambitions* which stated the key objectives to be:

- a well-informed public;
- a seamless service, working across boundaries;
- knowledge-based decision-making;
- a responsive service, sensitive to differing needs.

Between June and November 1996, the DoH produced *Choice and Opportunity: Primary Care: The Future* (DoH, 1996b) and *Primary Care: Delivering the Future* (DoH, 1996c) in December. Both White Papers set out proposals which were enacted in the NHS (Primary Care) Bill in February 1997. The Bill was rushed through Parliament to receive Royal Assent just before the May 1997 General Election.

The *NHS Primary Care Act* 1997

Three key features emerged from the legislation. First, the individual GP contract was no longer to be the only basis on which general medical services could be provided. Partly intended to encourage new recruits to a profession which increasingly faced a 'manpower' crisis, partly to enable the recruitment of GPs to areas where services were poor, the Act introduced an option for the employment of salaried GPs within primary care provider organizations. The salaried GP option could also open up flexibility in the roles and responsibilities of different professionals who made up a 'primary care team'. For example, nurse-led services could substitute for some traditional GP contractual responsibilities where, previously, the contractual responsibility remained solely with the GP who then employed other members of the primary health care team (Glendinning, 1998).

A second regulatory measure allowed the separate funding streams (provided by the GP services, community services and hospital services) to be pooled and allocated more flexibly according to the contracted responsibilities of the provider organization. GPs, who retained their traditional contracts, could receive extra payments from health authorities to address local health needs.

Thirdly, flexibility was also extended to organizational and budgetary arrangements to help health authorities place resources, as well as open up services, in areas of poor provision or high levels of need.

While in opposition, the Labour party supported the 1997 *NHS Primary Care Act*, in recognition of the need for organizational and funding changes. However, the responsibility for the implementation of the legislation was to rest on the outcome of the general election in May 1997.

10 NEW PATHWAYS FOR THE NHS 1990–1997: QUALITY HEALTH CARE AND THE USERS

Three factors were to play a key part in the developments of health care provision during the 1990s. First, the central role of contracts for health care soon underlined the need for quality assurance, auditing and evaluation. Secondly, the place of patients as service users became ever more significant. Thirdly, the new pathways were increasingly being engulfed in a mounting financial crisis.

THE ENTERPRISE SOCIETY

The new emphasis on quality in the National Health Service was part of a wider government initiative to improve standards of service across the public sector, although part of a society which encouraged ever more private enterprise. Under John Major's administration, as Conservative Party Leader from 1980 to 1997, the main features included:

- low taxation;
- individualism;
- enterprise initiatives;
- means-tested benefits;
- the continued selling-off of public assets to the private sector;
- accountability to public service users via charters (for Citizens, Parents, Patients amongst others) to establish national rights and quality standards;
- according choice to service users;
- competition within and between the public and private sectors which was intended to encourage enterprise initiatives across the health and welfare services.

QUALITY MATTERS

To ensure quality of service might sound like a positive new pathway but the first problem was to define the term. Definitions varied between the macro and micro levels of interventions, between the aspects of service focussed on, and the extent to which consumer views were incorporated (Ranade, 1994: 101). Underlying the King's Fund quality assurance initiatives that started in 1984, Maxwell (1984) argued that quality in health care had to include the following six dimensions.

1 *Acceptability:* to satisfy the reasonable expectations of patients, providers and the community.
2 *Accessibility:* for services to be readily available to the user within distance and time.
3 *Appropriateness:* for services to meet the actual needs of the individual or population.

4 *Effectiveness:* for services to achieve the intended benefits for the individual or population.

5 *Efficiency:* to avoid wasteful use of resources.

6 *Equity:* for the services to be shared to meet the needs of the population.

Such a comprehensive definition raised the question as to whether all elements carried a similar weight. Then again, whose quality was at stake, who would define quality: the purchasers, providers or users? Further, who was to be accountable to whom? Were the outcomes to be judged by the assessment of professionals, managers, politicians or consumers?

The commentary provided by the 1995/6 King's Fund annual review of health care (Harrison and New, 1996), on the concept of equity, showed just how complex all elements of quality could be. Equity could be interpreted to mean: to improve the health of the population as a whole so that everyone should have access to the services that the NHS provided where no group nor section of the population would be excluded. However, equity also contained the implication that services should be provided only when effective because, on equity grounds, no justification could be made for directing resources which resulted in no health improvement. The matter did not rest simply at this point: territorial equity between regions or districts was also relevant, as were issues of need, availability, eligibility criteria and health status.

Quality regulation

Nevertheless, the regulation of quality was important to ensure the effective delivery of health care. However, as Le Grand and Bartlett pointed out (1993: 197), various forms of quality regulation were already widespread in the health care, education as well as social care markets. Methods included self-regulation by professional bodies and accreditation and inspection by government watchdogs such as the Social Services Inspectorate and the Audit Commission. The levels of standard setting and monitoring were also of relevance to quality regulation. As Sale (1996) has shown (Figure 10.1), three main levels of standard setting could be distinguished: a universal or generic level, the purchasing level and the provider level. As standards were set so statements were required to include indicators of quality, appropriate to the populations and addressed in terms of what was *acceptable, observable, achievable* and *measurable.*

However, within the 'quasi-market' the problem of poor information and information asymmetry remained, particularly where the health care purchaser was large or unable to obtain information easily from the providers (Propper, 1993: 198). Under the White Paper *Working for Patients* (DoH, 1989a), the government had introduced two new mechanisms in quality regulation: the contracting process and medical audit – which will be reviewed shortly. A third mechanism had increasingly come to the fore: evidence-based medicine.

Evidence-based medicine

As Rivett (1998: 382) has described, health technology assessment was initially perceived as a threat to clinical freedom: doctors wished to retain the right to

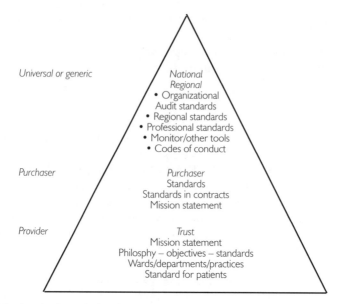

Figure 10.1   Levels of standard setting and monitoring.
Source: Sale (1996: 45).
Reproduced by kind permission of Macmillan Press Ltd.

decide what was effective, without the delays that could arise from cost containment or procedures which slowed down innovation. However, clinicians and purchasers of health care became increasingly interested in evidence-based medicine, which Rivett (1998: 382) defined as: 'the conscientious, explicit and judicious use of current best evidence in making decisions about the care of individual patients'. Evidence-based medicine became central to health service policy for both government ministers and clinicians. Previously the process of disease and use of treatment were thought adequate as a base of knowledge but, as outcomes rather than the process became examined by numerous trials, the expected improvements did not occur in some forms of care. However, even if most patients benefited from one form of treatment, there was no guarantee that every individual would do so (Rivett, 1998: 328). With quality regulation in the forefront, the DoH and NHSE soon made the improvement of clinical effectiveness a key priority which led to heavy investment in evidence-based medicine. For doctors to keep up with developments in medical practice, evidence-based medicine also had to be closely linked with continuing medical education. Subsequently, nursing also sought to be evidence-based (Jack and Oldham, 1997).

The quality assurance cycle

The importance of quality increasingly took centre stage within the contracting process, together with the issue of resources. Amongst the various terms used to denote aspects of quality, 'quality assurance' referred to activities designed to improve the quality of care overall. Sale (1996) assembled a map (Figure 10.2)

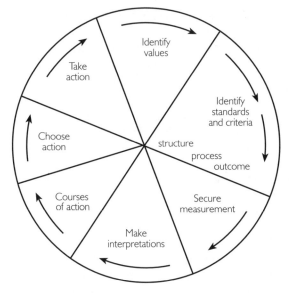

Figure 10.2 The quality assurance cycle.
Source: Sale (1996: 43).
Reproduced by kind permission of Macmillan Press Ltd.

which reflected the general agreement that quality assurance was a cyclical process with three essential stages. The first part of the cycle was to identify the values, philosophy and high quality of care to help patients or clients as well as to agree on expectations and to establish standards, criteria and goals. The second stage was to measure what was happening by auditing the performance and function of the organization. The third element was to take action to remedy any discrepancy between the first two stages. The cycle was based on a vision of continuous movement through the circle to ensure that the quality of care was protected or enhanced.

Quality improvement

To facilitate an effective outcome for quality measures, a clearly identified process was required. To further training in quality improvement, Barnes et al. (1994) set out eight steps which would be needed to further quality matters. The Quality Improvement Cycle covered the following sequence.

1 Organize.
2 Identify problems.
3 Prioritize.
4 Define and analyse.
5 Identify possible solutions.
6 Select a solution.
7 Implement.
8 Evaluate.

Increasingly, service specifications were assembled alongside pathways to assess quality improvement, guided by advice from the DoH, to respond to the quality standards that purchasers expected. Quality manuals and detailed standards (Ranade, 1994: 110) were assembled to include:

- appropriate treatment and care;
- optimum clinical outcome;
- clinically recognized procedures to minimize complications;
- treating patients with dignity and as individuals;
- ensuring patient safety, reassurance and well-being within a conducive environment;
- responding speedily to patients' needs with minimum inconvenience to them, their relatives and friends;
- involving patients in their own care.

Total quality management

Adapted from a Japanese industrial model, total quality management (TQM) became the next, broader, approach to quality improvement. Once again, the arena defied a clear definition. The different versions of TQM sought to achieve an integrated, co-operatively led programme of organizational change in order to sustain a culture of continuous improvement to meet a customer-oriented view of quality. The main features included:

- quality improvement structures to ensure accountability and staff commitment to TQM;
- staff empowerment to create a quality-aware, motivated staff skilled in process improvement;
- quality models and methods for systematic measurement and evaluation;
- the customer to come first, in the definition of quality and in order to meet users' needs and expectations (Joss et al., 1994).

Many health authorities sought to adopt a TQM approach to quality improvement. From 1989, the Department of Health funded 17 pilot sites; more were added later. An independent evaluation of the TQM pilot projects by Joss and Kogan (1995) found that much quality work was being undertaken throughout the NHS, some innovatory and determined; but a lack of cohesion between initiatives and difficulties in developing a corporate-wide approach were identified. Further, the link between attempted definitions and measurements of quality had not been made sufficiently with an appropriate, corresponding, organizational structure. Nevertheless, quality improvements *had* been made while the focus on the customer had become more apparent (Ranade, 1994: 113), but the commitment to an organization-wide strategy such as TQM was undermined by the lack of a shared view on the meaning of 'quality' (Ranade, 1997: 149). While conceptual confusions continued, quality issues were now high on the agenda of health service managers, professionals and politicians. Above all, quality requirements were routinely included in the contracts drawn up by purchasers for services from health care providers.

Sales' (1996) map shows the overall picture of total quality management in health care (Figure 10.3).

From the picture as a whole, the place of audit will be reviewed as a further innovatory process brought about by the government's recommendations in *Working for Patients* (DoH, 1989a).

Medical audit

As Packwood and Kober (1995: 25) have described, the development of audit in the 1980s was predominantly a professional, but medical, activity. The initial version of audit was intended to improve individual practice through collective knowledge. As wide variations in medical practice became manifest with the increasing pressures on health resources, so audit was seen as a way to persuade doctors to review efficiency and medical effectiveness in the light of value for money. New computer systems were seen as a means to serve as a data bank for audit. In *Working for Patients* (DoH, 1989a) medical audit was essentially concerned with the more managerial concept of effective resource use but was explicitly related to doctors. Medical audit was defined as: 'a systematic critical analysis of the quality of medical care, including the procedures used for diagnosis and treatment, the use of resources and the resulting outcome for the patient' (DoH, 1989a: 39).

The responsibility for medical audit lay with district management. To allocate resources for medical audit and to supervise the process a system of unit to regional level committees was created which included management represen-tation (DoH, 1991a).

Amongst the outcomes was, first, disappointment: there was little evidence that medical audit actually improved clinical care. Secondly, as Rivett (1998: 427) explained, part of the problem was that medical audit had two conflicting aims: for doctors to improve care as a result of an assessment of the work of medical professionals and for providers to show that the purchasers' contractual requirements were met. Thirdly, the implementation of medical audit was not helped by the challenge presented to clinical autonomy nor by differences in medical practice which offered valid alternatives for particular patients. Fourthly, as Allsop (1995: 86) pointed out, there was less acceptance of patients' evalua-tions of health status – or even of what patients thought important in medical care. Finally, in the monitoring of medical audit, clinicians felt the benefits of medical audit were low (Kerrison et al., 1993); the knowledge gained from audit could be gained by means other than the creation of a formal process and clarifi-cation of purpose was needed for audit to take on a greater significance.

Nursing audit

Nursing audit was well established in the NHS before the 1990 NHS reforms. Nursing audit set out to provide a detailed and systematic review of nursing records in order to evaluate the quality of nursing care (Sale, 1996: 126) and to promote quality assurance generally. Nursing audit has usually been run by nurse managers rather than as part of a peer group exercise. The results of nursing

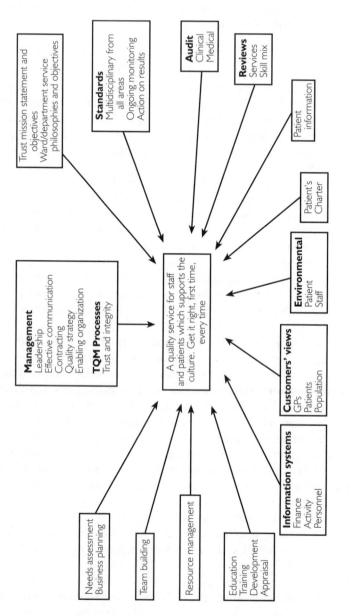

Figure 10.3   Total quality management in health care.

Source: Sale (1996: 35).

Reproduced by kind permission of Macmillan Press Ltd.

audit have always been available to managers which has enabled managers to introduce standardized, costed 'packages of care' together with a more efficient deployment of nursing resources (Ranade, 1997: 148).

Clinical audit

By 1993, the DoH (DoH, 1993b) introduced a change in policy. The development of audit was expressed in the shift from a uniprofessional to a multiprofessional system of clinical audit to form a wider quality management programme that would span all aspects of care in hospitals and in the community. As Packwood and Kober (1995: 27) explained, while funds were being allocated for the medical profession (the greater proportion) and for the nursing and therapy services, the provision of care in the NHS was a multidisciplinary activity and to audit each profession's contribution separately might not only be wasteful but also counter-productive. Contracts were therefore increasingly set up in terms of services for patients rather than services provided by individual professions. From 1994, funding was to be distributed to health authorities in accordance with weighted capitation principles but the audit programmes were funded in agreement with clinicians and managers. However, clinical audit was to provide a stronger role for non-clinicians; although professionally led, clinical audit might not necessarily be conducted by a doctor. Further, clinical audit was to be integrated into the main contracting and quality assurance programmes and linked with the evaluation of clinical effectiveness and patient outcomes.

Among the conclusions on clinical audit, Packwood and Kober (1995: 28) drew attention to the rising management controls over professional management activity (both in number and strength), the time that professional workers, (especially those in senior positions) have had to give to marketing, defining, costing and recording services and to controlling service activities, managing a budget, engaging in audit and quality assurance, all of which might be to the detriment of time available for patient care. However, although the concepts of quality were largely determined by health care professionals, managers were taking on an increasing role in this respect. (Ranade, 1997: 149). Once again, while the government insisted that consumer views should carry more weight, patients and their families continued to have the least influence over the kind of service they received.

Audit

Clinical and medical audit were placed on Sales' (1996: 35) map of total quality management (see Figure 10.3) under the wider heading of audit. As Norman and Redfern (1995: 8) have pointed out, in the UK literature the terms audit and quality assurance had become increasingly interchangeable to the extent that 'the audit cycle' began to replace the term 'quality assurance cycle'. Audit was originally seen as one stage, concerned with the assessment or measurement of quality, within the cycle of quality assurance. The broad use of the term then began to take the concept of audit beyond measurement to incorporate other aspects of the quality assurance cycle.

Medical, nursing and clinical audit have used a similar cycle of activity to focus on the delivery of care. Audit has essentially been based on a three-part cycle.

1 Define expectations.
2 Compare expectations with observed reality.
3 Bring about appropriate change in practice.

Audit is not a new idea: in the nineteenth century, Florence Nightingale drew up 'Forms of Enquiry' to reform workhouse nursing (Dunford and Smith, 1992). In the 1960s, an American pioneer of quality assurance in health care, Avedis Donabedian, influenced developments in the UK with the concept of quality modelled on a dynamic relationship between structure, process and outcomes (Ranade, 1994: 102). The audit cycle was therefore based on a tradition of measuring performance against standards set by experts. The purpose of audit was to improve the environment in which services were offered, as well as the process and the outcome of care for clients, by comparing existing practice with predetermined standards. Figure 10.4 sets out the Donabedian (1966) model of an audit cycle which brings the whole together in simplified form.

The use of an audit cycle was increasingly recognized as a marker of quality, which was essential to ensure that health care purchasing was not based on cost alone (Dunford and Smith, 1992). Nevertheless, in evaluating outcomes, the more economics-based approach to the different stages of the health care process of inputs, outputs and outcomes somewhat oversimplified the difficulties of assessment. Much depended on the measures of health outcomes. On a circum-scribed basis, audit might hold good. However, once measures were expanded to embrace elements associated with the quality of life (health status, pain, psycho-logical well-being, life satisfaction and morale; Norman and Redfern 1995: 17), so the equation became more complex. The matrix could be further classified under differing audit activities, such as the category (type of clinical activity), the

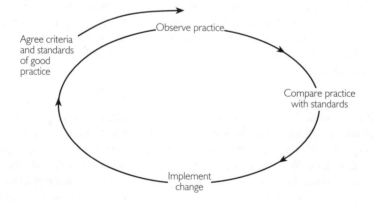

Figure 10.4 The audit cycle.
Source: Donabedian (1966).
Reproduced by kind permission of Blackwell Publishers Inc.

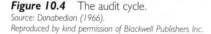

focus (the structure, process and outcome), the profession(s) (who were leading or involved) in the audit). Clarity of purpose and pathway were essential. As Norman and Redfern (1995: 13) contended, the challenge to health care professionals concerned with audit and quality assessment was to recognize the links, in terms of patients' experiences, between the three parts of Donabedian's (1966) framework in order to identify whether the component parts of high quality health care had been achieved.

More widely, but more critically, Michael Power (1997) argued that auditing was not a neutral process. Audit imposed its own values on the activities regulated. As a result, the process could have unintended and even dysfunctional consequences. The audit explosion across the public sector had been caused, in Power's (1997) view, by three factors: the need for fiscal restraint; an ideological commitment on the part of neo-liberals to a reduction in the size of the public sector; and, most importantly, for the 'New Public Management' which claimed to speak on behalf of taxpayers and consumers against the cosy cultures of professional self-regulation. Auditing had become an important means of regulating all the professions. While the roots of auditing were associated with political demands for accountability and control, the process of audit had come to affect almost every sphere of modern life.

THE PLACE OF NHS USERS

For those who received health care in Britain, a variety of terms could be used. The terminology covered a spectrum, from *patients*, who were treated and cared for by doctors and nurses in hospitals or in general practice; *users*, who engaged in the services of the NHS more widely; *clients* who, for some health care professionals, denoted a well customer who might come along, for example, for a health check-up; to *consumers*, who were regarded as those who received services within an NHS internal market even though consumer choice was limited, in the commercial market sense, as agents (such as GPs and health care purchasers) made decisions for referral and service selection on behalf of their 'consumers'.

The Patient's Charter

In July 1991, Prime Minister John Major launched the Conservatives' 'big idea' for the decade: the Citizen's Charter, which was intended to improve the quality and responsiveness of public services. Although the tools of Mrs Thatcher's previous government – competition, deregulation and privatization – were retained, the commitment to public services marked a shift in political emphasis (Timmins, 1991). The Citizen's Charter led to a series of specific charters in health, education, rail transport, etc., which, in turn, spawned local charters underpinned by four main themes: quality, choice, standards and value for money.

In November 1991, the Patient's Charter announced seven existing rights, three new rights and nine charter standards which were aimed at standardizing the best (DoH, 1991b) on behalf of NHS users. The three new rights created were these:

1 That patients had to be guaranteed admission for treatment within two years of being placed on a waiting list by a consultant.
2 That detailed information should be available about local health services including waiting times and quality standards.
3 That patient complaints should be fully and promptly investigated.

Other rights included:

- a named qualified nurse, health visitor or midwife to be responsible for each patient;
- after-care services for discharged patients to be ensured by hospitals;
- patients to have the right to complain about NHS services to the Chief Executive;
- patients to have an immediate assessment in accident and emergency departments.

The Patient's Charter was implemented in April 1992 but was revised and expanded in 1995 when an 18-month guaranteed inpatient waiting time was brought in amongst other elements, which emphasized the security and cleanliness of hospitals. Further, emergency admissions to hospitals through accident and emergency departments were to be reduced from 3–4 hours to 2 hours by April 1996 (Ranade, 1997: 154). Overall, the pressure was to focus on hospital waiting lists, patients' complaints and discharge arrangements between hospitals and the financially stretched local authority community care programmes. To comply with the requirement to assess patients immediately in accident and emergency departments, a quick solution was found – 'Hello nurses' who did greet patients straight away but further attention was often long in coming.

Charters were intended to be set up on behalf of service users to improve standards in the public sector. In 1993, the Charter Unit set up a Charter Task Force to examine how complaints should be handled in the public sector services in line with Charter principles (Allsop, 1995: 258). However, despite attempts to lift the level of public sector performance through the work of the Charter Task Force and, despite the introduction in 1993 of Charter Mark awards for excellence in delivering services, the general public remained 'ignorant' of the Citizen's Charter (Wynn Davies, 1993). In a 1992 survey undertaken by Mahon et al. (1993), over 40% of patients had never heard of the Patient's Charter.

In 1993 the Health Secretary, Virginia Bottomley, set up plans to introduce comparative information in the NHS – beginning with waiting times (Wynn Davies, 1993). The Complaints Task Force then published a list of principles with a checklist for managers to assess the performance of their organizations. In reviewing performance, managers were encouraged to consider the users' views of the service (Allsop, 1995: 259).

On the positive side, some regarded the Patient's Charter as a major step forward, if properly implemented (Baggott, 1994: 197). As Rivett (1998: 428) pointed out, the Patient's Charter did set standards for a patient to be seen in an accident and emergency department as well as for the length of wait for an operation. By 1997, further standards had been introduced which were related more closely to clinical performance. Hospital league tables had also been developed to show how far individual trusts had met Charter standards. The standards imposed also provided a benchmark of performance by which hospitals were judged. Subsequently the Charter was extended into primary health care.

Importantly, the Patient's Charter had opened up health care to greater scrutiny as well as to provide information, comparative data on performance standards and to set standards to improve quality while seeking to extend greater autonomy for the user (Allsop, 1995: 259). Then again, as Sale's (1996) map on total quality management has shown (see Figure 10.3), the Patient's Charter formed an important element in the overall delivery of health care.

On the more negative side, the rights set out in the Patient's Charter were not legal rights. Even some existing rights – such as the individual's right to a GP – were not necessarily upheld in practice. Baggott (1994: 197) has drawn attention to many homeless people, with no fixed address, who have had difficulty in registering with a GP. However, patients could ultimately take up complaints or any views about the denial of rights with the NHS Chief Executive. Baggott (1994) also contended that the naming of nurses responsible for each patient, set out in the Patient's Charter service standards, could be viewed purely as a 'cosmetic' exercise.

Waiting lists probably represented the most problematical aspect of the Patient's Charter. While the number of patients waiting 1–2 years started to fall significantly, the total number of patients waiting for treatment remained fairly constant at over 900 000 by the mid-1990s (Baggott, 1994: 197). Opposition parties maintained that the figures underestimated the real size of the waiting lists. Some hospitals manipulated the figures (Rivett, 1998: 428), often for political reasons. Other hospitals dealt with patients, with less costly minor conditions ahead of more serious cases, while there was some evidence of patients awaiting minor surgery who were removed from waiting lists altogether (Baggott, 1994: 198).

The perverse effects of the internal market on waiting lists were reflected in events at the neurological surgery department of the Radcliffe Infirmary, Oxford. The surgeon in charge of the department, Mr Christopher Adams, who had run one of the most efficient and cheapest neurosurgery departments in the country for 20 years, was told to create artificial waiting lists. David Wilson, chief executive of Radcliffe Infirmary, commented at the time that the waiting list for patients with sciatica had been forced on the hospital by purchasing authorities who said there was insufficient money to pay for speedy treatment, so the hospital should find a way to make patients wait. Mr Adams resigned in disgust with the comment that waiting lists solved nothing: except to delay the time that hard decisions had to be made. The health service changes had meant a rush to win patients at the lowest cost. Effectively money was chasing, rather than following patients, while efficient units were being penalized (Mihill, 1995).

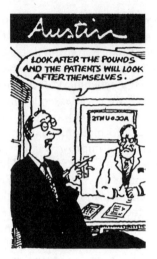

The Guardian, 8 December 1995.
Reproduced by kind permission of The Guardian and Austin.

Community health councils (CHCs)

The CHCs were set up under the 1974 NHS reorganization to represent patients' interests. Their role, which was to act as a public watchdog, had changed little. CHCs (one for each health district) continued to monitor local health services, to make recommendations for improvement and to provide information for the public. While appointed and funded by Regional Health Authorities, CHC membership consisted of one-half nominees from local authorities, one-third from voluntary organizations and the rest from RHAs: 18–24 in total.

CHC powers were limited to:

- the right to be consulted about service changes (if opposed to hospital closures, the decision would have to be referred to the Secretary of State);
- the right to information (CHCs could attend as well as speak at DHA public meetings, but had no right to vote);
- the right to visit health authority premises (but not GP practices), although the right was not automatic with regard to NHS trusts where visits had to be negotiated either via the purchasers' contract requirements or directly with the NHS trusts.

Despite the rhetoric in *Working for Patients* (DoH, 1989a) about the importance of consumer participation, there was to be no consumer scrutiny of purchasing decisions by GP fundholders, no formal role in monitoring the contracts set up for the provision of services nor any guarantee that CHCs would be able to monitor service standards and quality built into the contracts between GPs and service providers (Butler, 1992: 95).

CHCs were therefore another example where appointed/nominated members acted on behalf of NHS patients and users. No public voting procedure existed to place user representatives onto the local CHCs. Just how far CHCs were able to represent user views was a moot point, as the CHC role increasingly faced limitations.

- CHCs received little public funding in relation to the roles CHCs were expected to undertake.
- Full-time staff members were few, which created a reliance on voluntary commitment (Allsop, 1995: 246).
- In the reformed NHS, CHCs had to walk a tightrope between representing patients effectively and maintaining good relations with their respective health authority.
- Although local concern mounted over NHS trust deficits the CHCs could do little: muzzled as watchdogs by lack of money. Public petitions mounted – for example, to save Guy's Hospital in South London and the protective circle of thousands of pairs of hands from people around Glasgow's Stobhill Hospital in Scotland – the 'power of the people' did manage to shelve some NHS hospital closures across the country (Moore, 1995).
- If CHCs discussed priorities, the accusation of sanctioning NHS rationing could be made; refusal to discuss priorities could lead users to question the very purpose of Community Health Councils.

One widespread criticism of CHCs was just how far they truly represented health service users (Pollock, 1992). The consumerism of the 1990s, however, went further than to question the representativeness of collective bodies but to question the belief that consumers could exert an influence through such bodies at all (Mahon et al., 1993).

Accountability

Representative bodies offered one potential, but limited, route to user involvement in the NHS process. More tenuously on behalf of users, accountability could offer another. Both national and local accountability for health care provision have had a wider, more diffuse, target audience to address.

At national level, methods of accountability have included the following.

- The Secretary of State for Health, accountable to Parliament for all aspects of the NHS.
- Health Ministers, accountable to the House of Commons and outside through verbal and written replies to questions.
- A range of *ad hoc* committees and commissions of inquiry, reporting on various specific issues. Examples are: the DoH Standing Advisory Committees; within the House of Commons, both the National Accounts Committee and (from 1990) the Health Committee looking at various financial and policy issues the National Audit Office undertaking reviews on the effectiveness of public spending; the Audit Commission investigating public expenditure and assessing the promotion of good practice in the NHS and in local authority community care.

However, as Allsop (1995: 242) has described, most of the accountability activities at national level were the concern of national politicians; civil servants at the Department of Health and Social Security; the representatives of professional bodies; together with occasional union representation on behalf of health care workers. Despite pressure group activity on specific issues, the public had little chance to participate in the formulation of health policy at national or regional level.

At a more local level, local authorities no longer had the right to representation on DHAs under the 1990 NHS reforms which emphasized far more of a business approach to the whole system. As a result, there was no longer local community representation in any aspect of health service delivery. On the provider side, the non-executive NHS trusts board members were appointed by the Secretary of State. Amongst health care purchasers, contracts were to be based on an assessment of the service needs of the local population. However, there was no stipulation that contracting should involve consultation with relevant consumer groups from the local community or should establish a forum of accountability for the local population.

Patient choice

If locality representation was increasingly being limited, just how far was choice extended to the user within the NHS? Once again, choice was restricted within the monopoly-type service provided which offered two points of entry: GP referral or the hospital accident and emergency department (Allsop, 1995: 241). From the entry point onwards, choice would be determined by NHS professionals in response to resource availability. More widely, choice was also part of an uneasy political balance, between the principles established under the 1990 NHS reforms to pursue efficiency through market competition and the maintenance of previous values, such as universal, comprehensive provision, which commanded public support. Therefore to maximize efficiency might conflict with the promotion of choice for patients and with the principle of equal access (Butler, 1992: 43).

The introduction of a quasi-market, in Bartlett and Harrison's (1993: 91) view, was indeed more likely to restrict the extent to which individual patients or users were able to make choices about the health care received. The constraints faced by both purchasers and providers to make the system run smoothly and to limit the adverse effects of patient flow uncertainty on service delivery were likely to limit rather than enhance patient choice. However, as Bartlett and Harrison (1993: 91) reflected, individual users might place a higher value on certain aspects of quality, such as accessibility and service co-ordination, than on the means of making choices between services.

If choice was to be considered a crucial element to meet user needs, to what extent could the private sector offer choice? Any comparison was largely irrelevant as only a very small minority of people could afford private care. The private sector was therefore greatly aided by employers who included private medical insurance as an employee perk. By 1995 private health care had grown to 7% of total health care spending (Laing, 1995). The growth had been fuelled by supply and demand: the demand for access which resulted in the supply of services. Although the number of persons insured with private health insurance had fallen slightly in 1991 (CSO, 1994: 105), the figure was expected to increase from 6.23 million in 1995 to 9 million by the end of the century (Deffenbaugh, 1996). Although access to private treatment was quicker than NHS treatment, choice was also significantly limited in the private sector. For example BUPA (the British United Provident Association), the largest medical insurance organization in Britain, had always limited access to provision. Exclusions traditionally covered dental and oral treatment, cosmetic and reconstructive surgery as well as treatment for any condition arising from pregnancy or childbirth. Certain other conditions (e.g. AIDS/HIV) were addressed only under very specific circumstances. To meet the costs of some other forms of treatment, hospital accommodation and nursing care, the level of cover would depend on one of three payment scales selected by the private patient (BUPA, 1998). Although normally offering a faster route to treatment than in the NHS (emergencies apart), the private sector still curbed aspects of choice; nor could the Private Sector match the NHS intent to offer universal, comprehensive provision.

Consumer complaints in the NHS

If representation and choice contained limitations for NHS users, what mechanisms were available to protect the individual? Up to the mid-1990s, there were four main channels for handling complaints in the NHS.

1 FHSAs dealt with complaints about breaches of contract made by GPs, dentists, opticians and pharmacists.
2 DHAs handled complaints in the hospital and community health services under the 1985 Hospital Complaints Act.
3 Patients could seek redress from professional bodies (such as the General Medical Council) or the courts.
4 From 1977, the Parliamentary Ombudsman or Commissioner for the Health Service would investigate complaints about maladministration from patients who were dissatisfied about the way their complaints were handled locally, but no legal redress could be sought once a case was taken on by the Commissioner.

Rather more under the heading of inspection, although relevant to consumer complaints and quality of care, in 1969 the Health Advisory Service was set up to advise on standards of good practice for elderly people, children, people with mental illness or learning disability – essentially groups of patients who might not be able to protect themselves. However, as it had no powers of enforcement, the role of the Health Advisory Service was to be reviewed by 1997.

Taken all together, in a report from the National Consumer Council, the complaints procedures were criticized as being bureaucratic, complex and inappropriate from the user perspective (Mulcahy, 1995). In order to bring the NHS complaints systems in line with the principles laid down by the Complaints

Task Force of the Citizen's Charter Unit, the systems were reviewed by the Wilson Committee (1994), whose recommendations were accepted by the DoH (1995a). The changes to be implemented included a common system of complaints and written complaints to be acknowledged within two working days. A three-stage approach was taken to cover immediate response, investigation and/or reconciliation and referral to an independent panel. A report was to be sent to the complainant who, if still dissatisfied, could approach the Health Service Ombudsman. All stages were to be completed in three months.

Despite measures to address dissatisfaction within the reformed NHS, service users were increasingly making complaints about their particular experience of health care provision (Allsop, 1995: 252). Written complaints rose from 37 000 in 1990–1 to 58 400 in 1992–3 and shot up to more than 87 000 in 1994 (Cole, 1995). Furthermore, a major study on health service users, carried out for the NHS Executive, showed that only 40% of dissatisfied respondents actually made a complaint about their treatment (Mulcahy and Tritter, 1994).

Philip Hunt, former director of the National Association of Health Authorities and Trusts (Cole, 1995), attributed the increase in complaints to higher public expectations and greater openness within the NHS, but especially to the result of the Patient's Charter, which had focussed people's concerns while providing a benchmark by which to measure standards. Cole (1995) suggested that the rising number of complaints should be seen, not as an indication of falling standards but, as a sign of progress and rising consumer consciousness.

User views

In 1992, the King's Fund Institute undertook a survey of user views on the NHS. There were wide variations in satisfaction levels with specific services: 90% of people reported satisfaction with the GP services, 66% were satisfied with the NHS as a whole; but hospital services at 66% and outpatient departments at 57% received lower ratings. Striking regional differences were also found: residents in London and the south-east were consistently less satisfied than people in Wales, Scotland, the Midlands, East Anglia and the south-west, where the satisfaction level was the highest. Criticism of the hospital services predominated (waiting lists especially needed attention), but the quality of medical and nursing care was perceived as less in need for improvement (Solomon, 1992).

Similar user views on hospital provision were reflected in the Audit Commission's (1993c) report on the quality of hospital care, seen from the patients' perspective which showed that patients were satisfied with the care but not with the information received or in the manner it was given. Hospitals were urged to open lines of communication with more readily available written material together with more effective information systems for patients.

The *British Social Attitudes 11th Report* (November 1994) showed that the government's health reforms had taken the steam out of political controversy but the general public was not yet convinced that anyone was listening to their views. However, the consistent trend in public attitudes for increasing dissatisfaction with the NHS had now started to reverse. Women and older people were the most satisfied with the NHS. People were largely happy with the care in hospitals but not with the time taken to get there, via waiting lists, accident and emergency or outpatient departments. Only 58% were satisfied with the NHS dental service (Bosanquet, 1994), but dentistry was becoming increasingly privatized.

The user voice, NHS involvement and empowerment

Numerous groups existed to promote the voice of patients, carers, users and consumers:

- pressure groups for particular causes (e.g. Mencap, Mind, Age Concern, Multiple Sclerosis Society, Carers' National Association);
- organizations which represented alliances of patient groups such as the Long-Term Medical Condition Alliance, the Patients Association;
- focus and community groups.

To further the interests of patients and users as a whole, the Director of the College of Health called for changes to respond to patients' needs (Rigge, 1994). The main issue was for the Department of Health, the managers and the medical world, who had to deliver services within all too finite resources, to enable genuine patient choice based on information on the availability and quality of services.

At this point, a clear link could be seen with the work the NHS, as a whole, had sought to undertake on audit, quality and service evaluation. The problem was that the outcomes tended to remain in-house; the user was not readily informed. Shackley and Ryan (1994) even questioned whether it was either realistic or possible for consumers to fulfil the role envisaged by government policy, which carried an implicit assumption that greater consumer involvement was both beneficial and desirable. Barriers to consumer participation remained in that providers had considerable information advantage. Further, the acquisition of information was both costly and time consuming.

Overall, in the light of varying demands and constrained resources, the impact of the user voice faced limitations, especially where choice was concerned. However, Bartlett and Harrison (1993: 92) argued that, where patients could not express real choice, users, carers and community groups needed to be given a 'voice' to enable their involvement in strategic planning, setting performance measures and establishing priorities which required the development of an effective participatory framework.

User involvement in the NHS gradually began to be absorbed into the system. North Derbyshire's health authority was one example where the importance of listening and responding to the views of local people was enshrined in the health policy objectives for the locality. By allowing greater representation of local people in the decision-making process, of developing new ways of working with other organizations (especially with the voluntary sector) and of opening up two-way communications with local people, the authority became more responsive to the needs of local people (Layzell, 1994).

By the mid-1990s, a wide-scale evaluation of public participation in service planning and user involvement showed that progress had been patchy: 21% of health authorities were categorized as 'good', 57% were acceptable but 21% were deemed unsatisfactory (Donaldson, 1995). The study on health authorities, together with three case studies in Leeds, Bradford and Bristol, concluded that there was some way to go before a better match was established between what the public wanted in relation to the provision of health care and what they received – and before a more democratic, accountable system was achieved. The evaluation was based on the *Local Voices* initiative, launched by the NHS Management Executive (NHSME, 1992) three years previously. This programme, which encouraged health authority purchasers to take local people's views into account to establish priorities, develop service specifications and monitor services, was beginning to have an impact. Nevertheless, some confusion remained between the Patient's Charter, which was concerned with rights for people at the point of use and *Local Voices*, which was about wider public involvement (Donaldson, 1995).

The next step in user involvement was the bolder notion of *Power to the People* (Rodgers, 1994). The principle of empowerment was based on the view that if consumer involvement was to be more than notional, users needed to be empowered, not just consulted (consultation did not guarantee that any response would be made). Patient advocates and representatives were beginning to appear in some areas, including Brighton and Bristol. However, the case for user empowerment ultimately argued that more than simply notional consumer involvement was important: patients needed not only the right to choose, but the right to influence which choices were available in the first place. Without empowerment, consumerism was meaningless.

Meanwhile, Paton (1998: 159) contended that governments were never really concerned about genuine public participation but were more interested in legitimising inevitable decisions which emerged from health policy and funding levels. As the NHS headed into increasing financial turmoil, user empowerment was unlikely to be the first item on the NHS agenda.

11 FINANCING HEALTH CARE PROVISION IN BRITAIN AND ABROAD BY 1997

On Wednesday 8 May 1996, some 50 years after the legislation in 1946 which created the National Health Service, the British press reported: 'THE END OF THE WELFARE STATE' (Brindle, 1996b). Within half a century, the NHS had become highly regarded by both professionals and public alike, but latterly hospitals were heading towards 'MELTDOWN' in which 'CASH LIMITS [were] PUSHING NHS TO BRINK' (Mihill, 1996a). What were the factors that had contributed to rising costs? In this chapter the place of NHS expenditure is explored with regard to the financial outlay, the options to raise money and to curb costs. The second section reviews just how far health care systems abroad could point to more effective ways forward for the NHS.

FINANCING HEALTH CARE PROVISION IN BRITAIN 1990–1997

Cash crisis was a perennial feature in the NHS. By 1996 the causal factors, which had changed little over the years, included poor financial stability, growing waiting lists, an ageing population, advances in medical science, the mounting cost of drugs and the struggle to match the rise in demands with a modest growth in funding in real terms (NAHAT, 1996). Further elements covered more recent developments, such as the expansion of computer technology (Cross, 1995), increased expenditure on management; and confusion. By 1995, the NHS was unable to account for £422 million due to accounting complexities introduced by the internal market. As a result, auditors refused to approve the accounts of 84 health authorities, NHS trusts and GP fundholders (Hencke, 1995). Draining all available cash, the greatest financial pressure was to be found in the hospital sector. Disputes had broken out across the country as many contracts remained unsigned. One in ten NHS trusts expected to run into the red in 1996, with deficits of up to £3 million (NAHAT, 1996).

The press reflected the mounting anxieties:

- 'NHS NEEDS AN EXTRA £6 BN' (*The Guardian*, 25 June 1995);
- 'HOSPITALS ARE AT FULL STRETCH' (*The Times*, 19 June 1996);
- 'NHS SINKING LIKE TITANIC' (*The Evening Standard*, 24 June 1996).

Some health chiefs were even considering giving away cottage hospitals, which could not be closed due to public opposition, by inviting local people to run them as charities (Brindle, 1996c).

However, NHS spending in real terms had significantly increased even from the implementation of the internal market in 1991, when expenditure was £36 billion, to £43 billion by 1996 (see Table 11.1). The blunt fact was that demands had outstripped supply (Elliott, 1996).

To perceive NHS costs simply in relation to a financial crisis would be to

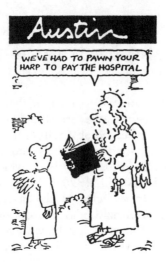

Source: The Guardian, 8 May 1996.
Reproduced by kind permission of The Guardian and Austin.

Table 11.1 General government expenditure in real terms: by function.

United Kingdom					£ billion at 1996 prices*	
	1981	1986	1991	1994	1995	1996
Social security	64	80	85	104	107	107
Health	28	31	36	41	42	43
Education	29	31	34	38	38	39
Defence	26	30	27	25	24	23
Public order and safety	9	11	15	16	16	15
General public services	9	10	13	14	15	13
Housing and community amenities	15	13	10	11	11	10
Transport and communication	9	6	8	7	9	8
Recreational and cultural affairs	3	4	5	5	5	5
Agriculture, forestry and fishing	3	3	3	3	4	5
Other expenditure[†]	46	41	28	38	44	37
All expenditure	241	260	264	302	315	305

*Adjusted to 1996 prices using the GDP market prices deflator adjusted to remove the distortion caused by the abolition of domestic rates.
†Includes expenditure on mining, manufacturing, construction, fuel and energy, and services, as well as all other expenditure not allocated to a specific function.

Source: Office for National Statistics (1998; 120).
Crown copyright material reproduced with the permission of the controller for Her Majesty's Stationery Office.

underestimate the complexity of the equation. As Appleby (1994b) questioned, how were the ongoing developments in medical technology and changes in treatment to be unpicked from the potential effects of the 1990 NHS reforms on waiting times and activity? How were the effects of the Patient's Charter, the comparatively large inputs of cash in the 1990s, changes in the GP contract and the continuing imposition from the centre of efficiency gains, to be disentangled from effects brought about by the NHS reforms? The contention that a burgeoning elderly population had led to rising health care costs was challenged by Hunter (1996a), who argued that the NHS suffered from too little effective management: to cover-up for the failure in management, the blame was placed on an ageing population.

Dobson (1994) pointed out that specific action for an individual high-risk patient could focus on the efficient use of resources more easily than in the field of health prevention and health gains, where results were neither as dramatic nor as easily pinpointed as the provision of a cure. Then again, in looking to tighten up on expenditure and efficiency, outcomes could be contradictory. For example, on the assessment of the 1990 NHS reforms by Robinson and Le Grand (1993), Robinson (1994) commented that, while the evaluation suggested only modest achievements overall, with little evidence of change in the key areas of quality, efficiency, choice and responsiveness, the official claims that NHS trusts had achieved greater efficiency were difficult to substantiate. As Klein (1999) reflected, on reviewing Charles Webster's (1998) book *The National Health Service*, the assumption that the NHS was underfunded might be true (particularly in terms of capital investment), but the case was not self-evident because no one had ever come up with a satisfactory formula for determining what the actual level of funding should be.

Funding options for the NHS

If NHS funding from taxation was perceived to be inadequate, what other options were there for raising funds? A number of proposals and financial developments took shape during the 1990s.

Hypothecated Health Tax

A separate NHS tax (an 'earmarked tax') to be used exclusively to fund health care provision had been favoured by the Liberal Democrats, the right-wing think tank, the Institute of Economic Affairs and the British Medical Association, amongst others. From the Office of Health Economics (OHE), Jones and Duncan (1995) produced an evaluation of the proposals. For an earmarked tax to be successful, seven criteria were identified, including equity, clarity as to who was pay, incentives for increased efficiency and a link between NHS taxes and spending. However, as the OHE director, Adrian Towse (1995) recognized, two key questions remained unresolved: first, whether a separate NHS tax would increase public willingness to pay tax; secondly, what mechanisms could credibly be used to set limits on an earmarked tax and NHS spending while, in practice, increasing responsiveness to public preferences as well as ensuring efficient provision? With few answers available, the idea of an earmarked tax went little further.

Shifting resources across public spending

One of the seven OHE criteria suggested that there was a case for flexibility and indeed argued against a separate NHS tax, to enable resources to be shifted between the NHS and other areas of public spending by the government to meet priorities more effectively. It could, nevertheless, be argued that the government was already undertaking a similar exercise through public sector financial adjustments between annual budgets.

However, as the Office for National Statistics (1998: 120) has shown (Table 11.1) the main financial pressure was to be found in the expenditure allocated to social security: the £107 billion accorded for 1996 represented 35% of the total. While expenditure on defence had generally been decreasing, social security represented one of four functions where expenditure had not fallen (the other three areas were health, education and agriculture, forestry and fishing). Acknowledgement was made of the consistently high level of support from the general public for increased government spending on health, in contrast to attitudes towards unemployment benefits which fluctuated according to the levels of unemployment, although culture and arts came bottom of the list in the level of support for public money. The problem, as to how to reconcile all the demands for resources across the public sector, remained.

Supplementary ways of financing the NHS

Given that raising taxes would run against the Conservative administration's principle of maintaining low taxation in an enterprise economy, another approach was to consider potential sources of income for the NHS which could supplement general taxation. Bailey and Bruce (1994) looked at a range of such measures which included: local taxation, earmarked taxes, patient charges (hotel, prescription and other charges for non-clinical items), a lottery, income generation, charitable donations and patients 'opting out of the NHS' with private insurance. The outcome, by the authors' own admission, was unexciting. Although decisions about the levels and quality of public service provision were ultimately matters of democratic accountability, the inescapable fact was that all alternative sources of funding were found to have both advantages and disadvantages. Rather than providing a panacea for the financial problems of the NHS, any new supplementary source of finance might simply replace one set of problems with another. Even though a diversity of income might allow greater financial flexibility, the various income sources could not substantially increase NHS revenue. As there were no easy solutions to the perceived funding problems in the NHS, central government would continue to finance the bulk of health care from general taxation.

In contrast, Professor Alan Maynard (1995a) put forward the view that prescription charges should be abolished, as the evidence showed such charges reduced patient demand, avoided tackling waste and did not facilitate spending controls. Instead of taxing the sick with user charges, which raised about £310 million a year, a more valuable policy would be to focus on the appropriateness of GP prescribing and to make more effective use of pharmaceutical skills. Allan Sharpe, a South Wales pharmacist from Newbridge, Gwent, also favoured the abolition of prescription charges. Mr Sharpe lodged an appeal when fined £550 by Mid Glamorgan Family Health Services Authority in September 1995 for selling prescribed drugs at far less than the prescription fee, in breach of a pharmacist's NHS terms of service. Doctors and pharmacists seized on the test case to demand an overhaul of the NHS charging system which had raised the prescription fee from 20 pence in 1979 to £5.25 by 1995. Allan Sharpe wanted the cost of dispensing medicines to be borne out of general taxation (Gow, 1995). The outcome was a technical victory for Mr Sharpe, in that the fine became void when the body which imposed the fine breached NHS regulations by hearing the complaint more than 13 weeks after the case had been made (Gibbs, 1997). Of further interest, a survey by Chester and Ellesmere Community Health Council had found that 74 of the 100 most commonly prescribed drugs cost less than the £5.25 fee (Gow, 1995). Charges for prescriptions, nevertheless, remained. Many groups of people continued to be exempted – such as those with specific medical conditions, those on family credit or income support, children under 16 and young people under 19 in full time education, people over 60, pregnant women and those who had had a baby in the previous 12 months and, those receiving a disability working allowance – altogether an extensive list.

Specific hospital charges

The Law Commission (1996) came up with a new proposal for charges. The suggestion was that drivers should pay the bill for crash victims on the road. The NHS would recoup the costs of treatment from the person whom the courts decided was to blame. The Law Commission estimated that the NHS could recover nearly £100 million a year by shifting the cost of treating accident victims from the taxpayer to motorists. The insurance companies warned the Law Commission not to single out motorists because motor insurance premiums would be likely to increase significantly under the Law Commission's proposals, if they were ever implemented.

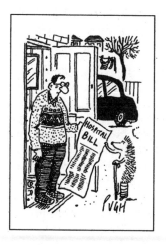

Source: The Times, 12 December 1996.
Reproduced by kind permission of The Times and Pugh.

A two-tier NHS

Twelve members of Healthcare 2000 (1995), who included Sir Duncan Nichol, former NHS chief executive, Patricia Hewitt, deputy director of the Institute of Public Policy Research and Linda Lamont, Patients Association director, acknowledged that there were no easy answers to the problems facing health policy markers. However, drastic action was needed if the NHS was to survive financially into the twenty-first century. The Healthcare 2000 (1995) report rejected arguments for hypothecated taxes and social insurance. While supporting a continued commitment to tax-based funding, the report favoured a two-tier NHS in order to meet the overwhelming health demands. The two-tier NHS would provide basic health care for all, but a higher level of service for those who paid. Free NHS treatment would be limited to a set of core services with a waiting list. Patients would be encouraged to pay for extra services or 'fast track' treatment. The report envisaged more competition for patients among purchasing authorities and provider hospitals.

Healthcare 2000 had effectively shifted the debate from *what* should be covered to *who* should be covered, which would destroy the universal principle fundamental to the NHS. Maynard (1995b) criticized the report for the advocacy of private rather than public finance for health care, which was not evidence-based health care policy. The weaknesses of dual-source funding had not been recognized, whereas international evidence had indicated that 'single pipe', or tax funding of health care, facilitated cost control. Further, Healthcare 2000 (1995) had advocated a difference in the quality of care available for rich and poor, which would be produced by the effects of private payments or private health insurance. In outcome, the Healthcare 2000 group had not provided an acceptable solution to the financial 'crisis' in the NHS.

Private funding for the NHS: creeping privatization

Throughout the 1980s a range of measures were encouraged to bring money into the NHS from the private sector which included:

- sub-contracting hospital laundry, cleaning and catering services through competitive tendering (Allsop, 1995: 165);
- income generation schemes;
- NHS partnerships with the private sector in co-operating on training, sharing equipment, selling off surplus NHS equipment and hospital wings to private medical bodies – and, more particularly in the 1990s, through treating NHS patients on a contract basis (although by the mid-1990s, health authorities and GP fundholders had contracted little acute work to private hospitals). However, commented Laing (1995), there was potential for growth, such as NHS-sited day surgery units, funded by private capital, with long-term contracts to provide NHS services. Even so, by 1996, the NHS had become the leading provider of private health care because of the rapid growth of pay beds in NHS trust hospitals (Brindle, 1996d).

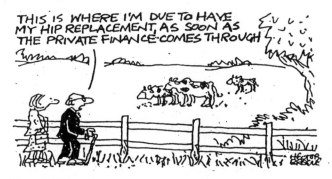

THIS IS WHERE I'M DUE TO HAVE MY HIP REPLACEMENT, AS SOON AS THE PRIVATE FINANCE·COMES THROUGH

Source: The Guardian, 23 July 1997.
Reproduced by kind permission of The Guardian and Hector Breeze.

The private finance initiative (PFI)

The private sector became increasingly drawn into joint enterprises with NHS trust hospitals which, under the private sector initiative inaugurated in 1992, essentially involved renting or leasing of capital owned by private contractors. All capital schemes were required to be tested for private finance before public funding could be considered. Amongst the 57 PFI projects at various stages of development by 1996, Treasury approval was accorded to two of the biggest ever privately funded and owned hospital building projects. A brand new £170 million Norfolk and Norwich Healthcare Trust hospital and Swindon and Marlborough Trust's £90 million replacement scheme were given the go ahead under the Conservative government's PFI scheme (Hunter, 1996b). By 1996, St James' University Hospital Trust and South Buckinghamshire Trust had also become involved in major PFI projects (Appleby, 1996a).

The benefit to the public sector of private investment was based on two assumptions. The first was that risk was transferred from the public to the private sector; the second was that the private sector had greater incentive to produce cost-effective solutions to capital schemes. A further case for PFI was based on the assertion that the private sector would be more efficient than the NHS in hospital construction (Appleby, 1996a). Further, Moks (1996) argued that the PFI philosophy was particularly appropriate to information technology services, where suppliers could readily develop economies of scale which would benefit the NHS.

However, criticisms of the PFI initiative significantly outweighed the claimed benefits. Whitfield (1995/6) stated that PFI distorted NHS priorities, weakened democratic control and risked destroying the public sector ethos of health care provision. Mihill (1996b) reported that the British Medical Association questioned whether PFI was not simply back-door privatization which could destroy the NHS. Although welcoming the initiative in principle, even the House of Commons Treasury Committee (1996) was concerned about the suitability of PFI for health projects. By December 1996, the government was set to bail out troubled PFI schemes by giving cash to NHS trusts who were struggling to get schemes off the ground (Cervi, 1996). As Ranade noted (1997: 199), PFI had not

Table 11.2   Methods of rationing NHS health care provision.

By exclusion:	By quantity:	By access:
Age-based Via treatment selection Via treatment denial	Care diluted Care thinly spread	Through GP gatekeepers Through waiting lists Through differing health authority priority decisions leading to postcode access
By the internal market:	**By priority setting:**	**By management approach:**
Through competition for contracted provision	According to need According to suffering According to quality adjusted life years	Haphazard Explicit
By deflection:	**By outcomes:**	**By deterence:**
Passing patients on to other sectors (to local authority community care; informal carers)	Cost benefit analysis Medical audit Clinical audit Nursing audit Evidence-based medicine Clinical effectiveness	Through charges Through pricing

measured up to the government's ambitions. Less than half of the £300 million cut in Treasury funding for NHS capital had been contributed by private capital since 1995. Nevertheless, by the November budget of 1996, the government was relying on investment from the PFI to grow from £65 million in 1996 to £166 million net (150% in real terms) by the following year (Appleby, 1996b).

Rationing

As the NHS had secured a lower level of resources than anticipated from the private sector, a different strategy was available in the form of rationing: instead of raising money, cutting back on NHS provision was a widely used alternative. However, the NHS has always had to ration health care. While the introduction of the PFI initiative sought to raise private sector funds for the NHS system, rationing approached the financing of the NHS from a different angle: curbing costs. Setting priorities locally, nevertheless, went against the basic NHS principle of maximizing health gain. As a result, there was unwillingness on the part of some involved in the management of the NHS to accept rationing, when what was needed was, in Allan Maynard's (1996) views, to ensure that the necessary rationing processes were efficient, equitable, open and facilitated the accountability of politicians, clinicians and managers (Maynard, 1996).

By the mid-1990s rationing had become complex. A variety of means and mechanisms had increasingly been introduced, some with local application, others with national implications. Table 11.2 attempts to give a succinct overview of some of the main methods employed.

Quality-adjusted life years (see Chapter 7) or rationing by some of the outcomes listed could be argued to be more potential than actual methods in use, but the possibilities remained. As the NHS budget was limited in response to demand, rationing seemed inevitable, but at least eight key issues emerged.

1. The internal market

The rationing of health care at the point of purchase in the internal market, rather than undertaken more informally by the providers, was a key theme of the White Paper *Working for Patients* (DoH, 1989a). However, as Paton (1998: 34) commented, the consequences of rationing by purchaser were not thought through.

2. Differing perspectives

In responding to government policy, the purchasers/commissioners of health care largely operated on a basis of process rather than outcomes, such as health achievements. In contrast, individual users might rate benefits rather differently (Paton, 1998: 160).

3. Decision-making

A NAHAT (1994) survey showed that health authorities appeared reluctant to make explicit rationing decisions. Most health authorities left the Department of Health to decide nationally which treatments should be excluded, while health authorities determined locally the extent of availability, which reflected the authority's view of their brief to tailor services to meet local needs. New and Le Grand (1996a) argued that the Department of Health had failed to provide any consistent national guidance to health authorities on what should, or should not, be regarded as universally available NHS provision. The result was that services, such as *in vitro* fertilization, were available in some parts of the country but not others. National policy should therefore override local discretion in setting out which services the NHS would provide.

However, after Berkshire Health Authority had controversially introduced a blanket ban on certain treatments (Crail, 1995), the Health Secretary, Stephen Dorrell, warned the move was unacceptable. In future, health authorities would be set targets for cutting out ineffective and unnecessary treatments; further, health authorities would agree specific targets to evaluate progress on clinical and cost-effectiveness, although the targets would vary between health authorities (Chadda, 1996b). By 1996/7, a list of ten procedures explicitly excluded by health authorities had been drawn up: the first two items covered such treatments as reversal of sterilization and sex change (Brindle, 1997).

4. Ageism

A Medical Research Council (1994) report showed that sick elderly people were being discriminated against by the NHS through exclusion from some treatments. The report stated that there was a widespread tendency, amongst both purchasers and providers of health care, to use age as a criterion for exclusion. Rogers (1995) subsequently reported on the continuing evidence of pensioners, regarded as too old to merit expensive surgery, who were being denied hospital treatment for debilitating heart conditions. Although most agreed that older people should not be at a disadvantage in the competition for resources (New and Mays, 1997), the apparent consensus on rationing was taken by surprise when leading health economist, Alan Williams (1997), suggested that age was an appropriate criterion to take into account, while priorities should favour the young.

5. Ethics
Further ethical issues were raised by Cambridge and Huntingdon Health Authority's decision to refuse to fund treatment with only a small chance of success for a 10-year-old girl dying of leukaemia (the Jaymee Bowen (Child B) case). An anonymous donor subsequently paid for the child to be treated privately. In the ensuing furore, Wall (1995) argued that a pluralist approach based on ethics as well as cost and efficacy of treatments was needed.

6. The inevitability of rationing
The case rested on the assumption that health care prices were irreducible. After ten years of attempting unsuccessfully to curb excessive expenditure on health care, one well-known example of rationing was introduced by the Oregon state government, USA, which saw rationing as the only way forward (Roberts, 1995). The public was asked to rank some 700 treatments in priority order. State administrators agreed to cover only the first 587 treatments with the funds available, although no attempt was made to examine the efficiency with which health care was delivered or the appropriateness of costs. The Oregon approach ran into problems as a result of allegedly untenable and unacceptable conclusions from the public ranking order: for example, dental capping came out higher than treating appendicitis (Paton, 1998: 160).

However, the need for rationing *could* be questioned. Another approach to the inevitability of rationing, put forward by Roberts (1995), started from an entirely different premise: that the price of health care need be neither fixed nor irreducible, but should always be rational, based on sound methods of assessing effectiveness. Hunter (1993) had pointed out that much could be done to make better use of resources before needing to deny treatment. Mullen (1995) claimed, on the basis of an extensive study of the relevant literature, that rationing was by no means inevitable; furthermore, the mechanisms suggested for use were a mass of contradictions.

7. Choices
Rationing was, above all, about choices: but who should make the choices and how should the choices be made? Klein (1996) called for health authorities to be more explicit about the implications of purchasing decisions. New and Le Grand (1996b) argued that only politicians could decide what had to be paid for and what should be on the NHS in the first place; clinicians were then best placed to decide how the treatment was to be administered and to whom. One development was rationing by postcode, whereby different health authorities varied in their decisions to pay for how many and for what types of specialized treatment. Some health authorities ruled out couples for *in vitro* fertilization by applying strict criteria (often age-based) as to who could receive NHS treatment.

8. Prevention and monitoring

The British Diabetic Association (1996) pointed to an alternative approach. The Association warned that the cost of diabetes could be expected to reach 10% of all NHS inpatient expenditure by 2011. However, 'huge' savings could be made if NHS managers invested more in preventive care and monitoring for people with non-insulin dependent diabetes.

In a wider context, Will Hutton (1995) pointed to the real pressure faced by the NHS: that it was increasingly difficult to run a tax-financed, universal, National Health Service in a profoundly unequal society. Universality, inclusion and equality, upon which the NHS was based, were under assault. There was no alternative to a tax-financed NHS, free at the point of delivery, that did not involve constructing a multi-tiered service which thereby destroyed the ethic of care for all.

The financing of the NHS therefore continued to be juggled between the political wish not to raise the basic taxation level above 25% (1992–6 which was indeed lowered to 24% in 1996/7) and the need to raise NHS charges, where possible, encouraging income generation schemes and privatization, more particularly with the private finance initiative development, underpinned by rationing health care provision. The combination did not necessarily solve the apparent financial crisis in the NHS. To what extent, then, could health care systems abroad point to more effective ways forward by the mid-1990s?

HEALTH CARE SYSTEMS ABROAD: A COMPARATIVE VIEW BY 1997

Comparisons in health care policy between the European countries and the United States continued to reflect significant philosophical and structural differences which would render application to Britain problematical. First, the USA still accepted what was unacceptable to most Europeans: that some 40 million US citizens had inadequate health insurance which indicated the absence of European-style solidarity. Secondly, the Americans' lack of support for universal health care was influenced by a dislike of any egalitarian implications. Quality health care was considered a privilege not a right. Thirdly, Americans' misgivings about the role of Government together with a blinding faith in the market place stood in contrast to the European outlook (Laetz, 1996). Then again, populations in European countries were generally ageing faster than in the USA. However, European countries and the USA had many forces in common that drove health care cost escalations, although differences existed between countries (Abel-Smith et al., 1995; Laetz, 1996). As all health care systems in industrialized democracies operated under financial constraints, all sought ways to disperse costs (Laetz 1996).

The European Union: the dreaded 'S' word – subsidiarity

The extensive forms of unification across Europe might suppose that effective ways forward for financing health care systems could be found. By 1993, the European Economic Community had been re-titled the European Union (EU). In 1994, the European Parliament voted to admit three new members: Sweden,

Finland and Austria. Bringing the total membership to 15 members (Austria, Belgium, Denmark, Finland, France, Germany, Greece, then comprised Ireland, Italy, Luxembourg, the Netherlands (Holland), Portugal, Spain, Sweden and the UK).

Across Europe, two main health care systems were in use: the taxation model (the UK and the Nordic countries) and the social insurance model (countries south of Scandinavia, see Chapter 7, and Ireland) which might contain government support schemes, often means-tested, for low income groups. Outside both systems access to private medicine was available, but self-funded. Through the EU, might there be an historic opportunity to work together to overcome some of the inherent financial problems in the respective health care systems? However, what had the EU had to do with health? In asking this question, Andrew Hayes (1998), President of the European Public Health Alliance, has shown that health ministers jealously defended the right of member states to run their own health care systems. More fundamentally, the fear of subsidiarity has played a part: that in defining the proper level for policy decisions (a definition of subsidiarity), Brussels might be seen to want to take over day-to-day problems such as hospital waiting lists and staff shortages. As the geographical centre of the EU Commission, the EU Parliament (also meeting in Strasbourg and Luxembourg) and the EU Council of Ministers, Brussels has always been perceived by Euro-sceptics as a threat to national interests and endeavours. Burkitt and Baimbridge (1994/5) also warned that the 1991 Maastricht Treaty imposed a new dimension of EU control over a nation's economic and political independence, as the key economic criteria for convergence towards economic and monetary union concerned the ability of governments to determine their budgetary policy.

In the context of public health, however, the EU has been significantly involved. Under the *Single European Act* of 1986, ratified in 1987, the EEC countries were encouraged to improve the working environment as regards the health and safety of workers. Article 129 of the 1991 Maastricht Treaty, ratified in 1993, required the EEC to contribute to a high level of human health protection amongst a range of public health measures which were concerned with the prevention of disease and the promotion of research. Programmes have been adopted by the European Commission on cancer, AIDS, drug dependence, health promotion, education, training and health monitoring. Questions have remained as to whether the EU should seek positive health gain for the population as a whole or be confined to a more narrow, regulatory approach. However, solutions to the financial problems of the individual member countries' health care systems have not been forthcoming. While the EU has been given a mandate to co-ordinate action in public health with the need to develop a coherent strategy to integrate public health into other EU policies (Mossialos and McKee, 1997), health care provision was left to the member states.

Convergence: internationally

In contrast to the seemingly separate, distinctive models in the different health care systems (such as the taxation, social insurance and private insurance models; see Chapter 7), a new phenomenon was becoming apparent: that of convergence.

By the end of the 1980s, Ham et al. (1990) had concluded from an analysis of health care reforms in Sweden, the Netherlands (Holland), West Germany, Canada and the USA that there was dissatisfaction with the funding and delivery of health services. All methods of funding had their weaknesses: there was no 'quick fix' to the problems faced by the health care systems of developed countries.

The experience of the United States demonstrated the shortcomings of a system which relied mainly on private insurance, such as unequal access to provision and inability to control overall expenditure. The real choice that faced policy makers was therefore between (compulsory) social insurance and tax funding. In both Canada and Sweden, universal, public tax-based financing had enabled the whole population to gain access to a comprehensive range of services where cost controls were also involved. Thus in Sweden, agreements between the national government and the county councils had led to limits on increased public spending. However, the ability to control expenditure had, in itself, given rise to problems where a health system was unable to provide sufficient services to meet the perceived needs of the population. Social insurance, as a middling way between tax financing and private insurance, was effectively an earmarked tax levied on a narrower base than general taxation Exemplars were the Netherlands and West Germany, where expenditure as a proportion of the gross domestic product had been stabilized, but concern remained over increased insurance contributions. Inequities could also arise when social insurance and private insurance operated in tandem – as in the Netherlands – or where social insurance was administered by sick funds which set different contribution rates, as in West Germany (Ham et al., 1990).

As all systems had difficulty in controlling costs, tendencies towards convergence were becoming increasingly apparent. Countries that had relied on competition were introducing regulation, while countries that had relied on planning and regulation were experimenting with competition. Resources were being shifted away from institutional care into community care as in the Netherlands, West Germany, Sweden and Canada where (as in the USA) moves were also taking place to introduce global budgets for both hospitals and doctors' fees. Overall, greater efficiency and effectiveness were high on the agenda in all three health care systems but, in contrast to the EU programmes, support for public health policy was surrounded by rhetoric, whereas the reality of health policy was dominated by the financing and delivery of health services (Ham et al., 1990: 101).

Convergence: between the two Germanies

A major form of convergence occurred between the former East and West Germany on the fall of the Berlin Wall in 1989. A unified Germany was absorbed into the former West German social insurance system for health care provision, but not without some cost. Differing arrangements between the two countries on access to abortion were eventually resolved through a transitional phase, in which the more stringent arrangements in West Germany eventually prevailed. Fierce debates were fought over the future of East Germany's polyclinics, the popularly esteemed group doctors' practices, funded by the state, which formed the cornerstone of East German health care but which became a museum piece of social medicine. Cross-funding of a poorer Eastern health insurance fund by a richer Western one was ruled out on unification.

The problem centred on inequality, on the significantly lower local income (60%) in the East than in the West. Convergence between two countries was therefore dominated by the wealthier partner where estimates suggested that East Germans would have to wait until 2007 before achieving the standards of living guaranteed by the constitution, financed by the German taxpayer (Sheldon, 1992).

Convergence: across the European Union

By the mid-1990s, convergence across differing health care systems, rather than between two countries, was moving apace. Across the EU the moves included separating purchasers and providers, widening choices (for insured people), population-based arrangements for distributing resources, mixed systems for paying doctors and moving towards market competition (Abel-Smith, 1995). Just before his death, Professor Brian Abel-Smith (1996), as Chairman of the European Health Policy Research Network at LSE Health, had assembled further issues in considering the international dilemma of health care costs. On convergence, more and more countries in the EU had been 'doing the same in whole or part, directly or indirectly'. Budgets provided one example: in countries without overall budget control (such as France and Belgium), each hospital was given budgetary control. In Germany, budgets were used to limit the total amount all doctors could receive for treating patients outside hospital; budgets, as in Britain, were also to be introduced for doctors' prescribing. Furthermore, to control costs in several EU countries, a range of methods were in place: rationed rights to install expensive medical equipment, the direct or indirect control of drug prices, user charges (at least for drugs) in virtually all EU countries (except the Netherlands). However, in most EU countries, technology assessment was uncoordinated; there was therefore a clear case for the EU to finance action collectively in order to co-ordinate the field of technologies (Abel-Smith, 1996).

A more fundamental question was whether there were any more effective solutions for Britain. Preventive interventions had clear benefits in terms of the reduction in human suffering but, despite great potential, prevention carried costs and risks, nor could prevention necessarily be assumed to be cheaper than cure. A second option would question whether there were ways to force health services to be more efficient. Competition was still widely debated in the USA; nor could the early gains in efficiency achieved through the internal market in Britain be determined, or justified, in terms of the extra administrative costs the reforms generated. Thirdly, 'a package of care' as in the Netherlands, to which everyone was entitled (low-priority care excluded), remained an unknown quantity in terms of outcomes or what patients would choose when given informed choice. A fourth option was to persuade people to adopt healthy lifestyles but, as Abel-Smith (1996) pointed out, changes in knowledge did not necessarily lead to changes in attitudes or practice.

Lilley (1997) concluded that, as European policies unrolled, convergence on health care entitlements was not more than 10 years away. Patient contributions to the cost of services were inevitable. The drive for value for money from health expenditure across Europe would become a common crusade wherein no immediate solutions were evident for the financing of the British NHS.

Health care expenditure: international comparisons

In comparing international experience, data from the Organization for Economic Cooperation and Development (OECD, 1996) compiled the proportion of the gross domestic product (GDP) spent on health services in the OECD countries by 1994, which has provided a means to place health care provision in Britain in context. Table 11.3 shows a number of OECD countries, relevant to the countries under present review. The range was considerable, from Turkey (which has been included as the lowest spender) to the USA as the highest (significantly so throughout the 1990s). The average for all OECD countries in 1994 was just under 8%. Sweden's percentage, as traditionally a top European spender, had dropped significantly from 9.1% of the GDP in 1982 to 7.7% by 1994, due to the transfer of the responsibility for nursing homes from the county councils to the municipalities as well as the implementation of various reforms – but, more particularly, through the determination of the

Table 11.3 The proportion of the GDP spent on health services in a selection of OECD countries, 1994.

Country	Percentage of GDP
USA	14.3
Canada	9.8
France	9.7
Germany	9.5
The Netherlands (Holland)	8.8
Italy	8.3
Finland	8.3
Belgium	8.2
Ireland	7.9
Sweden	7.7
Portugal	7.6
Norway	7.3
Spain	7.3
Britain	6.9
Denmark	6.6
Luxembourg	5.8
Greece	5.2
Turkey	4.2

Source: OECD (1996).

Swedish government to control health care costs. From 1985 onwards, health care expenditures had started to stabilize and some reductions occurred (Rehnberg, 1997: 65).

Health care reforms: moving towards convergence by 1997

In the mid-1990s Ham (1997), together with a team of international contributors reviewing outcomes in five developed countries (UK, USA, the Netherlands, Sweden and Germany), showed that all had undertaken major health care reforms for similar reasons. Health services in developed countries had faced mounting financial problems: new demands had arisen due to advances in medical technology, public expectations were rising, demographic changes had led to an increase in the ageing population and a decrease in the proportion of the working age population, and health care expenditure had risen (largely funded from public sources), which had put pressure on governments to control public spending. The consequence was that countries which had traditionally relied on a market approach to health care turned to regulation and planning mechanisms, whereas those countries which had relied on regulation and planning were employing a more competitive approach.

The USA

By 1992, the newly elected President Clinton had put health care reform at the centre of the Democratic agenda. As submitted to Congress, the proposals were a complex mixture of private financing, private delivery, managed care, competition, universal coverage, choice and cost containment. The intent was for everyone to be insured whatever their health risk, either by employers or by government funding (for non-workers). Small businesses would be gradually phased in. Three main factors killed off the proposals.

1 The first problem was the sheer complexity of the detail: as Kirkman-Liff (1997: 35) commented, if President Clinton had announced his proposal in a document no longer than five pages two weeks after his inauguration, instead of the White House Task Force document of 1000 pages one year later, the scheme might have succeeded.
2 The proposals faced overwhelming opposition from a vast lobby of powerful groups: the medical profession, corporate, bureaucratic health care management and the private health insurance companies amongst others (Ginsberg, 1992: 132). Critical TV advertisement campaigns by the insurance industry, stating 'There's got to be a better way', further undermined the proposals in conjunction with political opposition from the Republicans.
3 The implication that, the poorest Americans apart, everyone would pay more (which could lead to further demands from those who did pay more) also contributed to the failure of the Clinton proposals.

The scale of the health care problems in the USA therefore remained. In 1995, the USA spent $950 billion on health care, of which the federal government contributed 40% through Medicare (which catered for elderly people) and

Medicaid (for poor people). If government spending were to continue at such a rate, health care costs would overtake the USA's gross domestic product in less than 50 years (Cross, 1996). With the defeat of Clinton's health reform bill in 1994, a more modest bipartisan bill secured the support of a, by now, Republican Congress. Nancy Kassenbaum, a Republican from Kansas, and Edward Kennedy, a Democrat from Massachusetts, successfully introduced the Kennedy–Kassenbaum Bill, which prevented insurance companies from ending the health insurance of workers who changed or left their jobs. In August 1996, President Clinton signed the bill, which received support on the basis that the measures would improve the health insurance system in future years (Berliner, 1996; Walker, 1996). However, the bill did nothing for the 40 million or so Americans without health insurance.

The approach to health care reform over the previous 30 years in the USA was described by Kirkman-Liff (1997) as reform without reform. Piecemeal reforms had been defeated by powerful groups (physicians, hospitals, business groups, private health insurers) who had an interest in preserving the system. Furthermore, the public's faith had declined in the ability of the government to confront rising costs and poorer access to care for a large minority.

Health care reforms in Europe by 1997

In contrast to the 'reform without reform' in the USA, which reflected a highly pluralistic system of health care based on a more organic process of change, three approaches to reform in Europe were identified (Ham, 1997):

- the 'big bang' reform in the UK (through the 1990 NHS and Community Care Act);
- incremental reform in Germany and the Netherlands;
- bottom-up reform in Sweden.

Across the measures for reform, changes had been introduced for similar reasons: to contain costs, to increase efficiency, to raise standards and to improve performance.

Germany and the Netherlands

Essentially based on a social insurance system, by 1995 Germany was in the middle of a third reform in health care provision which involved the pooling of sickness funds and cost containment, with the power shifting away from state governments towards central government (Schwarz and Busse, 1997). Similarly, the Dutch system was based on compulsory social insurance (although a group of civil servants had their own mandatory scheme), while about 34% of the population – mainly self-employed and higher income groups – could buy private health insurance; a compulsory national insurance scheme also provided coverage for the whole population against catastrophic risks. The Dutch reforms from the 1987 Plan-Dekker, the 1990 Plan-Simmons and further reforms in 1995, sought to achieve a balance between accessibility/equity and market-oriented financial incentives/efficiency (van de Ven, 1997).

Sweden

In Sweden, five major reforms were undertaken during the 1990s, concerned with internal markets, family doctors, maximum waiting lists and the care of elderly people. The 'bottom-up' reforms were reflected in the decentralized nature of the system where policy variations existed between the county councils. A common principle in the reforms upheld the need to make politicians concentrate on the interest of citizens, by separating the purchaser and provider roles within the county councils. While the providers were to remain under public ownership, the purpose was to increase incentives, to use resources more efficiently, to enable competition between public providers and to open up new health care markets for new private providers. In all county council models with a purchaser/provider split, the reforms increased the individual's opportunity to choose providers which, in turn, gave rise to a co-ordination problem. Meanwhile, the principles of equity and equal access to health care continued to provide a major argument for maintaining the public financing of health care. In terms of efficiency and equity, outcomes could not be established in the time span available by the mid-1990s, more especially as the structure of the internal markets was also changing (Rehnberg, 1997).

What lessons for the future financing of the NHS in Britain?

Ham's (1997) conclusions were that cost containment had been more successful in some countries (Sweden) than in others (Germany). If the basic goals of access to health care for all groups in the population and equity in service provision were considered important, then the American approach was not a model to follow, despite the high standards of care for many people together with the outstanding examples of clinical innovation and excellence. As a result, from the European perspective, the emphasis on health care funding mainly through public sources was more appropriate, but reform efforts needed to be focussed more on the delivery of care than on the funding. Across Europe, the importance of the purchaser role in the contract model had not been fully recognized in that a countervailing force to the power of the provider was required. However, in learning lessons for the NHS, each model had advantages and disadvantages. Indeed Paton (1998: 170) has argued, in reviewing the continuum of health care systems from largely private to the more integrated public health sector reforms, that Britain should aim to preserve equity, increase efficiency in an appropriate manner, maintain the integrated nature of the NHS, but without adopting the diverse solutions from health care reforms elsewhere.

Although the international emphasis in health care reforms in the 1990s could be placed on rationing, priority setting, primary care, managed care, health technology, assessment and evidence-based medicine, the failure to evaluate the reforms represented a major missed opportunity (Ham, 1997).

Practitioners, managers and academics at a European Healthcare Management Association conference in 1995 considered that health care reforms across Europe had been driven by ideology and cost-cutting concerns that had concentrated on systems and structures rather than on improving the health of the population. In welcoming delegates, Hans Stein, Health Policy Officer in the German Federal Ministry of Health in Bonn, described the future of health care in Europe not as harmonization but as convergence. Co-operation could lead to common methodologies to assess outcomes, enable comparisons to be made and compare data on evaluating services, technology, medical devices and the results of a wide range of per capita spending (May, 1995).

Meanwhile, policy makers in some countries were already moving away from competitive strategies towards greater emphasis on accountability and contestability (Ham, 1997). The fashionable affair with market forces had started to fizzle out, claimed Ham (1998). There was an implicit acceptance that collaboration and competition could be used together. By early 1998, policy makers in the Netherlands, New Zealand and Sweden were all having second thoughts about the role of competition in the health services; alternative ways were being explored to improve performance. Why had there been a change of heart? The reasons included: the election of governments less convinced of the merits of competition, the failure of markets to deliver the promised benefits, the concerns over high level transaction costs involved in contracting and the challenge to equity placed by the competition model. Policy makers were now beginning to face a more sober reckoning for the future (Ham, 1998).

12

SERVICING CARE IN THE COMMUNITY 1990–1997: THE PLACE OF WORKING TOGETHER WITH THE NHS

In Britain by 1990, social reforms extended beyond health care. The 1990 *NHS and Community Care Act* encompassed both health (discussed in Chapter 9) and community care. The legislative changes will now be reviewed in the context of the community together with the involvement of the user. From the perspective of health care, one key element concerned how far the health and social services were working together, particularly over assessing needs and caring for elderly and mentally ill people, amongst other groups.

THE COMMUNITY CARE REFORMS 1990

In contrast to the speedily formulated NHS reforms contained in the 1990 legislation, the background to changes for caring in the community was comparatively extensive. In the mid-1980s, the Audit Commission (1985) provided a comprehensive review of the community care services which showed that services for elderly people were wastefully provided, inadequately managed and poorly co-ordinated between health, housing and social services. The Audit Commission (1996b) then reported that services for elderly, mentally ill, physically and mentally handicapped people were under-funded, fragmented between agencies and that the community care policies were in disarray (see Chapter 4). Both the Wagner Report (1988) and the Griffiths Report (1998), which officially reviewed the use of public funds to support community care, recommended that local authorities should continue to assume the lead role (see Chapter 6). The government's subsequent White Paper *Caring for People: Community Care in the Next Decade and Beyond* (DoH, 1989c) largely followed the Griffiths Report's (1988) recommendations, particularly in furthering a new policy objective: to provide a central role for the assessment of needs linked to the role of 'case' managers. Local authority social services departments would become managers, not simply providers, of care for elderly, disabled and mentally ill people and those with learning disabilities. Nevertheless, the government rejected Griffiths' proposal for specific community care grants to local authorities as well as the appointment of a Minister for Community Care to implement effective joint planning between health, housing and social security.

A key underlying motivator that led to the community care reforms in 1990 was the runaway social security budget which had become involved in assisting old people and others, who were in private residential or nursing homes but found themselves in financial difficulties. As a result the money allocated rose from £10 million in 1979 to over £2000 million by 1991. While the NHS was under financial pressure in response to the growing demands for geriatric facilities, the social security budget had unintentionally rescued families, local authorities and the NHS, all under budgetary restraint (Lewis and Glennerster, 1996: 3–4). Individualized choice in residential care, with little check on rationing or on how decisions were made, had caused an explosion in public expenditure. The outcome of the community care reforms was therefore largely prompted by the need to transfer the costs of residential care away from the social security budget and onto local authorities and users. Lewis and Glennerster (1996: 9) have argued that the reforms were finally hurried through to address a funding crisis. Improvements in services for elderly and mentally ill people were not necessarily sought, nor were ways forward furthered for the relations between statutory agencies.

The 1990 *NHS and Community Care Act* was essentially based on the White Paper (DoH, 1989c), which was signed by the Secretaries of State for Health, Social Security, Wales and Scotland. Six main objectives and seven key changes were set out.

Caring for People (DoH, 1989c): key objectives and changes

Key objectives:

1 To promote domiciliary, day and respite services to enable people to remain in their own homes whenever possible.
2 To ensure high priority to support carers.
3 To make assessment of need and good case management a cornerstone of policy.
4 To promote a 'mixed economy' of welfare through both independent and public services to enable a more flexible choice to users.
5 To clarify the responsibility of agencies to ensure accountability.
6 To secure better value for taxpayers' money.

Key changes:

- Local authorities would become the lead agencies (in collaboration with medical, nursing and other interests) to assess individual need and to appoint case managers to design individually tailored packages of care.
- Local authorities would be required to publish community care plans, in consultation with interested agencies (for health and housing). Joint planning was to be based on planning agreements to set out common goals for community care and funding arrangements.
- Local authorities would be required to establish inspection and registration units to monitor standards in both the public and independent sector residential care homes.
- To develop social care for mentally ill people through a new specific grant.

Most of the White Paper's proposals would apply equally to England, Wales and Scotland, although some would have to be adapted to the special circumstances of the Welsh and Scottish health and social services. A separate policy paper was to be published for Northern Ireland, where the health and social services structure was distinctively integrated.

Financing community care and demographic trends

Funding was the key issue. Under the White Paper's proposals for the flow of resources to community care (DoH, 1989c: 106), only support for mental illness was to receive a special grant via health authorities. The remaining local authority income would be gathered from the central revenue support grant, community charges, income from various charges and joint finance (with health authorities) amongst other elements. Expenditure had to cover not only caring for elderly people but also a range of services for domiciliary care, child care, social work support, care for mentally ill and disabled people and for those with learning disabilities. However, the government subsequently decided to ring fence the community care budget when the first allocation of funding was announced in November 1992.

The implementation of the community care plans was delayed until April 1993 when the additional funds, previously made available through the social security system, were capped and transferred to local authorities (the special transitional grant or community care transfer money; Audit Commission, 1997b: 11). Local authorities therefore had time to plan as 85% of the community care grant, which contained the social security transfer element, had to be spent within the independent sector, while the Department of Health was able to provide more policy guidance (DoH, 1990).

Nevertheless, local authority financial pressures began to mount in the light of the demographic estimates: numbers of people over 85 were projected to rise from 695 000 in 1986 to 1 146 000 in 2001 (DoH, 1989c: 62) – the group of very elderly people who were also most likely to be disabled and in greater need of community care. The community care transfer money did include a rise from £399 million in 1993/4 to £518 million in 1995/6 (DoH, 1992a), together with extra funds to cover the costs of setting up new systems of assessment and administration (Lewis and Glennerster, 1996: 29), but the transitional payments were to be absorbed into the general local government support grant by 1996 (later extended to 1999). Financial stringency then escalated, as the central revenue support grant was reduced in 1995, together with cuts in local authority education budgets in 1995/6 (Lewis and Glennerster, 1996: 42) which left social services departments ever more vulnerable in competing for local government resources. Nor was the situation likely to diminish into the twenty-first century, as demographic trends have shown for the dependent population by age in the UK (Figure 12.1). In 2011, those of pensionable age (as 65 for men and 60 for women) would form around 18% of the population but which would rise to constitute 24% by 2025 (Tinker, 1997: 14). Even more startling, in the long term, was the estimate of around 8000 centenarians in the UK by early 1998, which was likely to double in seven years to reach 100 000 in 2066 (Appleby, 1998a: 38–39).

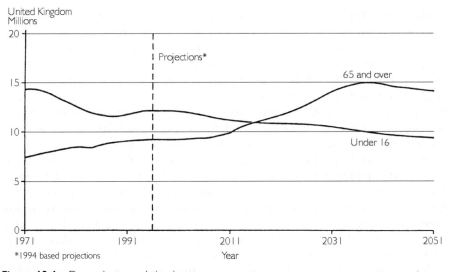

Figure 12.1 Dependent population by age.
Source: Office for National Statistics (1997: 27), Chart 1.1.
Crown Copyright material reproduced with the permission of the Controller of Her Majesty's Stationery Office.

COMMUNITY CARE INVOLVEMENT AND OUTCOMES FOR USERS AND CARERS: THE OLDER POPULATION

Probably the most important issue for elderly service users was the ambiguous question of charges for residential and nursing care in the community. Local authorities had long been charging for residential care under powers derived from the 1948 *National Assistance Act* which allowed for limited local discretion. The 1983 Health and Social Services and Social Security Adjudications Act also gave permissive, discretionary powers to local authorities to charge for domiciliary and day-care services. The government's view, confirmed in the community care White Paper (DoH, 1989c), was that users should be expected to pay if they were able to do so. However, as the Audit Commission (1996b: 26–8) found, the user income and capital taken into account varied between local authorities. With the transfer of financial responsibility to local authorities from 1993, old people who needed residential or nursing home places could normally obtain a 'free' place if their individual assets were less than £3000, rising on a means-tested assets basis to £8000, whereupon the full care costs had to be paid by the user. Meanwhile, some local authorities were using the household benefit threshold of £16 000 as the cut-off point for an individual to meet the full costs of residential care. By 1995, local authorities were more generally moving over to an increase in the means-tested limits to between £10 000 and £16 000; by 1997, all local authorities had moved onto the higher base calculation.

The outcome for elderly people was the risk of forfeiting a lifetime's savings or even their own homes to fund long-stay care which, in turn, could disinherit their children.

Ethical problems were also reflected in the quandaries within the system. Those with assets of £16 000 who had been prudent enough to save for their old age were not entitled to any state help to pay for care in nursing or residential homes. From the mid-1990s onwards, thousands of pensioners had to sell their homes to finance care. Their sense of injustice was aggravated by the lottery of illness, in which hospital care remained free on the NHS while nursing care in the community was not. By 1997, the annual cost of long-term care to the government was heading towards £7 billion, although some 30% of the 500 000 or so people in long-term care were paying for that provision.

On the other hand, the shift in the growth from public sector care to the private and voluntary sectors had given older users and carers a wider range of choice, had opened up the care sector to new ideas and fresh capital and exerted pressure on service providers to contain costs and improve quality (Audit Commission, 1997b: 15). A significant fall had taken place in the UK provision of care from 1983, when NHS beds and local authority residential care accounted for 59% of total provision, to only 20% in 1996 (Figure 12.2). The Audit Commission (1997b: 15) pointed out that, in order to improve services for older people, proper co-ordination with the independent sector was now required: some social services departments had been slow to come to terms with the mixed economy of care, but the independent sector needed to be more effectively integrated into the care system.

The regulation of residential care for elderly people

As business in the private and voluntary care homes escalated, the need for regulation became an increasingly important issue. Giant American health care companies were also buying into British firms to profit from the boom in private

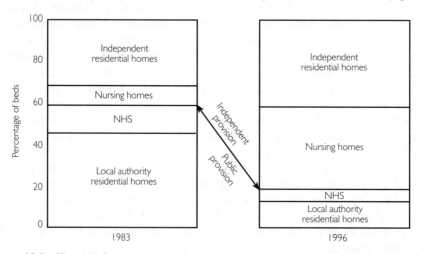

Figure 12.2 The shift from primary to independent sector provision of care. A legacy of the 1980s has been a significant shift from the public to the independent sector in the provision of care. Source: Audit Commission (1997b: 14). Primary source: Laing and Buisson (1977). Care of Elderly People: Market survey 1997. Reproduced by kind permission of the Audit Commission.

nursing homes brought about by the expansion of care in the community from 52 000 nursing home places in 1987 to 168 200 in 1993. American companies were realizing profits of around 20% on UK operations compared with 8% in the USA (Brindle, 1996e). Day et al. (1996) undertook a study of the 107 local authority inspection units in England which were responsible for the registration and biannual inspection of 12 000 residential homes for elderly and disabled people (with over 300 000 places) – including homes run by local authorities. The findings showed that considerable variations in standards existed, although both providers and inspectors agreed that overall standards had risen over the last decade in line with rising regulatory and societal expectations. Some confusion remained as to whether the regulatory system should aim to set minimum standards or improve existing standards. Regulators and the regulated had trouble in resolving disputes. However, the main recommendation to emerge was the need for national standards to be set which could prompt a move towards a national regulatory system.

Carers

For carers, important developments had also taken place by the mid-1990s. The *Carers (Recognition and Services) Act 1995* marked a significant milestone. From April 1996, the *Carers Act* recognized the importance of supporting those people who were responsible for others. Carers of older and disabled people were often themselves elderly. The 1995 legislation required local authority social services departments to assess the ability of carers to provide care. Local authorities were then asked to take the carers' assessment into account when deciding what services to provide for each person in need of care. A 'carer' was defined as someone who provided substantial care on a regular basis which included young people under the age of 18. In the aftermath of the legislation, new demands for services arose for night sitting services, planned respite care, provision of aids and adaptations and the provision of home care (NHS Health Advisory Service, 1997: 32; Tinker, 1997: 200).

McGlone (1993) examined the increase in informal family care between a 1985 Office of Population Censuses and Surveys survey and the 1990 *General Household Survey* on carers (OPCS, 1992). By 1990, some 2.9 million men and 3.9 million women were providing informal care – 15% of all people aged 16 and over in Britain. The total of 6.8 million carers reflected a 15% rise in numbers since 1985, which had occurred almost entirely among the 45–64 age group, largely accounted for by the growth in the numbers caring for parents and parents-in-law. McGlone (1993) pointed out that the continuing growth in the number of married women going out to work might reduce the potential pool of carers, while the rising divorce rate could make family care more problematic. However, as the Carers National Association (CNA, 1995a) recorded, informal carers undertook most of the caring in the community, which saved the Treasury some £35 billion per annum.

Meanwhile the Carers National Association launched their Fair Deal for Carers campaign in 1994 to help carers find their way through the community care system and to encourage health and social services professionals to take the needs of carers fully into account. The CNA (1995b) subsequently reported on the findings of the campaign's independent survey, which assessed the carers' own experience of the 1990 NHS *and Community Care Act*, to reveal that:

- 17% of carers questioned had not heard of community care at all;
- 74% had not had a social services assessment of the person for whom they cared;
- more than half of the carers did not know what an assessment was;
- 13% had noticed an improvement in services under care in the community (CNA, 1995b).

Twigg and Atkin's (1994: 148) study on carers (particularly for adults with a learning disability, mental health problems or physical disabilities) suggested that the key to successful local authority case management was clarity over the aims of community care services. The lack of clear aims or targets for provision had led to impediments in developing a more effective response to carers. Crucially, carers would continue to provide most of the care, but how carers were perceived by service providers would continue to determine the level and pattern of help received from health and social services. Indeed, some evidence suggested that service provision was biased against those who had resident carers (Parker and Lawton, 1994).

Community care: taking stock

By the mid-1990s, various assessments had been made on the outcomes of the community care reforms. The Audit Commission (1996b) had continuously monitored the implementation of community care in England. The main findings were that progress was evident but that most local authorities had to take action to keep control of expenditure, although priority to community care had been given: spending on community care was 7% more than proposed by the government. The numbers of people receiving care depended on the numbers who sought help as well as on eligibility criteria which were often complex and difficult to understand. Further, wide variations existed on eligibility criteria between local authorities: the terms 'dependency' and 'risk' were used in varying ways, often interchangeably with 'need'. Most local authorities were increasing charges but, again, wide variations occurred across the country, although most authorities needed better information to keep within budget. However, many local authorities were working hard to improve arrangements for both users and their carers, despite the financial challenges.

Lewis and Glennerster's (1996: 201) analysis showed that local authority social services departments were initially preoccupied with implementing the community care reforms in terms of structures and process: the care management schemes (care now used rather than case), the purchaser/provider splits and needs assessment. Lewis and Glennerster (1996: 206) considered that the profile of work with elderly people had been raised which would have a positive effect on services for the older client group. The reforms also held potential to promote greater choice, flexibility, responsiveness and higher quality services. However, the community care reforms were intended to provide a needs-led service not a user-led service. Care managers therefore had to define need in terms of a combination of risk, need and statutory responsibility which had led to the formalization of hierarchies of need in the face of constrained resources.

Despite the considerable progress in the first year of the community care reforms, the views of users and carers were intended to play a central role in helping to establish need and to determine the appropriate service response (Audit Commission, 1994a: 6). However, carers had not noticed much difference by the end of the first year (Warner, 1994). Despite considerable government rhetoric about the involvement of users and carers in community care planning, despite government pressure on local authority social services departments to consult with local voluntary organizations and service users on proposals and developments, the genuine involvement of users and carers in community care planning and service delivery was still relatively rare (Craig and Manthorpe, 1996).

As Lewis and Glennerster's (1996: 208) concluded, the finance of long-term care would become one of the key national policy issues by the turn of the century, in the light of the rising numbers of people over 80, those with learning difficulties who lived a full life span as well as the growth of long-term mental illness in the community.

Access to resources was only part of a wider picture for the future. More fundamentally, a deep structural and financial division remained at the core of the health and welfare system. As Age Concern (1994: 5) commented, the community care reforms did not address the deep-seated and long-standing problem that faced all policies for community care: the lack of a co-ordinated legal and administrative framework within which true 'community care' could be enabled to flourish.

WORKING TOGETHER FOR HEALTH AND SOCIAL CARE

Two major disjunctions lodged between the provision of health and social care in Britain. The first division occurred between largely free, centrally funded, health care and means-tested, locally funded social care. The second division contrasted a centrally directed NHS with a locally elected local government service for community care. Figure 12.3 shows the complexity of the services but the clarity of administrative division (heavy back line). A further distinction between the purchasing and provision of health services and social care in the community was introduced in the 1990s.

Historically, the divisions between the provision of health and community care had not been resolved across the century. The post-war arrangements inherited unresolved pre-war tensions and settings: the tripartite split between hospital provision, GP services and local (health) authority arrangements remained. When local authorities lost their health functions in 1974 the split deepened, although mechanisms were introduced to bridge the gap, such as Joint Consultative Committees and joint planning. However, the record on cross-boundary missions was generally regarded as disappointing (Webb and Wistow,

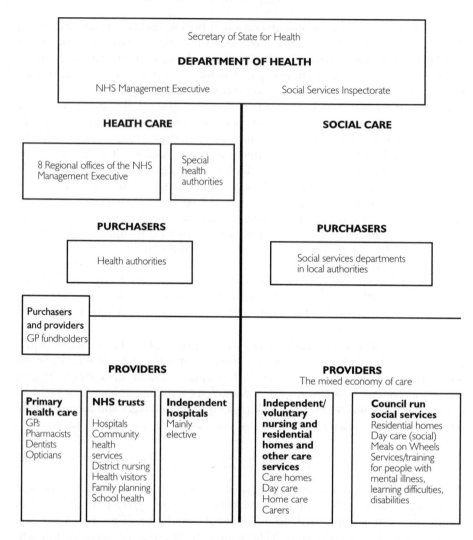

Figure 12.3 The structure of the NHS and community care services in England by 1996.

1986; Lewis, 1993). Good community care had therefore long been recognized to require collaborative planning and working (Glennerster et al., 1983). As the Audit Commission (1986) pointed out, the professional cultures and forms of accountability differed significantly between health and social services.

Collaboration between health and social services was, however, seen as a key initiative in the 1990 community care reforms. Local authorities were required to consult with health and housing authorities, voluntary organizations, users and carers and to produce community care plans. Joint commissioning was one way to emerge in which health and local authority social services sought to work collaboratively 'to ensure a more effective and efficient use of the available resources'

(Poxton, 1994: 4–5). In reviewing various joint commissioning programmes at both local authority borough and county level, Lewis and Glennerster (1996: 185) found that commitment from senior management and clearly established posts for joint commissioning were required to overcome the barriers to formal collaboration. Nevertheless, whether concerned with joint commissioning, or the more disparate forms of collaborative working between providers to produce seamless care, the programmes faced conflicts between agencies that were separately financed, administered and staffed (Lewis and Glennerster, 1996: 185–6).

By 1996, a review of the joint commissioning of health and social care over a period of three years at one of the King's Fund sites found 39 tangible and 15 intangible achievements (Poxton, 1996). Some achievements of joint commissioning included:

- multidisciplinary community mental health assessment;
- comprehensive services for people with learning disabilities;
- specific housing improvements;
- respite care in various settings;
- home bathing – generally considered a classic issue for joint commissioning;
- a 'one-stop shop' for information, basic advice and some basic provision for older people.

The King's Fund study showed that joint commissioning had helped to bring collaboration between health authorities and social services departments to the fore. Joint working at both strategic and operational levels was more common. Although the assortment of activity was encouraging and although joint working should continue to resolve health and social care boundary issues, the scale of change required and the complexities involved were making progress slow (Poxton, 1996).

Needs assessment

The 1990 *NHS and Community Care Act* had created a 'cascade of change', identified by the Audit Commission (1992a), which introduced the contract culture together with the assessment of needs. Local authorities were now given the responsibility to assess individual need in collaboration with health authority staff (DoH, 1989c). Behind the changes were two key aims. The first was to empower the service users and their carers through choice about the support provided. The second aim was to enable people to be cared for at home where appropriate. If the new approach was to work the agencies involved needed to work together to provide a 'seamless' service. Experience had shown that differences in priorities, organizational styles and cultures between the key agencies of health and social services had led to a reluctance to work together co-operatively (Audit Commission, 1992c: 2).

As the voluntary and statutory sectors struggled with the various forms of collaboration required by the 1990 legislation (Lewis, 1993), the assessment of needs introduced a range of complex issues. First of all, whose needs were to be met? The White Paper *Caring for People* (DoH, 1989c) provided an answer for the community care services: not everyone needing care in the community. People with exclusively health care needs would continue to have direct access to and receive services directly from community and primary health services. Slight needs could be met by information and advice. Local authorities would have to decide when a formalized assessment became necessary where people's needs extended beyond health care to social care. In other words, the advice indicated the potentially very fine dividing line between health and social care provision.

Lewis and Glennerster's (1996: 152) analysis of community care services in four boroughs and one county council concluded that, while a needs-led approach to assessment had widespread support among staff, the implementation proved difficult. The difficulties were explained by the cultural shift needed to think first about needs then about the existing services that might be offered rather than, as previously, to consider the services first. Even so, deciding on eligibility criteria for assessment and services posed major problems. Priority for assessment tended everywhere to be by urgency and risk (Lewis and Glennerster, 1996: 163).

Paton (1998: 125) queried whether needs assessment by experts would produce different priorities from those established by consultation with users. Meanwhile, local authorities set about needs assessment and community care plans meticulously. The details on care set out by Wandsworth Social Services Department (1993/94) represented one example. Individual assessment and care management procedures were worked out in minute detail: assessment of need and an agreed care plan would be offered to people in serious risk of self-neglect or abuse, where existing care arrangements were in danger of breaking down, or to people who required help because they could not manage personal care or domestic tasks. The objective was to develop a system which ensured that assessment was needs-led, involved maximum user choice, which included full consideration of racial and cultural needs as well as carers' needs. Although Wandsworth Council had the lead responsibility, the arrangements were to take account of the role of health agencies both in assessment and in providing community care services.

From a health care perspective, assessing need for localities within districts was not straightforward for health authorities. From the outset of the 1990 NHS reforms, data on health needs and service utilization were difficult to collect, while methods for assessing needs had yet to evolve. Questions also arose as to how quality, health outcomes and health gains should be assessed and by whom (Allsop, 1995: 179). As Young and Haynes (1993) have discussed, easily available quantitative data indicating need (as contained in the national census) could be useful in health service planning, but was mostly based on tightly defined geographical areas. Young and Haynes (1993) argued that, in describing a district within Norwich Health Authority where community nursing and paramedical staff were organized in a system of GP attachment with a commonly dispersed patient population, the problems of assessing population needs would be reduced and multidisciplinary teamwork enhanced if teams could be organized to work within explicit geographical boundaries.

Primary health care was becoming increasingly involved in health needs assessment which should be seen, according to Hopton and Leahy (1997), as a process to be integrated with the commissioning of health care. Health needs assessment was thus described as a systematic review of the potential alleviation of any health-related issue against service provision, in order to further priority setting and planned change (Hooper et al., 1997: 15). Such assessment therefore sought to move from reactive service-driven care to proactive needs-led care (Hooper et al., 1997: 15). The data and methods for locality health needs assessment varied, given the diversity in size of areas and populations. The key methodological issues were largely concerned with the problems of defining localities in terms of resource allocation, interprofessional working and assessing the needs of the local population. A major pitfall in primary health care needs assessments was to find the resources, once the needs had been assessed. Further, different localities tended to develop different approaches to the assessment of health needs.

Localities had long been seen as a focus for interagency and intersectoral co-operation. However, one factor remained unclear: how the NHS localities based on general practices would co-ordinate resource management and service development with local authority personnel and social services, to seek ways forward outside the health sector (Hopton and Leahy, 1997).

The key question for users was how far joint working through needs assessment actually addressed consumer views of health and social care. The lack of effective collaboration between health and community care services over long-term care increasingly presented a major problem at both national and local level. On the other hand, multidisciplinary teamwork was starting to make a positive impact on the care of mentally ill people and those with learning disabilities.

Long-term care for elderly people

Difficulties in the co-ordination of hospital discharge and long-term care for older people in the community really tested the principle of collaborative working. First, with complex medical problems and social needs, elderly people did not fit easily into either the health or the social care system. Secondly, how primary and secondary care should collaborate to support both older people and their carers, through seamless care, raised a challenge for the management of care. Thirdly, ambiguities existed as to which patients should remain in hospital. No nationally agreed eligibility criteria existed for long-term care, nor any commitment to underwrite funding for the future. Fourthly, local authorities and health authorities differed in their approaches to assessment: with responsibilities for care management, local authorities were required to purchase packages of care for *individual* clients (children, elderly and disabled people, etc.), while health authorities tended to plan and purchase care according to the clinical needs of *populations* and client *groups* (people with cancers or those who required mental health services). As a result, incompatibility in service planning processes occurred (NHS Health Advisory Service, 1997).

The financial changes brought about by the 1900 NHS and Community Care

Act led to a significant difference between the continuing care facilities purchased by social services departments (which were means-tested) while continuing NHS care which was free at the point of delivery.

In February 1995, the Department of Health (DoH, 1995b) attempted to clarify the responsibility of the NHS with regard to continuing care. Collaboration with local authorities was considered crucial to ensure effective and integrated delivery of care. The introduction of the new community care arrangements, in April 1993, further strengthened the need for joint working; in particular, health authorities, GP fundholders and local authorities needed to work together. While the guidance did not provide definitions nor national eligibility criteria, certain obligations were placed on health purchasers and providers which included the need to improve hospital discharge for frail patients with continuing social or health care needs and to collaborate with local authorities to define their responsibilities for continuing care.

In July 1996, the third report of the House of Commons Health Committee (1996) on long-term care stated that, despite considerable uncertainty about future payment for long-term care, the situation was more manageable than many commentators had suggested: that there was no immediate crisis. The Health Committee supported the argument for means testing of both assets and capital in respect of access to long-term care in the community. However, local authorities, health authorities and housing agencies were advised not to lose sight of the fact that preventive services could play an important role in delaying or reducing the demand for long-term care. The Health Committee concluded that more effective liaison was needed between housing, social services and health authorities.

The Secretary of State for Health (1997a) then put forward ideas for consultation on financial schemes to tackle long-term care. The argument advanced was that by creating a partnership between the state, individuals, families and relevant financial institutions, the costs of caring for elderly people could be kept within reasonable limits. Schemes for immediate needs annuities, 'top-up' resources (to be disregarded by means-tested residential care) and a partnership scheme based on indemnity insurance were put forward but received little further attention due to the political changes ahead .

The outcomes of assessing and arranging care for older people were then reviewed by the Audit Commission (1997b: 17). Older people had experienced care services that were poorly co-ordinated: health and social services often failed to agree on their respective responsibilities, which resulted in confusion and delays in discharge from hospital. Access to information about services had been patchy and staff did not have the flexibility to tailor services effectively. Where initiatives *had* taken place, some improvements in services and choices available had occurred. Recommendations for the way forward included mapping needs and services, strengthening of management information, working with service providers and developing better monitoring arrangements to ensure effective and high-quality service. Above all, both agencies needed to work together.

More radical proposals were put forward by Lewis and Glennester (1996: 209) to move towards a fully integrated service by creating separate, centrally funded, long-term care agencies with health and social care staff. Another option was to transfer all forms of long-term care (both health and social) to local authorities.

In the interests of health and social care integration and democratic account-ability, a further proposal was to transfer the health commissioning budget to local authorities (AMA, 1994). Christine Hancock (1994), General Secretary of the Royal College of Nursing, dismissed the integration approach on the basis that 'two into one won't go'. While greater co-operation between health and local authorities was essential, integration was not the answer as it could lead to the end of a *national* health service. Social services chiefs subsequently backed Department of Health officials in opposition to extending Northern Ireland's model of integrated health and social services to the mainland for three reasons.

1 Social services chiefs favoured the social model of care but not the medical model, which might dominate in any shift.
2 The different legislative frameworks and funding regimes of the two sectors limited opportunities to share resources effectively.
3 Social services would wish to see the current lines of democratic account-ability to local populations maintained (*Health Service Journal*, 1998).

The structures thus remained unchanged.

Multidisciplinary teamwork for mentally ill people

In 1975, a government White Paper (DHSS, 1975) described a model to replace care in large psychiatric hospitals with a range of accommodation and services in the community (see Chapter 3). The 1983 *Mental Health Act* remained the key legislation in regulation of the care and treatment of patients who were detained or liable to be detained in hospital, but the legislation continued to pose problems of interpretation, construction for discussion, comment and occasionally for resolution by courts (Secretary of State for Health, 1995: 21).

The creation of NHS trusts, under the 1990 *NHS and Community Care Act*, introduced significant changes in the delivery of care for people with mental illness. Hospital units were closed or inpatient provision reduced, accompanied in most cases by an increase in the community provision of psychiatric services, in social support and in the development of multidisciplinary community mental health teams together with the provision of community residential facilities. A care programme approach (CPA) for the assessment, co-ordination and review of care for individuals was introduced, together with a specific grant to local autho-rities for social care for people with serious mental illness to provide further support for people in the community. The CPA was later supplemented by supervision registers, designed for those most at risk of harming themselves or others, or of self-neglect, who needed particular care and follow-up. Subse-quently, the Mental Health Act Commission found that, while many long-stay and elderly mentally ill patients had been successfully relocated into community settings, there was a core of patients for whom community care was not appro-priate (Secretary of State for Health, 1995: 134).

In 1992, mental illness was chosen as one of five key target areas in the government's Health of the Nation programme (DoH, 1992b), which aimed to improve the health and social functioning of mentally ill people and to reduce suicide rates. The policy in Wales differed slightly in form, although based on similar principles. The strategy for mental illness services also made community teams the focus of the service but was updated by the 1993 *Protocol for Investment in Health Gain* (Welsh Office, 1993). Other goals included reduction of the impact of socio-economic factors on mental distress and reduction of the stigma attached to mental health problems.

The programme in Britain moved rapidly: old long-stay institutions were reduced in number (130 in 1960 to some 92 by 1994) while residents were resettled in the community or acute-care hospitals (Audit Commission, 1994b). The number of community-based teams increased significantly throughout the 1980s and into the 1990s. Key professionals involved in the multidisciplinary community health teams, which provided assessment, treatment and care for individuals and groups outside hospitals, included:

- psychiatrists, who worked both in hospitals and increasingly in the community;
- psychiatric nurses (the most numerous professionals in mental health care);
- community psychiatric nurses (usually registered mental health nurses);
- clinical psychologists, who had a key role in assessment and carried out a wide range of treatment such as behavioural therapy and cognitive therapy;
- occupational therapists, who worked both in hospitals and in the community;
- social workers, some of whom specialized in mental health; approved social workers received specialist training in mental health, had to be approved by the local authority and had statutory responsibilities when people were compulsorily admitted to hospital;
- psychotherapists, psychoanalysts and counsellors, who offered 'talking treatments';
- GPs and primary-care teams: the main providers of care for people with less severe mental illness.

In 1994, the DoH (1994) underlined, once again, the importance of collaboration and partnership between disciplines in mental health care and emphasized the need for clear protocols for the relative involvement of the various professions. The DoH (1994: 5) vision for the future of mental health services placed mental health nurses in the vanguard of practice – to build on existing expertise, to develop disciplinary teams and to respond directly and appropriately to the needs of service users. The Audit Commission (1994b) provided a visual circle of the range of services needed to meet individual needs (Figure. 12.4).

So what were the outcomes of the various policy initiatives? On the down side, the Audit Commission (1994b) reported that, despite progress in policy:

- good comprehensive community care for people with mental health problems was slow to develop;
- users needed more practical help with employment, housing and benefits;

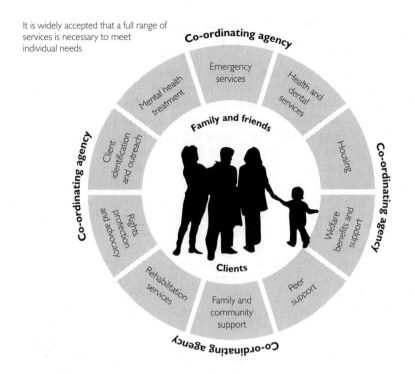

It is widely accepted that a full range of services is necessary to meet individual needs

Figure 12.4   The elements of an appropriate service.
*Source: Carson and Sharma (1994) In-patient psychiatric care. What helps? Staff and Patient Perspectives, Journal of Mental Health, **3**, 99–104. Adapted in Audit Commission (1994: 17). Reproduced by kind permission of the Audit Commission.*

- carers and relatives of people with mental illness complained about the lack of information on services and treatments;
- the needs of ethnic minority groups were not well addressed.

Concern was also caused by the lack of policy implementation. Further, two-thirds of expenditure was still locked up in hospitals, while only one-third was available for community care. The Mental Health Act Commission (Secretary of State for Health, 1995: 132) found that problems included poor recording of care plans (particularly for unmet needs), scarcity and lack of variety in the range of services in the community. The principles of community care had not been easy to achieve due to the restrictions imposed by lack of resources.

Incidents such as disturbed individuals climbing into the lions' den at London Zoo and, in 1992, the fatal stabbing of Jonathan Zito by Chrisopher Clunis (a diagnosed schizophrenic) led to popular perceptions that community care was not working. Mentally ill people in community care were generally considered a danger to the public. However, although some criticized the shift to community care settings for people with mental illness, others argued that the programme had not gone far enough to secure an adequate resource base (Audit Commission, 1994b: 7).

In a report on London's mental health, Johnson et al. (1997) found that facilities were poorly provided for mental health teams in the community, that unacceptable delays were experienced by patients, their families and staff in the provision of basic services, that services in the community were insufficient to deal with the demand, that the need for better information systems remained and that the services for ethnic minorities (despite the development of specific services for the many and diverse ethnic minority communities) were limited in meeting the full range of needs. Equity of service provision in London compared with other parts of the country therefore was in doubt. The crisis in inner London was not due to meanness among purchasers nor out-dated attitudes among the providers, but to greater needs. Services in outer London were comparable with those in other English cities. However, inner London's mental health services were unable to meet the demands imposed by inner city deprivation where the needs exceeded the socially deprived areas of other cities.

On the positive side, the Audit Commission (1994b: 7) found that users supported the policy of community care: people who received services in the community hardly ever wished to return to hospital. The Mental Health Act Commission (Secretary of State for Health, 1995: 136) expressed satisfaction with the ability of approved social workers to handle the often complex elements involved with the care of psychiatric patients. The King's Fund report (Johnson et al., 1997) acknowledged the good features of London's community mental health services, which included many examples of innovative services, user participation in service planning and the introduction of multidisciplinary teams in most areas.

The way forward, according to the Audit Commission (1994b: 8) was to strengthen the leadership and management of the community mental health services. The government needed to reaffirm the commitment to comprehensive local services and to co-ordinate the responsibilities of the Departments of Health, Environment, Education, Employment, Social Security and the Home Office. The requirements for a comprehensive service needed to be drawn together at a strategic level, for which the Audit Commission (1994b) provided an early model (Figure 12.5) for inter-agency working.

In 1997, the Secretary of State for Health (1997b) (then Stephen Dorrell) acknowledged once again the importance of service co-ordination for the delivery of a comprehensive range of primary and specialist mental health services. The need was to ensure an effective partnership between the health and social care providers (in both the statutory and independent sectors) and other agencies, such as housing, education, employment and benefits agencies and the criminal justice system. To improve co-ordination four policy options were put forward:

- a new mental health and social care authority;
- a single authority responsibility;
- a joint health and social care body with a shared budget;
- agreed delegation of responsibilities.

Political developments overtook further action.

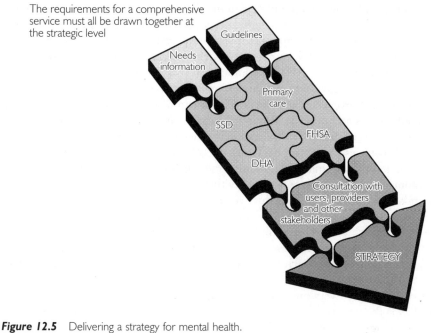

The requirements for a comprehensive service must all be drawn together at the strategic level

Guidelines

Needs information

Primary care

SSD

FHSA

DHA

Consultation with users, providers and other stakeholders

STRATEGY

Figure 12.5 Delivering a strategy for mental health.
Source: Audit Commission (1994b: 55) Exhibit 26.
Reproduced by kind permission of the Audit Commission.

Overall, tensions between the professions in community mental teams were reflected in racism and sexism; nor was interprofessional collaboration easily achieved (Leiba, 1994). However, partnership working was at the centre of the government's policy to ensure that comprehensive services were commissioned and provided in the best interests of the users. Further, interprofessional approaches could contribute to the prevention and management of conflict in mental health settings (Leiba, 1994).

A strategy for people with learning disabilities

Community teams for people with learning disabilities (sometimes called community mental handicap teams) were established earlier than mental health teams. Most team members worked in the community rather than in hospital. The range of services were more fully developed in the community than those for mental health, largely due to the fact that local authorities had taken a fuller role in the provision of services for people with learning disabilities. The 'ordinary life' and 'normalization' philosophies (Brown and Smith, 1992) provided a fundamental set of principles which accounted for the high level of integration in many community teams but which also unified members while allowing professional differences to exist without undermining the team (Ovretveit, 1993: 11).

The impact of the 1990 NHS and Community Act introduced care management and a new context for community teams. The services that a team provided now depended on managers and contracts with purchasers. More than careful planning and setting up a team were required; teams had to be managed, reviewed and evaluated. Various team models emerged to suit the local circumstances (Ovretveit, 1993: 209). In some areas only social workers were case co-ordinators of social care who might not necessarily be in a community mental handicap team; however, where mental handicap health and social services were integrated, nurses and other staff might be care managers.

To what extent were multidisciplinary team approaches for people with learning difficulties effective? McGrath (1991) undertook a study of different models of multidisciplinary community mental handicap teams in Wales. The disadvantages were mostly concerned with the inherent difficulties of teamwork (time taken to work together, dual loyalties to a profession/organization) but which were largely outweighed by the advantages. Positive factors included the more efficient use of staff resources through collaboration with professionals, a more satisfying work environment for staff and more effective service provision through the holistic approach to client needs, the encouragement of preventive work and the overall service planning and goal orientation. Group efforts were also more likely to give a more accurate assessment of needs.

By 1995, the government had placed a strategy for people with learning difficulties onto the Health of the Nation agenda (DoH, 1995c). The system for supporting people with learning disabilities was recognized as complex. The agencies involved included local authority social services departments, housing departments and housing associations, education authorities and schools, health services in primary care, hospitals and community health services, voluntary and private organizations. Collaboration and partnership between agencies were considered important in working towards meeting the needs of those with learning disabilities and using resources effectively. Working together for better health required alliances between all the agencies involved as well as with the people with learning disabilities, their families and carers.

The government's strategy for people with learning disabilities underlined the breadth of a programme that extended beyond health care provision to offer an integrated social welfare support programme.

13 HEALTH PROMOTION AND PREVENTIVE POLICIES: GENDER, RACE AND INEQUALITIES

Health and community care provision in Britain by the mid-1990s had demonstrated the width and depth of the programmes in hand. The breadth could be further seen in the development of health promotion initiatives and the New Public Health movement. However in turning to the place of gender and race, further demands and issues arose underlying the whole context, continuing inequalities in health remained but demonstrated the potential extent of the health care spectrum.

PROMOTING HEALTH FOR ALL

In the early 1990s, health promotion and preventive policies in Britain were influenced by the World Health Organization's (WHO) strategy of 'Health for All' and the subsequent Healthy Cities campaign.

Ashton (1992: 4) attributed the start of New Public Health to the work of McKeown (1976), who sought a synthesis between the environmental, personal, preventive and therapeutic eras. The emphasis was on public policy, individual behaviour and holistic health but within an ecological context. Further momentum was provided by the publication of the Lalonde Report (1974), which argued that improvements in health depended more on environmental and lifestyle changes than on health care and medical sciences.

From the Alma Ata declaration on primary health care in 1977, the World Health Organizsation furthered the New Public Health outlook through a series of initiatives based on the WHO's *Global Strategy for Health for All by the Year 2000* (WHO, 1981). The WHO's crusade, under the slogan Health for All by the Year 2000, emphasized five basic message for countries all round the world.

1 Within the resources available, the need to concentrate on first things first: to manage for results in terms of health status which meant, for example, public health and simple proven medical remedies.
2 To recognize the need for cross-sectional action: that health did not depend solely on medical care, so health had to be pursued through collaboration with other services.
3 The need to make individual and community participation real. Any other strategy was bound to fail because health was strongly influenced by personal and communal behaviour.
4 The need to pursue equity by reducing the wide disparities in health care and health status that typically existed between the poor and the rich, both because that was in line with justice and because that was how the greatest gains in health could be made.
5 The need to knit the levels of health services (primary, secondary and tertiary)

closely together in a mutually reinforcing network of referral and support and to do as much as possible on an ambulatory rather than an inpatient basis.

A European strategy for health was then formulated by the (European Regional) WHO (1984) Committee. Targets were endorsed by all the member states in 1985. The themes covered elements such as equity in health, health promotion and disease prevention, community participation, multisectoral collaboration, primary health care and international co-operation (WHO, 1985). The initiative to encourage 'Health for All by the Year 2000' much influenced developments in Britain.

The New Public Health

Within the NHS, which had taken more account of WHO statements than many other health care systems (Maxwell, 1988), the implications would point to strengthening cross-sectional action, individual and community participation and furthering referral and support networks, in order to remedy inequalities in health care and health status. Ashton and Seymour (1998) claimed that interest in public health had begun to revive in Britain. Disillusionment with the return on expenditure for hospital services, alongside growing recognition that most influences on health lay outside the medical sector, had switched attention to health promotion and public participation to improve many aspects of ordinary life. The New Public Health recognized the importance of social aspects of health problems (which were caused by lifestyles) but sought to avoid blaming the victim. Many health problems were thus seen as social, rather than individual, to be approached by local and national public policy. The New Public Health therefore sought to bring together environmental change and personal preventive measures with appropriate therapeutic interventions, especially for elderly and disabled people (Ashton and Seymour, 1998).

Healthy cities

The rationale for focusing on public health in towns and cities was a reflection of the rising numbers of people (some 75% of Europeans and a majority of the world's population) who would be living in cities by the year 2000. Following a meeting in Lisbon, of representatives from 21 European cities in 1986, the Healthy Cities Project adopted specific interventions aimed at improving health, based on Health for All principles (Ashton, 1992: 6–9). At local level in Britain, Oxford Regional Health Authority attempted to create a coherent health promotion strategy by setting up miniature projects based on the Healthy Cities approach (Griffiths 1991a, b). Healthy Liverpool (Ashton, 1992) and Healthy Sheffield (Witney and Moody, 1992) used the principles of locality planning and locality groups to enable multisectoral collaboration to establish a community health agenda based on a collective response to health needs. Similarly, Healthy Harlow sought to encourage community participation from voluntary organizations, local authorities and health educators to empower individuals to express their needs. Newcastle Healthy City brought together over 40 agencies and parent groups to work on a child accident prevention strategy (Ranade, 1997: 181). Locality planning was sporadic elsewhere, but had taken initial shape in Pimlico, London; Exeter, Devon; and Sittingbourne, in Kent where locality groups had set out to develop a partnership between the state and the community, between elected officials and local activity, to further health and welfare in the community (Heginbotham, 1990).

Assessing outcomes and achievements almost defied definition, given the complexity of the programmes across Europe although, in terms of health outcomes, good progress had been made in achieving many of the targets, albeit undermined by widening inequalities. The importance of the Health for All and Healthy Cities strategies had more to do with the process rather than the goals, in developing new approaches to health which cut across traditional functions and agency boundaries, to create coalitions and partnerships through working with local communities (Ranade, 1997: 184).

Developments in health promotion

Health promotion had formed a key concept in the strategy of Health for All through promoting health education, prevention of illness and health protection. Taken together with the importance of health promotion in the New Public Health, the approach sought to involve the population actively in the setting of everyday life rather than focussing on contact with medical services. The concept was also directed towards the causes of ill health. The aim was to promote lifestyles conducive to health but linked to prevention, rehabilitation and health services. The emphasis on health promotion continued with the recommendations of the Acheson Report (1988), on the future development of the public health function, setting out to improve the organization, as well as the availability of trained manpower and resources which, in turn, led to the appointment of directors of public Health and the production of annual reports on the local population's health.

By 1990, the NHS reforms also had important implications for public health, health promotion and the prevention of illness through the split between the purchasing and provision of health care. The purchasing authorities now had the responsibility to assess the health needs of their populations and would determine the importance of health promotion.

In 1991, the Conservative Prime Minister, John Major, brought together a group of health experts who produced a consultative document on a national health strategy (DoH, 1991c). Although the consultation paper (DoH, 1991c) acknowledged the Health for All strategy and targets, the outcome fell short of WHO's principles (Ranade, 1997: 186): neither equity in health nor the place of health inequalities and their causes were given serious consideration. However, as a result of extensive consultation, the White Paper *Health of the Nation* (DoH, 1992b) did emerge.

Health of the Nation

The aims of the *Health of the Nation* (DoH, 1992b) programme were:

- to promote health and prevent illness;
- to improve diagnosis, treatment and rehabilitation; and
- to maintain and improve environmental quality.

The overall goal was 'to add years to life and life to years'. The intent was to combine public policies, healthy surroundings and lifestyles with high quality health services. The strategy of health gain was also identified as important in achieving the goals set by the government. The concept of health gain was perceived as a useful tool by which to assess the policy or programme to pursue – which then raised the question of priorities in cost-benefit terms (Allsop, 1995: 232). Much would depend on monitoring people's health as well as on research into ways of improving health, especially in tackling variations between groups.

The criteria for choosing areas for action were that areas should be major causes of premature death or avoidable ill health and amenable to effective intervention, within which it would be possible to set objectives, targets and monitor progress. The five key areas identified for action were:

- coronary heart disease and strokes;
- cancers;
- mental illness;
- HIV/AIDS and sexual health;
- accidents.

Support for Healthy Cities was to be promoted by government assistance of the Health for All 2000 network in order to increase localities. The list of healthy environments to promote was extensive: healthy schools, healthy hospitals, healthy workplaces, healthy homes, even healthy prisons.

A ministerial cabinet committee, drawn from 11 government departments, was established to oversee health strategies in England as well as to co-ordinate health policy across the UK (the Scottish and Welsh Offices were responsible for the arrangements in Scotland and Wales). In looking at the outcomes, while some Health of the Nation initiatives contained flaws, the strategic emphasis on 'healthy alliances' was an important development.

Healthy alliances

The government clearly identified joint action within 'healthy alliances' as an important way to develop strategies for preventive health. Inter-sectoral arrangements were envisaged at two levels. The ministerial cabinet committee would operate at one strategic level, to enable the government to produce guidance on policy appraisal and health and to ensure that the consequences of policies were taken into account in further developments. The Department of Health would consult with the 'wider health' working group to prepare and consult on guidance about promoting healthy alliances. At a further level, a range of organizations were identified as crucial to healthy alliances (the NHS, the Health Education Authority, local authorities, voluntary organizations, the media) in settings that would contribute to the nation's health – such as schools, cities, the work place and homes.

By 1993, the DoH was promoting a positive view (*Working Together for Better Health*; DoH, 1993c) in order to meet the 'challenging' targets set by the Health of the Nation programmes. Commitment of time, energy and resources were envisaged to lead, through healthy alliances, to the more effective use of resources, broadening responsibility for health, to break down barriers between partners in the alliances, to promote better knowledge and understanding of partners, to improve the exchange of information and provide the opportunity to develop accessible, seamless services.

Wistow and Fuller (1986) had cautioned that aspirations and motivations of economic benefit and responsive community-based services could conflict with each other and that the objectives of health, social services and housing departments and voluntary organizations could compete. Alan Beattie (1994: 119) later pointed out that partnerships in professional work, rather like partnerships in families and private lives, very much rested on the making of bonds and the formation of attachments. What were intended as healthy alliances could easily become 'dangerous liaisons'.

The Health of the Nation appraised

Overall, the White Paper (DoH, 1992b) was well received as the first clear intention to give the NHS a positive direction in a health context, while providing a detailed strategy for implementation. The Department of Health and the NHS Executive had pursued the *Health of the Nation* programmes; progress had been made; information had improved. Further extensions of the programme were also made for particular groups such as those with learning difficulties (DoH, 1995c). However, flaws began to surface.

First, the five targets contained limitations. The chosen areas tended to reflect particular government concerns at the time, such as the incidence of coronary heart disease (the death rate in the UK continued to be the highest in the world; Smith and Jacobsen, 1988). Next, by June 1992, of the nearly 6000 people who had been reported as having AIDS, over half had died (CSO, 1993: 100). Many other areas of health were omitted from the targets. Ranade (1997: 189) has cited the increasing incidence of asthma as one major omission which affected one child in ten.

Secondly, the government stopped short of a ban on tobacco advertising and undertook no comprehensive approach to tackling smoking and ill health. Various programmes were suggested: an inter-departmental task force to set up and implement a comprehensive strategy to reduce smoking, for the DoH and the Health Education Authority to develop proposals for a major health education programme on smoking. Under the target to address cancers, the strong association between a number of illnesses and smoking made the activity an ideal target for prevention policies. However, the programme did not involve the tobacco industry which would have raised a number of problematical financial and political issues.

Thirdly, some have pointed out that the policies for prevention remained focussed on individual behaviour, while locked into the structure and culture of the NHS (Allsop, 1995: 232) dominated by medical definitions of health.

Fourthly, but more fundamentally, the idea that social deprivation could be responsible for ill health was missing from the *Health of the Nation* programme. Such a flaw, argued Limb (1992), shirked the acceptance of an explicit connection between ill health and poverty which would justify demands for concerted economic action to reduce social deprivation. The White Paper (DoH, 1992b) did briefly address the subject of health inequalities between sections of the population, but attributed health discrepancies partly to increases in 'risk behaviour', while commenting that the reasons for health variations were by no means fully understood in the light of the complex interplay of genetic, biological, social, environmental, cultural and behavioural factors.

The *Health of the Nation* approach was effectively a government response to the Health for All WHO initiative, but trimmed onto a targeted basis. Despite the flaws in the proposals, the *Health of the Nation* did present a strategy to improve the nation's health. The next question was: how far would the strategy make a positive impact on the nation's health?

ISSUES OF GENDER

In the UK, men outnumbered women in each age group until the mid-forties, when the numbers were approximately equal. Women then increasingly outnumber men until, at the age of 89, there were some three women to every one man (Office for National Statistics, 1998: 32).

One major implication of the gender ratio was that the increasing problem of caring for people in old age was, more particularly, an issue of caring for elderly women. Then again, women were more likely than men to consult a general practitioner. In 1996/7, the proportion was 19% for females and 13% for males, while those of 4 and under or 65 and over consulted a GP more than other age groups (Office for National Statistics, 1998: 135). Whether a reflection of the proportionate numbers involved it remains that women's health issues tended to dominate press reports, especially over cancer screening programmes.

Causes of death vary considerably with age and gender. Circulatory diseases were the main causes of death in men aged 35 years and over but breast cancer was one of the most common causes of death for women aged under 65 in the UK. Here was one targeted element of the 1992 *Health of the Nation* programme, so what had been the outcome? The NHS breast screening programme had already been introduced between 1988 and 1990. Women aged 50–64 were invited for screening every three years; the screening was also available to women aged 65 and over on request. Similar programmes had also been set up in Wales, Scotland and Northern Ireland. In 1995–6, 1.5 million women were invited for screening in the UK: the uptake was 76%; cancers were detected in just under 6000 women screened. Uptake had increased from 71% in 1991–2 (Office for National Statistics, 1998: 134–5). Further, more than a million women each year were screened and recalled every three years, in the 50 to 64-year age group. Significantly by 1996, deaths in the UK from breast cancer were falling by about 10% in all age groups – and in the screening group by 13% (Boseley, 1999a).

Nevertheless, the death rate due to breast cancer remained higher in Britain than almost anywhere else in the world, while the quality of breast cancer services varied greatly across the country. Concern about cancer treatment prompted the Calman-Hine Report (1995). Amongst the recommendations to improve services, one particularly reflected the *Health of the Nation* outlook, with the focus on collaboration in commissioning future cancer services, while encouraging professionals to work together across the different sectors and levels of care.

However, headlines subsequently proclaimed: 'OUTRAGE AT BREAST SCREENING DOUBTS' (The *Guardian*, 12 March 1999). Anxious women jammed the phones of the National Screening Programme after a Swedish study claimed that regular mammography did not prevent deaths from breast cancer. Michael Baum, from University College, London, who was one of those who had set up the screening programme, believed that the programme was flawed, while much of the annual £34 billion cost could be better spent on treating cancer patients (Boseley, 1999a).

A separate screening programme also existed for cervical cancer. In England, of the 3.8 million women screened in 1995–6 who had a result from tests (not all tests contained suitable material for analysis), over 94% were negative (Office for National Statistics, 1998: 134). All women aged 20–64 were intended to be screened at least once every five years. The acceptance for the programme was about 86%, although only half of those invited came forward in some inner city areas. More headlines declared: 'POSITIVE RESULTS VARY FIVE-FOLD IN TESTS FOR CERVICAL CANCER' (*The Times*, 21 February 1996). The percentage of women diagnosed with early warning signs of cervical cancer was five times higher in some parts of England than in others. The wide variation could not be accounted for by variations in the incidence of the disease, which meant that some women at risk of cancer were being missed while others were being needlessly worried. Confidence in the screening programme had been dented by a number of cases of smears being improperly taken or wrongly diagnosed (Laurance, 1996). On the more positive side Sir Kenneth Calman, then Chief Medical Officer of Health, claimed that the cervical screening programme was one of the best in the world, but improvements in the new guidance given to hospitals on reading smears could help to avoid repetition of previous mistakes (Mihill, 1996c).

On coronary heart disease, another *Health of the Nation* target, the male death rate had been falling significantly (to 68 deaths per thousand population in the UK by 1996: Figure 13.1). Although death rates from heart disease and breast cancer were gradually falling amongst women (Figure 13.1), both causal factors continued to be the most common causes of death for women under 65 (Office for National Statistics, 1998).

The reduction in HIV/AIDS cases in the UK could be seen as a further positive outcome of the *Health of the Nation* targets on sexual health. The number of AIDS cases had dropped from 24 per million in 1991 to 16 in 1996, the lowest number since 1988. However, the rate of new diagnosed cases of AIDS had also been declining across the European Union since the peak in 1994

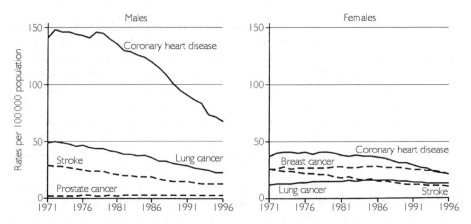

Figure 13.1   UK death rates (per 100 000 population) for people aged under 65: by gender and selected cause of death. Rates age-standardized to the 1971 population level.
Source: Office for National Statistics (1998: 136).
Crown copyright material reproduced with the permission of the Controller of Her Majesty's Stationery Office.

for various reasons, which included the discovery of preventative measures (Office for National Statistics, 1998: 129).

The *Health of the Nation* programme had also identified prevention of pregnancy among girls under 16 as a priority, with a target to reduce the rate of conceptions from 9.6 per 1000 (1989) to 4.8 per 1000 by the year 2000. Although conception rates in England and Wales had fallen from 9.3 per 1000 girls under 16 years in 1991 to 8.5 per 1000 in 1995 (Office for National Statistics, 1998: 54), Dickson et al. (1997) argued that the target for 2000 was unlikely to be met. Preventing and reducing the adverse effects of unintended teenage pregnancies require co-ordinated education, contraceptive and counselling services. However, the teenage conception rates and burden of pregnancy were higher in more deprived areas, while a key factor associated with deferred pregnancy was a good general education (Dickson et al., 1997), which pointed to one aspect of inequalities in health.

Human fertilization, embryology and abortion

Amongst the targets not covered by the *Health of the Nation* programmes was the issue of infertility – an aspect of sexual health of immense importance to a minority of women. After six years of debate (see Chapter 6) in the light of the Warnock Report's (1984) recommendations on embryo research and related elements, the 1990 *Human Fertilization and Embryology Act* was eventually passed. More banner headlines accompanied the breakthrough: 'MPs BACK CONTINUED EMBRYO RESEARCH: HUGE MAJORITY ENDS SIX-YEAR BATTLE AFTER EMOTIONAL DEBATE' (The *Independent*, 20 April 1990). MPs voted by a majority in favour of continuation of embryo research, which helped to sway the Commons against restricting abortion (Brown, 1990).

The 1990 *Human Fertilization and Embryology Act* prohibited bringing about the creation, keeping or using human embryos outside the body in the treatment of infertility (amongst other conditions), except under a licence from the Human Fertilization and Embryology Authority. The 1990 legislation accepted the Warnock Report's (1984) case for embryo research to be allowed up to a 14-day limit. Further, after a marathon series of votes on changing the 1967 *Abortion Act*, the 1990 *Human Fertilization and Embryology Act* also included a change in the abortion time limit. The upper time limit for most abortions was to be brought down from 28 weeks to 24 weeks' gestation. Two exemptions substantially liberalized the abortion law. One permitted abortion, without any limit of time, where there was substantial risk that the child would be born seriously physically or mentally handicapped. The second exemption similarly permitted abortion, without limit of time, if the birth were to cause grave permanent injury to the mother's physical or mental health.

The Times (1990) reflected on a question of tolerance in considering the outcome of the 1990 legislation. Law did not determine the morality of an action but sought to interpret morality where society had concluded that regulation was needed. What then remained was tolerance. The task of drawing a line in a matter which some people regarded as of life and death would never be uncontroversial: human fertilization, embryology and abortion thus represented the more controversial aspects of health promotion and prevention.

Had infertility treatment on the NHS been subject to a target of any sort, substantial inequalities would have been revealed. Infertile couples who sought *in vitro* fertilization faced a financial lottery. NHS costs varied widely across the country (Revill, 1997; Friend, 1998a). A report from the Human Fertilization and Embryology Authority (1995) revealed variations in the success rates of the UK IVF clinics, both private and NHS. Furthermore, the amount of infertility treatment funded by health authorities was falling significantly and was based on eligibility criteria such as age, number of previous children or simply funds available (National Infertility Awareness Campaign, 1999).

Health promotion for men

Towards the end of the 1990s Viagra, the pill against impotence, brought men's health into the headlines: 'HEALTHY' MAN, 65, HAD HEART ATTACK AFTER TAKING VIAGRA' (The *Guardian*, 18 September 1998). The introduction of Viagra had two immediate effects. First, the place of health promotion for men and the somewhat overlooked aspect of men's health generally came more into public focus. Secondly, Viagra immediately raised the issue of NHS rationing. The estimated cost of Viagra on the NHS was between £50 and £150 million a year. A ban on the NHS prescription of Viagra was designed to act as a holding measure while the Department of Health could work out the implications. Viagra tablets were to be available on private prescription from pharmacies (Boseley, 1998a) although this was later to change (see Chapter 15). However, by 1999, the government continued to spend eight times more on women's health than on men's, when doctors called for men's health issues to be taken more seriously and treated more sensitively (Hall, 1999b).

ISSUES OF RACE

Health care provision for black people and ethnic minorities

By 1996–7, ethnic minorities represented 6% of the total population of Great Britain (3.4 million people). However, ethnic groups had various backgrounds: Black Caribbeans, Black Africans, other black groups, Chinese and other groups. Over two-fifths of the Pakistani/Bangladeshi group were aged under 16, while only 3% were aged 65, in contrast to the white population of 16% aged over 65 and only one-fifth aged under 16 (Office for National Statistics, 1998: 34). Overall, the needs and backgrounds of all ethnic groups varied significantly.

By November 1991, the King's Fund acknowledged, in the newsletter *Share*, that the NHS had become more sensitive to the needs of minority groups. A steady stream of position papers had been produced by health authorities on good practice and on ethnically sensitive health care provision. Mohammed (1991) also welcomed the main thrust of the 1990 reform package in the split between the purchasing and providing roles of health care. A range of opportunities could be opened up to black people on the new boards of the trust hospitals; trusts could also become more responsive to the needs of black and ethnic minority users. The need for fundamental change was pressing as most black people still received a qualitatively and quantitatively worse service than the white population. The response of the health services had been either to neglect or to marginalize the needs of ethnic minorities.

As one illustration of the problems that faced the non-white population, Val Durham (1993), from the Hammersmith and Fulham Council for Racial Equality, pointed out that the Tomlinson Report (1992) on London's health services had avoided the contentious issues of inequality of access and implicit racism. No link had been made between social deprivation, ill health and the ethnic minority communities – who were often concentrated in the poorest sectors of the community, with inferior housing, unemployment, homelessness and poor working conditions, all of which contributed to the high rate of illnesses among these populations. Consultation and accountability were also conspicuous by their absence in the Tomlinson Report (1992); the black community was thus denied an opportunity to express any views on the proposed health changes.

The (then) Secretary of State for Health, Virginia Bottomley (1993), expressed her determination to ensure equality of opportunity in the NHS for the employment, training, promotion and equality of access to services for all sections of the community and to tackle racial disadvantage in NHS employment. Even so, the discriminatory barriers which faced black and ethnic minority health workers continued (Ling, 1993).

One way forward, in Ranger's (1994) view, was ethnic monitoring. Such a method could ensure that effective systems were in place to establish epidemiological patterns to help purchasers with needs assessment as well as to assist in providing more accessible and appropriate services.

By 1995 the King's Fund team, who undertook a major survey of inequalities in health (Benzeval et al., 1995: 127), acknowledged that those who classified themselves as belonging to a minority ethnic group had a high probability of experiencing particularly acute forms of disadvantage which exacerbated health inequalities. Racism and discrimination needed further investigation. However, for all relatively neglected groups, determination was required to examine the factors that inhibited good health and to identify and promote interventions that would improve health status.

INEQUALITIES IN HEALTH

In acknowledging the significance of health inequalities, Benzeval et al. (1995: 125) drew attention not only to ethnic differences: gender differences were also linked to the way health was affected by deprivation. However, more research was needed to understand social inequalities in health among women.

Some 13 years after publication, Douglas Black (1993) felt the need to defend his controversial report on *Inequalities in Health* (Black Report, 1980). The main findings were reiterated once again: the undeniable importance of poverty, which had been aggravated in the intervening years by fiscal policies, together with increased levels of unemployment. A prime recommendation of the Black Report (1980) was that children of poor families should be given a better start in life.

Social class inequalities

Whitehead and Drever's (1997) survey revealed that the gap between upper and lower social classes had widened. The nation had become more unequal under the Conservatives in the 1980s. In the period 1987–91, men could expect to live an average of 72.3 years and women an average 77.9 years but, although the figures were continuing to improve at the top end of the social ladder, the figures had stopped doing so at the bottom. Between 1982–86 and 1987–91, life expectancy in the social classes 4 and 5 – semi-skilled and unskilled occupations, respectively – fell from 69.8 years to 69.7. However, the overall life expectancy in Britain was close to the European Union average. Nevertheless, Benzeval et al. (1995: 128) demonstrated clearly that people with low income had poorer health status than those who were more affluent.

Unemployment

The Office of Population Census and Surveys (Smith, 1996: 22) compared data from the 1970s and 1980s which showed that mortality among unemployed people was significantly higher than that in the general population of men of working age. Despite repeated studies which revealed the impact of unemployment on health (OHE, 1993), ministers were reluctant to accept that joblessness caused illness and early death (Brindle, 1996f), although the causal links between unemployment and poor health have been disputed (Benzeval et al., 1995: 133). Nevertheless, the latest evidence suggested that people with poor health were more likely to be forced out of the labour market, while unemployment also led to avoidable morbidity and premature mortality, poverty, low self-esteem and social isolation.

Homelessness

Homeless people represented another vulnerable group with greater health needs than other groups. In research examining the distribution, health use and funding implications of London's homeless populations, a King's Fund Institute study (Sheuer et al., 1991) found that homeless people used planned acute hospital services 2.5 times more than other people in London. In a further study on homeless people and health care in the London area, Shiner and Leddington (1991) found that mainstream services tended to exclude homeless people by failing to take account of their personal circumstances. Homeless people preferred services to be located within the landscape of their homelessness: only 9% of the people interviewed were using the mainstream GP services as a major source of health care, when a relationship with a sympathetic doctor had usually been established. Although homeless people had more negative feelings about hospital accident and emergency departments than any other aspect of the health services, the main attraction of access to health care via the emergency section was the ability to be seen without an appointment – which, in turn, led to persistent 'inappropriate' use of such departments by a small group of people. Wall (1991) reported that in some areas of Swindon homeless people were victimized, while some GPs were reluctant, or refused, to register homeless people – who were seen as a mobile, poorly motivated population, unlikely to comply with immunization and screening programmes, which would affect practice targets. Accident and emergency departments were used as a substitute for the inadequacy or non-availability of GP services.

A King's Fund report advised on how the needs of homeless people could be incorporated into contracts but stressed that homeless people should not be discharged from hospital unless housing and support had been organized. Health needs should not be seen in isolation but met in collaboration with local authorities and the voluntary sector (Maxwell, 1992), a view supported by commentary on the earlier King's Fund study (Sheuer, 1991).

By 1996, Shelter had undertaken a major review of the use of the accident and emergency department at University College Hospital, London which showed that only 30% of the homeless attenders were known to be registered with a GP, while 57% of visits could be classed as 'inappropriate' (North et al., 1996). Many who had visited the department could easily have been treated in general practice. The study revealed a picture of the health of homeless people – the prevalence of illness, the inability to get help from primary providers while forced to use accident and emergency access to health care. The report identified another dimension of the costs of homelessness – that health was a housing issue. Emergency health care facilities were patching up the problem caused by a failed housing system (North et al., 1996).

The main determinants of health

In seeking to address the place of inequalities in health, the model, set out by Benzeval et al. (1995), illustrated the complexities of the arena. Figure (13.2)

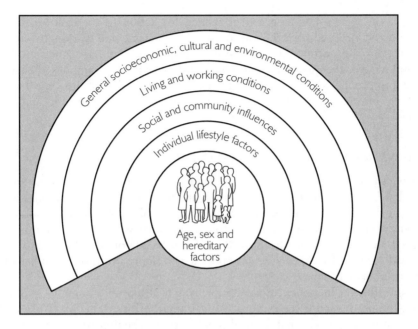

Figure 13.2   The main determinants of health. Benzeval et al. (1995: 23).
Source: Dahlgren and Whitehead (1991) Policies and Strategies to Promote Social Equity. Figure 1, Stockholm: Institute for Future Studies.
Reproduced by kind permission from the King's Fund.

sets out how layers of influences have made an impact on an individual's health: from individual lifestyle factors which then stretched across to social and community influences, living and working conditions to a range of wider conditions in society. For example, the place of women in society or attitudes to minority communities could influence their standard of living and socio-economic position (Benzeval et al., 1995: 23).

In seeking to tackle inequalities in health, Benzeval et al. (1995) came up with a series of recommendations which included:

- improving educational opportunities for the most disadvantaged young people;
- examination of the factors that inhibited the prospects of good health among ethnic minorities and other relatively neglected social groups;
- furthering understanding, through research, about social inequalities in health among women, although measures of socio-economic status needed to embrace the experience of both women and men;
- recognition that pre-school education was essential for making the most of formal schooling and raising educational standards in deprived areas;
- addressing unemployment, amongst other social deprivation factors, through taxes, benefits, wage subsidies, new patterns of work and entrepreneurship.

Overall, the King's Fund's practical agenda for action to tackle inequalities in health was concerned with the improvement of housing and working conditions, the social and economic influences of income, wealth and levels of unemployment, the quality of social relationships and social support, the barriers to adopting a healthier personal lifestyle and preventive health care (such as smoking prevention) and access to appropriate, effective health and social services.

NEW WAYS TO IMPROVE HEALTH PROMOTION

The width of the health inequalities agenda also reflected the broad span of intended health promotion programmes. By the mid-1990s, the *Health of the Nation* pathways could be seen more clearly in the place of health promotion and preventive health care. As has been shown, outcomes were mixed in terms of the original aims. However, Thornton (1996), on behalf of the Health Promotion Network, argued for an even wider approach to the health promotion agenda of health authorities (Figure 13.3).

To be effective in influencing and improving health promotion in local communities, the need was for the outlook of health authorities to be broad-based. The argument presented was that for health promotion to be limited to the level of the individual was flawed, as such an approach failed to acknowledge the root causes of ill health: social, economic, political and environmental. As Figure 13.3 shows, the model suggested that a health authority-led health promotion activity needed:

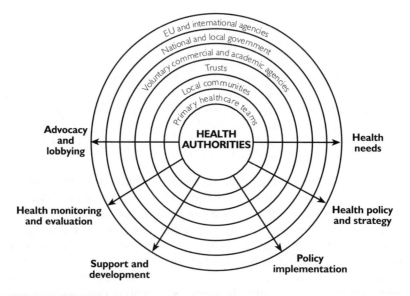

Figure 13.3   A model for health authorities to promote health.
Source: Thornton (1996).
Reproduced by kind permission of the Health Service Journal.

- to encourage fundamental structural, cultural and environmental changes at macro level;
- to ensure health-enhancing policies at a city, town or country level as well as to develop supportive environments;
- to strengthen local communities' capacity for community action;
- to strengthen individuals by developing their knowledge, skills and coping abilities;
- to lobby to improve access to existing health services and resources through programmes of advocacy.

Upholding the model was a strategy for implementation, based on advocacy, on support and development programmes to meet health needs and on programmes for the monitoring and evaluation of health promotion policies (Thornton, 1996).

The Health Promotion Network recognized that little progress could be made without stronger government support. Although a number of NHS Executive initiatives, such as the *Health of the Nation* programme and the pursuit of a primary care-led NHS, had focussed on health improvement as well as on the health authorities' responsibility for delivery, nevertheless, more guidance was needed to give greater prominence to health promotion. Furthermore, the interface between the health promotion role of local authorities and health authorities required co-ordination with other central government departments (Thornton, 1996).

However, any further potential developments, whether concerned with health promotion, illness prevention, the place of inequalities or the wider structure and delivery of health and social care, were all held in suspence as Britain prepared for the general election of May 1997.

14 NEW LABOUR: THE NEW NHS

On Friday 2 May 1997, Britain woke up to a political earthquake. New Labour had won a landslide victory, to capture 44% of the vote, 419 seats in Parliament; the Conservatives gained only 31%, with only 165 seats, while the Liberal Democrats had secured a significant increase with 46 seats and 17% of the vote. As *The Guardian* (1997a) commented, 1997 joined 1945 and 1906 as the third great progressive electoral landslide of the twentieth century. After eleven years of Mrs Thatcher's Conservative administration, from 1989 to the Cabinet coup in 1990 which brought in John Major as successor, whose one abiding legacy was likely to be the introduction of a national lottery, the New Labour leadership clinched the most decisive election landslide since 1931. The country had grown tired of a party which appeared to be arrogant, uncaring and non-listening.

The victory was three-fold. First, Tony Blair, the youngest Prime Minister since Lord Liverpool in 1812, brought in principles, objectives and hard-headed idealism. Secondly, the Labour party had undergone a change in political culture whose professionalism had opened up a new political era. Thirdly, the British public's priorities were those which New Labour had set out to meet: middle-of-the-road economic management, no higher taxation; better run public services, a limited, but pragmatic, agenda (Young, 1997).

What would be the impact on the Welfare State? What were the outcomes to be for health care provision?

NEW LABOUR'S VISION FOR A RENEWED WELFARE STATE

A stakeholding society

As New Labour approached the general election in 1997, Mr Blair's big new idea was to encourage a stakeholding society. The catchphrase stressed the notion that everyone would have a stake in society. Key elements for individuals and businesses to become more dynamic and innovative included: economic investment, harnessing technology, helping small businesses to succeed, building on science, research and a modern transport system, as well as developing people. New Labour welcomed competitive markets as the most efficient means of meeting consumers' needs, through offering choice and stimulating innovation, but a market that would be regulated in which inequalities had to be addressed. Rather than centralized 'statist' solutions to socio-economic problems, New Labour's aim would be to enable people to work together to achieve for themselves and for their fellow citizens. The job of government was to set the right framework (Mandelson and Liddle, 1995).

Blair's (1996, 1998) vision of a stakeholder economy was to create an education system for all, to ensure full employment, to encourage in industry an ethic of long-term partnership and co-operation, to return to the founding principles of the Welfare State and to reform the system in order to assist people out of welfare dependency. A stakeholder economy was to enable a fair and inclusive society.

Applied to Community Care, Alan Milburn (1996), when shadow Social Services Minister, outlined stakeholding for users and carers who would have a fuller stake in determining community care standards. New Labour would wish to see agreed, enforced national standards to overcome unacceptable variations in community care.

Applied to detailed complexity of health care provision, stakeholding implied the replacement of the internal market with a system based on co-operation and efficiency. Reversing the rise in emergency hospital admissions would be a high priority, together with a greater emphasis on bed management. A moratorium on closing mental health beds would be introduced; fundholding would be replaced with a flexible GP commissioning model. Innovations included a ban on tobacco advertising, the appointment of a Minister for Public Health and the creation of a foods standards agency. No promises were made about resources, but Labour's health policy would seek the essential foundations of good health, a modern, high-quality NHS, resources prioritized for front-line services and health care facilities accessible to patients whatever their background (Davies et al., 1996). Beds, not bureaucracy, was a major priority in New Labour's political manifesto (Labour Party, 1996). Under the banner of *Stakeholder Welfare* (Field et al., 1996), those with an interest in Welfare State reform increasingly took up the challenge of thinking the unthinkable.

The vision and the reality by 1997

With a new team in office, New Labour lost no time in establishing the political, economic and welfare agenda. Cabinet appointments of relevance to social welfare included John Prescott as Deputy Prime Minister, Gordon Brown as Chancellor of the Exchequer, Jack Straw as Home Secretary, David Blunkett as Education and Employment Secretary, Harriet Harman as Social Security Secretary and Frank Dobson as Health Secretary.

All was speed and action. Mr Blair pledged a shake-up for the Welfare State as the first Labour government's programme for nearly 20 years was presented in the Queen's Speech in mid-May. The government's main bills were to cover the following areas.

- *Education:* reduction of class sizes, raising teaching standards through training.
- *Devolution:* referenda would be held for a Scottish Parliament and Welsh Assembly.
- *Law and order:* all handguns would be banned and the punishment of young offenders speeded up.
- *Local government:* creation of an elected mayor and new authority for London.
- *Lottery:* redistribution of funds for education and health projects such as keep-fit clubs in healthy living centres.

- *Finance:* a windfall tax would be imposed on privatized utilities to enable 250 000 young people to move off welfare and into work.
- *Health:* plans to outlaw tobacco advertising were outlined.
- *Employment:* a national minimum wage would be set.
- *Business:* small firms would be allowed to claim interest on debts.
- *House of Lords reform:* while not included in the Queen's Speech, New Labour was committed to scrapping the voting and sitting rights of hereditary peers.

New Labour's approach, in the first Queen's speech, was more evolutionary than revolutionary. However, Mr Blair made plain that the drive to modernize the Welfare State and to tackle the £90 billion social security bill were two of the main priorities. All the new measures sought to represent an alliance between progress and justice. The mandate was clear: to modernize what was outdated; to make fair what was unjust; and to do both by the best means available (Webster, 1997). The era of neat phrasing, political catchphrases and buzz words had truly arrived. The most telling of all was: The Third Way.

The Third Way

By March 1998, the distinctive features which characterized Tony Blair's ambition to reform the Welfare State had become clear. The main thrust of Mr Blair's reforms was to shift the balance away from financing pensions and cash benefits towards the provision of better public services – above all, through the education and health systems, through new support programmes for disabled people, for single parents and for retraining unemployed people. The Tory attitude of free-market individualism had wanted to roll back the boundaries of the Welfare State by reducing both taxes and public spending but encouraging people to buy services from the private sector through cash benefits rather than by providing public sector services. Mr Blair's attitude stood in contrast. The pillars of the new Welfare State were to be the publicly managed health and education services, generously financed by taxes and equally accessible to all. High-quality public services were identified as the hallmarks of a modern Welfare State. Mr Blair's political project was to drive between free market capitalism and nineteenth-century Utopian socialism from which his inspiration had been drawn. Tony Blair defined a new blend of collectivism and individualism as New Labour's Third Way (Kaletsky, 1998).

In March 1998, Tony Blair went to Paris to address the French national assembly on Franco–British co-operation and the need for a new political vision of Europe. 'Je vais vous parler en français', said Mr Blair to applause, having gained French language skills as a young man working in a Paris bar (Hoggart, 1998). The real issue was to redefine the role of government in order to provide security in a world of change. Four guidelines were outlined: prudent financial and monetary policy; a shift in the role of government from regulation to equipping people for economic change through education, skills and technology; high-quality infrastructure; and a Welfare State that promoted work. Mr Blair

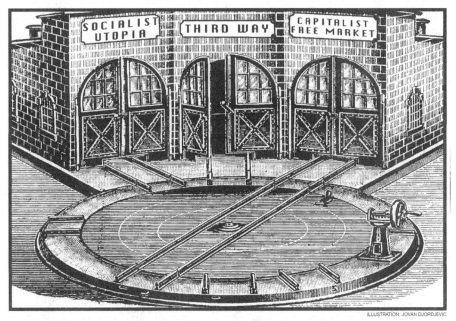

ILLUSTRATION: JOVAN DJORDJEVIC

Is there such a thing as a Third Way in politics?

Source: *The Guardian, Saturday Review, 23 May 1998.*
Reproduced by kind permission of *The Guardian* and *Jovan Djordjevic.*

then defined The Third Way: 'La Troisième Voie' was not *laissez-faire* nor state control and rigidity, but active government linked to improving the employ-ability of the workforce, based on a political and economic framework in touch with ordinary people (Riddell, 1998).

In September 1998, Tony Blair travelled to New York to attend Hilary Clinton's Third Way conference. However as Robert Reich (1998) argued, The Third Way needed courage to follow. The First Way involved redistribution of income and the creation of generous social safety nets. The Second Way (via President Ronald Reagan and Prime Minister Margaret Thatcher in the 1980s) rested on deregulation, privatization, free trade, flexible labour markets and fiscal austerity. The Third Way argued for economic growth, spurred on by free-market policies, to be shared widely, but to succeed required a political movement based on a social contract and furthered by an activist government.

How was The Third Way to apply to health policy in Britain? As health care managers might ponder on the relevance for the immediate action needed in the NHS to clear waiting lists, Professor David Hunter (1998a) felt that little of lasting or added value was likely to accrue for the health sector. Although the main themes of The Third Way were clear, inconsistencies between communitarianism and strengthening the role of central government made predictions difficult. For many, the concept remained elusive. However, by the July 1997 budget, Chancellor Gordon Brown had made an extra £1.2 billion available for the NHS and £1 billion for schools (*The Guardian*, 1997b).

THE NEW NHS

From the election of New Labour in May 1997, changes in the provision of health care were widespread. The next section will therefore look at the key moves as they emerged in the early stages with, amongst other initiatives, the NHS league tables and targets for waiting lists. The main points of the White Paper *The New NHS: Modern and Dependable* (Secretary of State for Health, 1997c) and the separate implications for Scotland, Wales, Northern Ireland and London will be reviewed, followed by an analysis of the outcomes in Britain. The renewed emphasis on inequalities in health will also be considered, together with the place of social exclusion and social care.

The newly appointed Secretary of State for Health, Frank Dobson, acquired a strong team at the Department of Health. With wide experience, both as a health authority member and Founder Director of the National Aids Trust, Baroness Jay became Health Minister in the House of Lords; the very able Alan Milburn was appointed Minister of Health with a remit to cover management, financial and structural issues as well as training and primary care. Tessa Jowell, with long-held connections in social services and in mental health, as Assistant Director of Mind among other appointments, became Public Health Minister; while an up and coming politician, lawyer Paul Boateng, took over responsibilities for mental health and social care as Junior Health Minister. Within 20 months, due to various unexpected political events elsewhere, Paul Boateng had moved to the Home Office, Alan Milburn, regarded as a young Blairite modernizer, was promoted to a Cabinet post as Chief Secretary to the Treasury (White and Hencke, 1998) and Baroness Jay became Leader of the House of Lords. Across the first year and three-quarters, a spate of changes and innovations were announced from the Department of Health.

The first 100 days in office

During the first 100 days of office a number of measures were taken, charted by Crail (1997), which included:

- *Day 19:* the eighth wave of GP fundholding applications was deferred while new models of commissioning were developed.
- *Day 21:* Frank Dobson said that management costs were to be cut by £100 million and £10 million was to go to breast cancer services.
- *Day 50:* a review of London's health services was to be led by Professor Sir Leslie Turnberg and was to advise particularly on St Bartholomew's hospital.

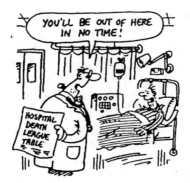

Source: Nick Newman's Week, The Sunday Times, 14 June 1998.
Reproduced by kind permission of The Sunday Times and Nick Newman.

- *Day 67:* Tessa Jowell announced plans for a Green Paper on public health and a review of health inequalities to be conducted by the former Chief Medical Officer, Sir Donald Acheson.
- *Day 69:* Baroness Jay announced that clinical indicators would be used as measures of hospitals' performance in NHS league tables that would be introduced in 1998. Measures would include deaths within 30 days of surgery and emergency re-admissions, despite criticism that the proposed indicators told little about the quality of care received by patients (Walshe, 1997). Subsequent data published by CHKS Ltd, a private health care information company, showed massive variations in clinical outcomes between English trusts, based on the 15 clinical indicators the government planned to introduce in 1998 (Chadda, 1997).
- *Day 76: The Private Finance Initiative (PFI) Act 1997* received royal assent.
- *Day 90:* Frank Dobson and Alan Milburn signed the first PFI contract to build a new hospital at Dartford in Kent.
- *Day 99:* Reports suggested that the Secretary of State for Health wanted to encourage pharmacists to expand their role to include diagnosing illness, counselling patients and recommending medicines. The last item represented a development of special interest, given the largely neglected role of pharmacists in health care provision.

However, by June 1999, pharmacists were moving into new arenas. Under the increasing threat to business from supermarkets, such as the Asda–Kingfisher merge which brought together a super-drug chain and Asda's aggressive health care pricing policy, pharmacists started to fight back. As one example, Boots (the chemist chain) added a range of new services, from chiropody and dental hygienists to internet shopping, as well as expanding abroad (Finch, 1999).

Waiting lists

In contrast to all the change and innovation, waiting lists represented an age-old problem. Effectively a technique to ration NHS provision in the light of constrained resources (whereas the private sector was financed to meet demand head-on), by November 1997 hospital waiting lists were growing by 1000 a week. Unable to prise any more money from the Treasury to address the problem, Health Secretary Frank Dobson scraped together £5 million from savings on NHS red tape, to set up new units to oversee greater efficiency by health authorities and action teams to co-ordinate good practice and tackle rising waiting lists. The intention was that, by March 1998, nobody would have to wait longer than 18 months for treatment (Murray, 1997).

New Labour was elected on the promise to cut the waiting list by 100 000. Figures released in November 1997 showed that, between May and September 1997, NHS waiting lists had grown more than 150 000 to 1 207 500 – the highest figure ever. The number of people waiting more than one year increased by 11 000 (24%) to 57 700 (Murray, 1997). Only three English regions had met the Patient's Charter guarantee that no one should wait longer than 18 months for treatment (Snell, 1997). Some offered different solutions; Weston (1997) described how orthopaedic consultants had led a campaign to reduce patient waiting limits by involving GPs in reorganizing referrals. Other doctors urged an NHS scoring system to dictate how soon patients would be treated (Brindle, 1998a). Dr Peter Homa, then chair of the National Patient List Action Team, believed that the NHS could not cut waiting lists merely by calling on staff to work extra hours (Crail, 1998a).

By March 1998, the government announced a £500 million budget increase aimed at cutting NHS waiting lists to below 1.1 million by April 1999 (Milburn, 1998). In August 1998, some argued that the claimed waiting list fall of 45 000 in the previous four months had been produced by sleight of hand (Brindle,

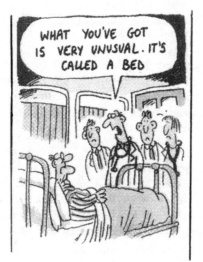

Source: Nick Newman's Week, The Sunday Times, 10 January 1999.
Reproduced by kind permission of The Sunday Times and Nick Newman.

1998b). Although the waiting lists had dropped to 1 162 000 by January 1999, which was close to the level at the time of the general election, Health Secretary Frank Dobson anticipated that the winter flu crisis would dent waiting list hopes and improvements (Murray, 1999a). However, the record monthly fall in March 1999 delivered the lowest NHS waiting lists for two and a half years, which took the total down to 1 073 999 in England. Frank Dobson (DoH, 1999a) commented that the government's promise to bring the waiting lists by April 1999 to below the level that the government had inherited in May 1997 showed that New Labour's commitment to get waiting lists down to 100 000 remained on course. Waiting times had also improved: for those waiting over 12 months down by 25 000; the average waiting time was just 2.96 months.

Nevertheless, as debates on radio and television reflected, matters remained problematic. Questions persisted about how patients were actually placed (or not) on a waiting list in the first instance (which could produce a 'fiddled' list); further, some doctors considered that the emphasis on waiting lists distorted clinical priorities. By May 1999, hospital waiting lists had risen slightly (by 3500) to 1 096 100 – a second successive monthly increase (Brindle, 1999a), which prevented ministers from proclaiming that the government's pledge had been achieved (Brindle, 1999b), although Mr Dobson insisted that the pledge would be met during 1999. In July 1999, the government published a second annual report on New Labour pledges and achievements (The Cabinet Office, 1999). Pledge 53 aimed to cut NHS waiting lists by 100 000: the report stated that waiting lists had been cut by more than 60 000 since New Labour had come into power and that the commitment was therefore on course. No comment was made on the recent slight rise in waiting lists, nor on the possible regret that officials might have on the target ever having been set in the first place. Waiting lists therefore continued as a challenge but one which represented only part of a wider picture of significant change and innovation to be introduced by New Labour from 1997 onwards.

The New NHS: modern and dependable

The White Paper *The New NHS, Modern – Dependable* (Secretary of State for Health, 1997c), which appeared in December 1997, was intended as the flagship for the future. In a foreword, Tony Blair stated that the NHS needed to modernize to meet the demand of today's public. The purpose of the new NHS was therefore to begin a process of modernization in order to provide new and better services to the public. The key features of the new NHS were (Secretary of State for Health, 1997c) as follows.

- To re-affirm the government's commitment to the historic principles of the NHS to provide a universal, comprehensive service with help for those ill or injured, where access would be based on need alone – not on the ability to pay.
- To construct a sustainable system to deliver better and more responsive health care for which additional resources would be provided annually.

- To replace the internal market by a system of 'integrated care' based on:
  - partnership driven by performance;
  - swifter health advice and treatment in local surgeries and health centres with fast, seamless entry to specialist hospitals;
  - harnessing new technology;
  - spreading best practice;
  - emphasizing quality.

At the centre of the programme for modernization, entitled 'A New Start – what counts is what works', was The Third Way. The New NHS was to chart a Third Way between the command and control of the 1970s and the fragmentation and bureaucracy of the internal market earlier in the 1990s. The new approach was to be founded on partnership and collaboration.

Six key principles underlined the changes proposed for the new NHS.

1 Renewing the NHS as a genuinely *national* service with consistently high-quality, prompt, accessible services.
2 Making the delivery of health care against national standards a matter of responsibility.
3 Breaking down organizational barriers to enable the NHS to work in partnership and to forge stronger links with local authorities.
4 Driving efficiency through a more rigorous approach to performance by cutting bureaucracy.
5 Shifting the focus on quality of care so that excellence was guaranteed to all patients.
6 Rebuilding confidence in the NHS as a public service, accountable to patients.

Underlying these principles, the White Paper (Secretary of State for Health, 1997c) aimed to move the NHS away from competition between providers and to bring in new measures to improve equity, efficiency and clinical quality. However, despite the intention to replace the internal market with 'integrated care', the separation between planning/commissioning and provision was to remain although the end of GP fundholding was confirmed. Along with a pledge to cut waiting lists, the developments were intended to chart progress to a quicker, more responsive NHS.

To drive change forward in the new NHS, new roles and responsibilities were envisaged for a number of groups.

Primary care groups
Primary care groups (PCGs) would bring together GPs and community nurses, to commission the bulk of health services, but would work closely with local authority social services, to serve populations of around 100 000 people with a single unified, cash-limited, budget through funds allocated by health authorities on an equitable basis (but management costs would be capped). PCGs would also decide how to use the resources allocated within the framework of local health improvement programmes.

Four models of commissioning groups were set out for future options.

1 At a minimum, acting in an advisory capacity to the health authorities in commissioning services for the locality's population.
2 Assuming devolved responsibility for managing the budget for their area formally as part of the health authority.
3 Becoming established as free-standing bodies accountable to the health authority for commissioning care.
4 As above, but with added responsibility for the provision of community health services for their population, to be known as Primary Care Trusts (PCTs).

For PCTs who qualified for such a status, legislation would be brought forward in 1999. Both PCGs and PCTs would monitor performance against targets by NHS trusts and develop primary care by joint working across practices. The GP Commissioning Group pilots were to begin in 1998 with an early transition to the new PCGs, to be formally launched on 1 April 1999.

Health authorities

Health authorities were expected to give strategic leadership in the new NHS by leading the development of local health improvement programmes (HImPs) to identify the health needs of local people. Health authorities also had to address certain key tasks such as: to decide on the range and location of health services (to flow from HImPs); determine local targets and standards in the light of national priorities and guidance; to support the development of PCGs; to allocate resources to PCGs and to hold PCGs to account. Health authorities would have a statutory duty to improve the health of their population as well as to work in partnership with local authorities and others to identify how local action on social, environmental and economic issues would make the most impact on people's health. Health authorities would also have to ensure that the local NHS worked in partnership to co-ordinate plans for the local workforce, while local education consortia should ensure appropriate training and education arrangements.

Amongst a further range of powers and responsibilities, health authorities were required to co-ordinate information and technology plans across primary care, community health services and secondary care, to produce joint investment plans with partners agencies for continuing and community care services and, significantly, to become involved with even closer working between health and social services through the pooling of budgets. To equip health authorities for their new role, the government also intended to clarify the revised, formal responsibilities, to align the accountabilities of NHS trusts and PCGs with those of health authorities, to provide for local authority chief executives to participate in health authority meetings and to work with health authorities to streamline their administrative functions.

Health improvement programmes

The first HImPs were introduced in April 1999 to begin to form the basis for a local strategy to improve health and health care. HImPs would cover the most

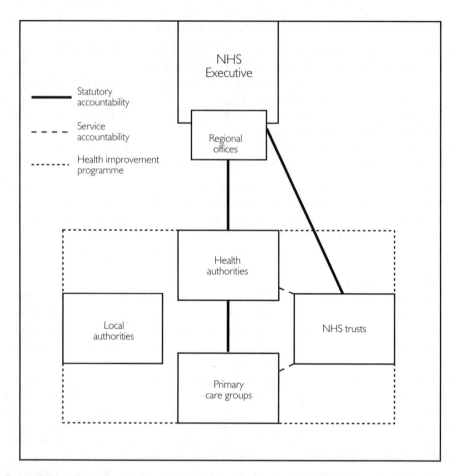

Figure 14.1   Financing and accountability arrangements in the new NHS.
Source: Adapted from Secretary of State for Health (1997c: 21).

important health needs of the population, the main health care requirements of local people and the range, location and investment required. The health authority would monitor the implementation of the HImPs in which NHS trusts, PCGs and local authorities would be involved in formulating the programmes. Figure 14.1 shows how the financing and accountability arrangements would map out in the new NHS to enfold HImPs.

Health action zones

Health action zones were to blaze the trail in modernizing the NHS. From April 1998, an initial ten health action zones set out to bring together all those in a health authority area to improve the health of the people. Once again, the emphasis was on partnership and innovation to find new ways to tackle health problems and to reshape local services in areas of pronounced deprivation and poor health.

NHS trusts

NHS trusts would create agreements around care groups, have new standards for quality and efficiency in local agreement with health authorities and PCGs (to which they would be accountable for service delivery), have to publish and benchmark the costs of treatment offered and, once again, have a new statutory duty to work in partnership with other NHS organizations. However, long-term agreements would replace annual contracts between purchasers and providers, while the extra-contractual referral system would be abolished.

Quality and performance

The Department of Health would further integrate policy on public health, social care and the NHS in order to provide a clear national framework together with similar local service developments. New evidence-based *National Service Frameworks* would set out to address health improvement, fairer access to services, effective delivery of appropriate health care in order to improve efficiency, patient and *carer experience* and health outcomes of NHS care. A *National Institute for Clinical Excellence* would give a lead on clinical and cost-effectiveness. Explicit quality standards would be included in the long-term service agreements to replace contracts. In addition, a new *Commission for Health Improvement* would have powers to support clinical improvements or intervene where problems had not been addressed.

Integrating health and social care

This was to be included in the various new measures at virtually all points of the programme for the new NHS. The government would consult on ways in which a closer relationships could be brought about through joint planning and budget operations. To modernize the NHS, specific new features would include the following.

- NHS Direct, a new 24-hour telephone advice line staffed by nurses, piloted in selected areas in March 1998 and intended to cover the whole country by 2000.
- Every GP and hospital to be connected to the Internet via NHSnet, with demonstration sites to be established in every region by the end of 1998, while everywhere to be covered by 2002.

However, the White Paper (Secretary of State for Health, 1997c) concluded overall that constructing a modern and dependable NHS would be a tough and challenging programme.

THE NHS IN SCOTLAND

By the autumn of 1997, Scotland's resounding 'yes' vote for a devolved Parliament with tax-raising powers gave the green light to the development of a health service which could look radically different from the English NHS in the course of time. Devolution offered the opportunity for a fundamental revision of the Scottish health service which could expose the arrangements to greater public accountability. Although Scotland spent more per head on health care than in England (making up almost one-third of the new Parliament's budget), within a devolved system the health service could face many competitors for the limited resources available. Under devolution, elected bodies in Edinburgh would have the power to decide how resources were allocated to health care within their budgets, whereas previously the Scottish Office made resource decisions within their block grant.

On a wider scale overall, the powers devolved to Edinburgh covered: home affairs and the judiciary; health; housing and local government; education; and social services, as well as the implementation of European directives. The powers retained by London included: employment law; economic and monetary policy; social security benefits and pensions; passports and immigration; negotiating with the European Union; and foreign affairs (Hetherington, 1999).

Regarding health care, in December 1997 the Secretary of State for Scotland (1997) produced the White Paper *Designed to Care*. Up to 1997, the arrangements for health services in Scotland had travelled along lines similar to those in England (Turner, 1998), with differences of detail in the implementation according to Scottish relevance. The two new White Papers for England (Secretary of State for Health, 1997c) and Scotland (Secretary of State for Scotland, 1997) reflected similar themes: of co-operation and partnership in the place of competition encouraged by the internal market, of long-term arrangements between purchasers and providers rather than short-term contracts, of abolishing the internal market (though not the purchaser/provider split), as well as harnessing new technologies to improve the reliability and effectiveness of patient care.

Amongst the differences was the radical shift in Scotland with the end of fundholding, when GPs would have no responsibility for the commissioning of hospital care. South of the border, GP fundholding had become so widespread that GPs could not feasibly nor politically be removed from the commissioning process. A further difference reflected the new NHS structure in Scotland which was to come into operation in April 1999. Fifteen health boards would remain, much as before, to oversee strategy and planning, while operational management would be the responsibility of acute hospital trusts and primary care trusts, who were to be responsible for mental health services, GP practices grouped into local health care co-operatives and community hospitals. Meanwhile, the health boards would prepare rolling five-year health improvement programmes (HImPs) to cover issues such as health promotion, needs assessment and resource allocation (Turner, 1998: 99). One interesting feature of the Scottish proposals was the creation of joint investment funds to encourage co-ordination of services at the interface between primary and secondary care (Hazell and Jervis, 1998: 52). No equivalent to England's National Institute for Clinical Excellence was to be installed but work on promoting clinical governance in Scotland would continue to be led by the clinical resource and audit group which would be strengthened to provide a stronger strategic direction (Woods, 1998). In March 1999, Lord Patel was appointed to chair the new Clinical Standards Board to develop and run a national system of quality assurance for clinical services (Millar, 1999a).

For the future, Jervis and Hazell (1998) suggested that devolution could highlight anomalies in health spending while professionals feared that devolution would fragment UK-wide policy networks. However, the NHS in Scotland's chief executive, Geoff Scaife, warned that NHS managers had to try harder to understand and to respond to the context in which their partners, such as local government and the voluntary sector, worked and shared ideas (Millar, 1999b). Nevertheless, the Scottish Parliament would have significant law making powers to include overall responsibility for the NHS in Scotland as well as for the education, training and terms of conditions of Scottish NHS staff.

The Scottish Parliament would still depend on block funding from London, although powers were available to vary the basic rate of income tax by up to 3% (Hazell and Jervis, 1998: 32).

THE NHS IN WALES

Unlike Scotland, devolution in Wales was only secured by a narrow margin of 0.6%, based on a 50% turnout in September 1997. The vote was just sufficient to ensure a May 1999 election to create a 60-member Welsh Assembly. The Welsh Assembly would have responsibility for a £7 million budget but no tax raising nor primary legislation powers as had been granted to Scotland.

By January 1998, the Secretary of State for Wales (1998a) had presented a White Paper in both English and Welsh: *NHS Wales: Putting Patients First* (*NHS Cymru: Rhoi Cleifion yn Gyntaf*). The Welsh Office had been told that the government wanted a 'national' health service that was recognizably the same institution across the UK. Devolution legislation also reserved various health policy matters for decision and action at UK level (the regulation of professions, abortion, human fertilization and embryology, amongst other matters (Jervis and Hazell, 1998)). Many similarities with the new NHS in England therefore remained: to scrap the internal market but to retain the separation of the commissioning process from the provision of services, to give GPs and primary health professionals an increased role, to improve cancer services, quality and openness and to set national standards for services under the direction of two new bodies: the National Institute for Clinical Effectiveness and the Commission for Health Improvement.

Significant differences, however, included local health groups to be established (rather than primary care groups as in England), to be co-terminous with the 22 unitary authorities established in Wales in 1996, together with a governing body which would reflect the range of health professionals' interests within the locality. Health authorities would be given a major role in the development of local health groups over time; as experience was gained, cash-limited budgets would be given to local health groups for a full range of services. Since the Welsh Assembly was to take over the Secretary of State's responsibilities for the NHS in Wales from 1999, the Assembly would eventually monitor the health of the Welsh population as well as respond with policies to promote health and tackle ill-health. To address such problems, the new vision for NHS Wales was to stress collaboration, increase local responsiveness and remove obstacles to integrated care.

Amongst the comments on the future of the NHS in Wales, health professionals were dubious that the Welsh Health Minister's claims (to save £50 million by removing the internal market paperchase) could be realized (Whitfield, 1998a). The proposals to halve the number of NHS trusts in Wales (from 29 to 11 on 1 April 1999) met hostility from those who wished to retain locally based trusts (Whitfield, 1998b). Nevertheless, ministers were planning to create a statutory responsibility for the NHS and local authorities to work together. Local authorities were to have a place on local health groups to advise the principality's five health authorities on priorities and objectives (Butler, 1998). However, the Welsh Institute for Health and Social Care (1998) had some doubts about the effectiveness of the proposals, as health authorities needed to be made more accountable both to local health groups and to the democratic process. Although local authorities wanted to be more involved in health matters, better partnerships were needed as well as clear lines of responsibility for running the NHS. The Welsh Office (1998) suggested that Community Health Councils should refocus their activities on NHS trusts or health authorities to help to develop services locally. Ways were outlined for the NHS in Wales to establish genuine partnerships with the public and the users. Nevertheless, much would depend on the election of the first Welsh Assembly in May 1999, as to how the views of the NHS would be received by the new members. With three potentially very different national health services in Scotland, Wales and England, the concept of a UK-wide NHS might be undermined.

Northern Ireland

Following the 1998 Good Friday 'peace agreement', fundamental changes were envisaged in the health service. An intended local assembly with local ministers, with an input to health and social services, would put Northern Ireland on a par with Scotland and Wales. The consultative document *Fit for the Future* (Department of Health for Northern Ireland, 1998) set out the Northern Ireland Office's plans for health and social services which the document made plain would continue to be integrated. A Belfast-based minister would take daily control in place of a London minister from Westminster. Apart from the basic principles of equity, health promotion, quality, a local focus, partnership, efficiency, openness and accountability, everything was up for debate. Although GP fundholding was likely to last one year longer than in the rest of the UK, the long-term plans could prove more radical than anywhere in the UK (Healy, 1998a).

Subsequently, although managers and staff welcomed the principles set out as the basis for reshaping health and social services, neither of the two models proposed in *Fit for the Future* were considered acceptable. The chief executive of the Northern Health and Social Services Board, Stuart McDonnell, contended that the way health and social services worked together in Northern Ireland was unique: changes should not be contemplated which would disestablish existing multi-agency networks. However, if arrangements were to be changed, even further integration was needed with other services such as education, probation

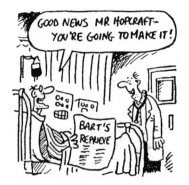

GOOD NEWS MR HOPCRAFT—
YOU'RE GOING TO MAKE IT!

BART'S
REPRIEVE

Source: Nick Newman's Week, The Sunday Times, 8 February 1998.
Reproduced by kind permission of The Sunday Times and Nick Newman.

and the police (Healy, 1998b). Whichever way for the future, as Healy (1998b) commented, progress seemed a long way off.

LONDON

A new London region was one of a series of recommendations put forward in Sir Leslie Turnberg's (1998) strategic review of the capital's health services. Amongst the recommendations, two routes were offered to keep St Bartholomew's hospital open: either to make it into a specialist research centre or, backed by the Turnberg panel, to give it a role in decanting patients until a new hospital was built at Whitechapel through the private finance initiative. Barts was to be temporarily reprieved to focus on a small number of tertiary services together with a continuing need to fulfil teaching and research responsibilities but, in the interim, rational, efficient and acceptable services were needed to be ensured across the two sites.

The new London region was part of nation-wide changes to redraw the NHS regions in England from April 1999. The previous eight regions would become ten: North West, Northern and Yorkshire, West Midlands, Trent, Northamptonshire, Eastern, South West, Hampshire, South East, London. The new London region would have the same boundary as the proposed greater London authority, to cover all 32 London borough councils and the capital's health authorities. The new arrangements were intended to support joint working between NHS organizations and other agencies.

One of the striking features of the NHS over the previous 50 years was the constant introduction, drawing and redrawing of boundaries – whether for regions (14 to 8 by 1994 but back to 10 in 1999), or different health authorities (AHAs in 1974, out by 1982; DHAs in 1982; mergers from 1991 onwards). One might be tempted to argue that boundary changes could be seen as hyperactivity to camouflage lack of resources. Rather differently, Exworthy and Moon (1998) argued that the planned reconfiguration of NHS regions, together with the pan-London region, would strengthen the power of central government in terms of policy and resources.

By January 1999, Nigel Crisp had been appointed as the NHS Executive's new London region's director. Some of the Turnberg (1998) recommendations were to feature amongst the priorities: targets to improve GPs premises, to develop primary care groups and performance-management measures, as well as to improve of the links between primary and community care (Donnelly, 1999a).

Parliamentary legislation was drawn up to create London's mayor and greater London Assembly. The question would then be how to develop an appropriate relationship between the London region's director and London's mayor. In December 1998, the King's Fund called for London's directly elected mayor, when eventually in office, to be a given a much stronger role in promoting health. The Public Health Minister, Tessa Jowell, stressed that the mayor would have a duty to promote improvements in health, a role that would depend crucially on a partnership between the mayor and the NHS Executive London regional office. However, little support existed for the idea that the mayor and assembly should manage and provide health services (Healy, 1998c).

THE NEW NHS: SOME OUTCOMES

Although evolutionary in context, the proposals for the New NHS heralded the most profound structural change in the history of the NHS (Baker, 1998: 14). However, Glennerster (1998) considered that *The New NHS* (Secretary of State for Health, 1997c) was essentially a good compromise document, high on generality, but into which many people could read different things, although the Department of Health's paper on setting quality standards (DoH, 1998a), together with the work of the National Institute for Clinical Excellence, was an encouraging start for the next half century.

Certainly by the late 1990s, whether from policy documents or new initiatives, all ventures had to have buzz words. The new NHS buzz word was modernization. The fundamental principles of the New NHS emphasized effective health care, quality, public accountability, efficiency and patient empowerment – but, above all, joint working instead of confrontation. However, as NHS staff had been encouraged to behave competitively for much of the 1990s, Baker (1998: 17) wondered just how far the new policy of working together could realistically be achieved. Nevertheless, the key theme was integration of the work of health and local authorities as partners in delivering the new health agenda. Professor Mark Baker (1998: 18) went so far as to suggest that such a strategy required that a statutory duty should be placed on local authorities to take an interest in health matters, since no duty had existed previously. Joint working, partnerships and pooled budgets were all mechanisms introduced to try to overcome the deep structural divisions between the health and community care services. It remained to be seen whether the new NHS notion of integrated care (one continuous process of care, based on an effective strategy for human resources and communications) would be sufficient to overcome the historical hurdles which had impeded joint working between health and local authorities.

NHS Direct: initial evaluation

Following the government's commitment to a new 24-hour telephone advice line in the 1997 NHS White Paper (Secretary of State for Health, 1997c), NHS Direct aimed to provide clinical advice to support self-care and appropriate self-referral to NHS services, and to give more general advice and information. Staffed by qualified and experienced nurses, who suggested best courses of action if and when people were anxious about ill-health, NHS Direct started in three pilot areas in March 1998: Preston, Milton Keynes and Northumbria. A second wave of 13 pilot sites was launched between January and April 1999. From April 1999, over three million people were covered by NHS Direct (DoH, 1999b).

The interim evaluation, undertaken by the Medical Research Unit at Sheffield University, published in March 1999, showed a 97% satisfaction rating for NHS Direct. Callers had particularly appreciated the professionalism of the staff and the quality of advice given (DoH, 1999b). In February 1999, the Secretary of State for Health (1999a) announced that, from the extra £21 billion invested in the NHS, 60% of the country would have access to NHS Direct by December 1999.

As NHS Direct expanded, one former GP fundholding practice in Hertfordshire introduced a telephone triage system to reduce pressure on staff, which proved of benefit to both the patients and health professionals involved (Vorster, 1999). In contrast, at the 1999 annual conference of representatives of Britain's 30 000 GPs, criticism was made of NHS Direct, whose merits claimed to be unproven but investment in which diverted scarce NHS resources from the urgent and serious to the relatively trivial, with variable advice and uptake across the country Brindle (1999c). Certainly the Department of Health's plans to specify a single software system to be used for a national service by 2000 would cost millions of pounds (Dudman, 1999).

Outcomes for Primary Care Groups

The master plan for health care commissioning was to shift to a network of PCGs which would evolve into Primary Care Trusts (PCTs). By August 1998, local decisions had to be made as to which of the four options (see pages 234–5) would be selected by each group in order to start work in April 1999. The greater majority of groups chose the level two pathway to take devolved responsibility for managing the health care budget formally as part of, and accountable to, the health authority. By February 1999, a Health Bill had been introduced into Parliament to end GP fundholding and to give the Health Secretary powers to establish primary care trusts. As the Health Bill would not be law by 1 April 1999, the Bill had to allow for a residual fundholding scheme to run alongside primary care groups until the legislation was passed. The Health Bill would apply to all parts of the United Kingdom, although Part II set out separate legislation for Scotland.

PCGs received a mixed reception from GPs. Some GPs were keen to start; others lacked confidence or had had enough of upheavals; some wanted to do what 'they felt they had been trained for'; others were anxious that they might be set up to take the blame for rationing (Brindle, 1998c). Fundholding was abolished due, in part, to the perceived effect of 'two-tierism' but many GPs had *chosen* to become fundholders and had given much commitment to the system, a fact often overlooked. The new primary care developments required all to become involved – there was no choice. In February 1999, a group of Leicester-shire GPs boycotted engagement with PCGs, because of the amount of time PCG work would involve and the loss of fundholding benefits (*Health Service Journal*, 1999a). In contrast, other areas were racing ahead with potential initiatives. Birmingham's primary care groups, for example, had found backing for a supra-PCG, supported by GPs, the health authority and the local medical committee, to monitor standards, provide management support and engage in strategic city-wide planning and clinical governance. Significantly, Birmingham was a city area where GPs and the health authority had previously worked closely together with total purchasing and multi-fund projects (Smith et al., 1999a).

From a collaborative perspective, by August 1998 the pace gathered momentum as the NHS Executive (1998a) issued a circular, one of many, on the development of primary care groups. Of significance, first, the PCG boards were to include:

- four to seven GPs;
- one or two community or practice nurses;
- one social service officer nominee;
- one lay member;
- one health authority non-executive;
- one PCG chief officer/manager (as a full *ex officio* member).

Secondly, the involvement of local authorities in the governing of PCGs clearly underlined the establishment of a new partnership between primary and social care in order to achieve better integrated local care.

The nurses were disappointed in PCGs. By February 1999, only two of the 481 primary care groups in England were chaired by nurses. On each case, the reasons were largely because local GPs were reluctant to take on the role due to the workload involved. Unison national officer Steven Weeks commented that PCGs were dominated by one professional group (GPs) although nurses represented the largest single occupational group in the community services. One of the two elected nurse chairs, Elizabeth Powell in St Helens North, suggested that the government should therefore look at a 'different' model for the board of primary care trusts (McIntosh, 1999a).

Would PCGs deliver all that was expected? Would PCGs actually work? As a former Family Health Services Authority general manager commented (Wilcox, 1999), PCGs would not be allowed to fail. At what cost had not been calculated, nor had the exclusion of mental health and learning disability services from primary care groups been fully addressed. By December 1998, however, the Department of Health indicated that *Modernization of Mental Health Services* (DoH, 1998b) would have a firm base in primary care. More widely, PCGs also had to work closely with specialist teams to integrate service planning and delivery, to develop a multi-agency approach and to involve local people – but just *how* was unclear (Peckham, 1998). Based on a modern framework of law, reform would be aided by new investment – £700 million over three years.

Quality matters: CHIMP, NICE and clinical governance

The performance of mental health services was to be monitored through the new performance assessment frameworks for health and social care, as well as by external inspection through the Social Services Inspectorate, the joint reviews with the Audit Commission and the new Commission for Health Improvement (CHIMP). Whether for mental health or health care as a whole, quality was to be at the heart of provision under the New NHS. New evidence-based national service frameworks were to ensure clinical and cost-effectiveness, taking into account the views of service users to determine provision. The new performance framework would focus on health improvement, fairer access to services and better quality and outcomes of care (Secretary of State for Health, 1997c: 18–20).

In a follow-up consultation document (DoH, 1998c) the government emphasized the need to shift the focus onto the quality of care and move away from measures which simply counted activity or financial performance. A further consultative document (DoH, 1998a), then set out an ambitious agenda. CHIMP (or CHI) was to be a new statutory body, responsible directly to the Health Secretary, to undertake regular inspections of all NHS trusts, to assess their local arrangements for clinical governance, to lead a programme of service reviews, to monitor local progress in implementing national service frameworks and guidelines, to check the competency of health units and to publicise those that fell below acceptable standards. However, although the government's key quality body would be set up in 1999, until the Health Bill – which was to incorporate CHIMP – became law, no launch date could be given.

The National Institute for Clinical Excellence (NICE) was established from 1 April 1999 as a special health authority, charged with providing national guidance to the NHS on effectiveness and quality. The purpose of NICE was to bring together responsibility for current work on health technology assessment, national service frameworks, clinical guidelines and national clinical audits. Importantly, the advice given by NICE would carry semi-statutory force (DoH, 1998a). In November 1998, Professor Michael Rawlins, chair of the Committee on Safety of Medicines, was appointed as chair-designate of NICE. However, while NICE would start work in April 1999, the new advisory body would not be an independent adviser to the government but would work within the Department of Health's budgets. Would NICE be the start of centralized control over doctors (Boseley, 1999b)? To make good progress, NICE would have to establish credibility. Nevertheless, by April 1999, Andrew Dillon had been appointed as NICE chief executive, which augured well as Mr Dillon had been an effective chief executive at St George's Healthcare trust in south-west London (McIntosh, 1999b).

Clinical governance

NHS trusts had a legal duty to ensure quality, complemented by a new framework of clinical governance for which the chief executive would be ultimately accountable. The initiative was to introduce a systematic approach to raise standards and to address poor performance. Clinical governance applied equally to primary and community health care and the acute sector, all of which was included in the 1999 Health Bill. The White Paper *The New NHS* (Secretary of State for Health, 1997c) also stated that all health care sectors would stipulate quality measures so that patient services met demanding targets for responsiveness.

The implications of clinical governance were considerable.

- Government policy had now seriously addressed clinical quality in health care, but no precise definition of clinical governance could be pinned down (other than working according to commonly accepted standards). However, the Department of Health (1998a: 33) consultative document *did* introduce clinical governance as a 'framework through which NHS organizations are accountable for continuously improving the quality of their services and safeguarding high standards of care by creating an environment in which excellence in clinical care will flourish'.
- Hospital consultants, immune from management strictures since the start of the NHS, could find that clinical governance transformed relationships with chief executives (Tyndall, 1998).
- A survey of board members showed that, by April 1999, many NHS trusts were simply not geared up for clinical governance (Health Quality Service, 1999).
- An Institute of Health Services Management survey also found that only 6% of top health care professionals were confident that managers had sufficient powers over health care teams to tackle poor clinical practice; more resources and more information were needed to enable clinical governance to function effectively (Donnelly, 1999b).
- In a King's Fund report, Dewar (1999) pointed out that the 1999 Health Bill gave chief executives only limited responsibility for making arrangements to monitor and improve the quality of health care. The wording established responsibility for the process rather than the outcome of clinical governance, without the extra resources needed. Ministers had made clear that no extra funding would be available for the clinical governance reforms. Meanwhile, managers and doctors were struggling to reconcile top-down guidance with bottom-up service that sought to respond to local staff and patient needs.
- Partly as a result of serious medical blunders in the NHS which had made big headlines, doctors and managers were increasingly developing monitoring systems aimed at preventing clinical malpractice (Moore, 1999a). A new system of competence checking would eventually be imposed on doctors. However, as Phillips (1999a) discussed, in order to bring about change effectively in long-held patterns of behaviour, recommendations had to be owned and incorporated into practice.

In primary care, clinical governance was to focus on prescribing, referrals to specialists and clinical care in practice. However, as so little was known about what happened in consultations, Baker (1998: 115) felt unconvinced that much progress would be made without radical changes. At a conference on clinical governance, held at Kingston University in May 1999, members came from a wide variety of backgrounds – from the medical and nursing professions, speech and language therapists, public health representatives and social workers – for whom the question remained: just how far could and should clinical governance be extended?

In a King's Fund policy review of the New NHS, Gillam (1998: 72) concluded that mechanisms for monitoring and managing clinical performance would prove controversial but success, in the short term, would hinge on adequate resourcing of the new structures and systems.

Clinical performance

In June 1999, another aspect of assessing the NHS trusts' performance was the government's publication of the first comparative figures for deaths among patients in England who had undergone surgery (DoH, 1999c). The first tables showed how trusts were performing against six clinical indicators which not only swept away the previous system of hospital league tables but were intended to underpin the NHS performance assessment framework launched earlier in 1999. Despite doubts about the validity of some of the data, health service leaders acclaimed the greater openness in the NHS. Similar clinical indicators had already been made available in Scotland and Wales. Most attention tended to focus on death rates but the DoH cautioned against regarding the clinical indicators as league tables. On the BBC Radio 4's programme *Any Questions* (18 June 1999) the chief executive of the King's Fund, Julia Neuberger, pointed out that, although the medical profession had largely welcomed the development of clinical indicators, the way of producing the figures remained simplistic as much hospital work was conducted in teams which needed to be disaggregated. Nevertheless, clinical indicators did provide a way in which patients and users could access information on NHS performance – for example through the Internet (www.doh.gov.uk/indica.htm).

Joint working

If quality concerns were one key focus of the New NHS, joint working was certainly another. The third of the six principles in the White Paper (Secretary of State for Health, 1997c: 11, 27) was to underpin partnership between the NHS and local authorities; the principle was further expanded in terms of health authorities who were to work more closely with local social services and other partners on planning for patients. Interprofessional and inter-agency approaches were not a new idea (Leathard, 1994, 1998): various initiatives had been tried over the years. The difficulty was to ensure effectiveness, commitment and continuity. The 1999 Health Bill specifically emphasized the duty of NHS bodies to co-operate with each other; the theme of partnership continued with the requirement that NHS bodies should also work with local authorities to secure and advance the health and welfare of the people of England and Wales.

Hudson (1998a) constructed the potential for partnerships in the light of the New NHS. Five pathways were perceived, for:

- programme partnership;
- professional partnership;
- administrative partnership;
- performance partnership; and
- governance partnership.

However, there was little scope for local democratic accountability in the NHS, although the NHS had to make health bodies more representative of local communities which did involve re-establishing a local government presence in the NHS governance. As Baker (1998: 109) commented, Community Health Councils had received scant attention in the White Paper (Secretary of State for Health, 1997c). Hudson (1998a) concluded, overall, that the proposals for joint working were less well developed than those for performance; that whether collaborative activities were discretionary or mandatory remained unclear. However, although effective joint working was not easy to secure, localities were far more likely to take inter-agency collaboration seriously when the government also took the matter seriously.

The challenge for the future was to make joint working effective across the different health and social care agencies and organizations involved. Recent studies, particularly on team working (Jones Elwyn et al., 1998; Poulton and West, 1999), and on collaborative partnerships across agencies and professions (Hudson, 1998b; Maddock and Morgan, 1999) had shown that certain basic requirements were needed to overcome the barriers to inter-agency and inter-professional collaboration. The criteria for joint working included:

- clearly defined, attainable and agreed objectives which evolved and were reviewed;
- clarity over roles and tasks in which management and practitioners shared the same agenda on quality and funding issues;
- clear procedures with agreed protocols based on staff participation and involvement;
- regular communications and high levels of information;
- adequate resources and a common budget;
- mutual respect and trust which acknowledged differences;
- effective leadership;
- constructive appraisal;
- appropriate performance measures which supported change, innovation and staff development;
- the need to overcome problems of different cultures and different patterns of accountability which could be helped by networkers who could blur organizational and professional boundaries.

Only time would tell whether the vision of joint working had actually produced the intended outcomes. Meanwhile, joint working, partnerships and service integration were increasingly to be taken aboard between the NHS and other agencies in the wider developments for health and social welfare, now reviewed.

Health improvement programmes: some early research

HImPs, which were anticipated to encourage innovative cross-sectoral working, including pooled budgets and integrated provision, represented one of several initiatives to be closely involved in joint working. Indeed, health authorities were to have a statutory duty of partnership which obliged health authorities to work with other NHS bodies and local authorities. Each HImP was expected to assess local needs, map resources, identify priorities and develop strategies for change. However, the future success of integrative developments in health care could well depend on the success of HImPs in practice.

From an initial piece of research from the King's Fund on the first year of HImPs in London (Arora et al., 1999), the perceptions and contributions of four health authorities, eight local authorities and 17 primary care groups towards HImPs were reviewed, as were the experiences of partnership, approaches to priority setting, accountability and public involvement. Welcoming the opportunity to work together, the contributors were largely positive about the HImP initiative although, due to the new demands, primary care groups were not in a position to make a significant contribution. Nevertheless, HImPs had been a good vehicle for setting up partnerships. However, as Anna Coote (1999), director of the public health programme at the King's Fund, pointed out, health authorities needed to make sure that local authorities really felt ownership had been shared, even though the process remained the responsibility of health authorities. Cultural barriers remained on language between primary care groups and local authorities. Then again, no one had addressed how to enable local people, especially marginalized groups, to have an effective voice in developing HImPs.

Although the government had envisaged that HImPs would focus on areas of inequality and social exclusion, the health authority of relatively affluent Kingston and Richmond (but with deprivation blackspots in Norbiton) showed how co-operation was the key to a successful HImP (Healy, 1999d). However, organizing a health improvement programme was an immense task as Avon – the second largest health authority in the country – had found, although the process provided opportunities in bringing people together from different organizations as well as forming new partnerships (Ewles, 1999). A study by Birmingham University's Health Services Management Centre of seven HImPs found that, although health authorities had tried to involve a wider range of stakeholders, management costs could hold back the development of HImPs. In the longer term, the concept of HImPs needed to be underpinned by genuine health improvement (Whitefield, 1999).

Overall, the early findings, particularly from the King's Fund assessment (Arora et al., 1999) of the government's key strategy on health inequalities, pointed to lack of funding. HImPs would only work if health authorities and local councils shared funds which required the NHS to provide money to local authority social services departments. Anna Coote (1999) argued that greater flexibility was needed to enable transfer of NHS funds into housing or social services or improving the environment. Some concerns lingered for the future, as local health promotion issues could be overshadowed by NHS priorities to perform on waiting lists (amongst other priorities) or questions over the lead in policy issues as primary care groups became more powerful (Ward, 1999). The King's Fund report (Arora et al., 1999) showed that HImPs could make a difference but that much work and commitment were required. HImPs represented a classic case for joint working: the formula for effective outcomes (as indicated under joint working) was known, but to cut across historical, cultural and financial boundaries would never be easy.

Healthy living centres

Lottery-funded healthy living centres were announced in the summer of 1997 to meet clear objectives for improving health and fitness among their target populations. Healthy living centres were to promote good health, both physical and mental, to help people get the most out of life. The centres were likely to be concentrated in the most deprived areas of the country which could involve a consortium of GP practices and primary health care teams, community groups, local authorities, health authorities and trusts, voluntary projects, businesses and schools – offering health promotion, healthy eating, relaxation and stress management, physical activity, education, equipment, advice and support, self-help groups, arts and health projects and places to meet. Greater Glasgow Health Board in Scotland was already involved in a prototype – the Eastbank Health Promotion Centre. In Newcastle, the West End Health Resource Centre was sest up by a partnership of GPs, voluntary sector groups, the local authority, Newcastle University and Newcastle City Health Trust. The centre was run as an independent charitable trust where, every month, over 1700 people used the health and fitness facilities and community services. The company secretary in Newcastle, GP Chris Drinkwater, considered that the healthy living centres initiative was long overdue (Millar, 1997). In July 1998, the *Lottery Reform Act* was passed, which affirmed the government's intention to create a network of healthy living centres for which £300 million of lottery money was earmarked, to be distributed through the New Opportunities Fund.

Health action zones

By April 1998, the first formally designated health action zones (HAZs) were extended to 11, to be supported by £5.3 million start-up costs for a seven-year life span. HAZs were to be concentrated in areas of pronounced deprivation and poor health to reflect the government's commitment to tackle entrenched inequalities. Each HAZ would be required to develop clear targets, agreed with the NHS Executive, for measurable improvement every year (Secretary of State for Health, 1997c). The purpose of the new initiative was to bring together all

Table 14.1   Health action zones (in alphabetical order).

Wave I	Wave 2
Bradford	Brent
East London and City	Bury and Rochdale
Lambeth, Southwark and Lewisham	Camden and Islington
Luton	Cornwall and Isles of Scilly
Manchester, Salford and Trafford	Hull and East Riding
North Cumbria	Leeds
Northumberland	Leicester City
Plymouth	Merseyside
Sandwell	North Staffordshire
South Yorkshire Coalfields communities	Nottingham
of Barnsley, Doncaster and Rotherham	Sheffield
Tyne and Wear	Tees
	Wakefield
	Wolverhampton
	Walsall

those who contributed to the health of the local population and to set up a locally agreed strategy for health improvement. Once again, the emphasis was on innovation and partnership to break down barriers between hospitals, GP services and the community as well as to involve local authorities, voluntary bodies and local businesses in working together to build on successful area-based regeneration schemes. HAZs were also to act as hothouses for new ideas in health and social care, while the potential for advancing a public health agenda could establish links with housing, health and education (Glassman, 1997).

The NHSE (1997) sent out an extensive invitation to bid from health authorities, in partnership with local authorities and other local agencies, to become HAZs. Key elements in the assessment criteria included: a clear purpose, realistic bids with a strategic approach, an indication of outcome measures, accountability arrangements, a commitment to increasing the effectiveness, efficiency and responsiveness of services and – above all – the development of partnerships across the statutory, voluntary and private sectors, to respond to social exclusion.

By January 1998, four times more bids for HAZ status were expected than the government's plans for the first wave of 11 HAZs to start work from April 1998 (Chadda, 1998). A second wave of 15 HAZs was then selected to begin work from April 1999 (Table 14.1), based on a further £30 million funding programme. In announcing the first wave, the Health Secretary particularly emphasized the East London's HAZ programme which planned to cut unemployment among under 25-year-olds from ethnic minorities (Whitfield, 1998c). Other initiatives included:

- new deals for lone parents keen to return to the labour market;
- area-based initiatives to regenerate blighted urban areas;
- improving educational standards in poor areas.

The HAZs varied considerably in size of population – the largest was Merseyside with 1 400 000 population, the smallest Luton, with 180 000. The starting point for all HAZs was the need to develop effective partnerships at local level to be linked to the national policy context. Partnership structures were expected to reshape the health and social care system, to empower local communities and to address the root causes of ill health in order to improve the population's health and reduce health inequalities. All programmes were to be evaluated, both locally and by a national evaluation team at the Personal Social Services Research Unit at Kent University, where one of the top priorities for evaluation was to look closely at the partnership and governance arrangements as well as the nature of the community involvement adopted (Judge, 1999).

Early indications revealed certain challenges across the programmes:

- little had been discussed on ways to achieve effective HAZ management (Hunter, 1998b);
- nurturing partnerships took time, with the danger that a hierarchy of partnerships might emerge with those underpinned by statutory duties (such as for youth offender teams) nearest the top (Peck, 1998);
- collaborative working might be tested by the legal constraints on the delegation of powers, in which health authorities were in a better position to delegate than a local authority (Owens, 1998);
- the DoH placed great stress on local accountability but NHS bodies were at best only indirectly accountable to the local public (Owens, 1998);
- the pressures to deliver might mean that targets were not always as radical as intended – or, as Donnelly (1999c) reported from Plymouth's HAZ, the challenge was to take developments forward in an effective way without controlling or stifling innovation.

Other commentators pointed out that HAZs were largely new programmes covering previous initiatives such as the Healthy Cities movement which had adopted a similar community development approach for the past five years. HAZs were simply another attempt to put local government centre-stage in the creation and protection of public health (Peck, 1998). Joan Higgins (1998) argued that HAZs were part of a long tradition of area-based social programmes. Lessons from the earlier health and social welfare approaches should be heeded to avoid past pitfalls: most had been only a marginal success. While HAZ programmes were to rely on partnerships between organizations, previous experience suggested that partnerships were often difficult to achieve. To mount a collaborative bid over a short period of time, as a 'trailblazer' in the new NHS, was relatively much easier than to sustain that level of enthusiasm and commitment over five to seven years. Was HAZ to become short for HAZard?

HEALTH INEQUALITIES REVIEWED – *OUR HEALTHIER NATION*

Further initiatives on working together were identified, by February 1998, in the consultation paper *Our Healthier Nation* (Secretary of State for Health, 1998a). To be fit for the twenty-first century, two key aims were set out for England.

1 to improve the health of the population as a whole by increasing the length of people's lives and the number of years people spent free from illness;
2 to improve the health of the worst off in society and to narrow the health gap.

Four priority areas were selected as targets for improvement by 2010.

- *Heart disease and stroke:* to reduce the death rate from heart disease and stroke-related illnesses amongst people under 65 by at least one-third.
- *Accidents:* to reduce accidents by at least one-fifth.
- *Cancers:* to reduce the death rate from cancer among people under 65 years by at least one-fifth.
- *Mental Health:* to reduce the death rate from suicide and undetermined injury by one-sixth.

The one missing target from those listed by the *Health of the Nation* (DoH, 1992b) was sexual health which was to be addressed in a separate policy (Baker, 1998).

Significantly, the way was open for further joint working between health and local authorities, in the field of public health, to implement the contracts for health. Contracts for each of the four priority areas and for each setting were set out for possible action by the government and local organizations. Some examples of the potential for contracts are set out below.

- A *contract for health* would involve the government and national players to tackle the root causes of ill health, for local players and communities to provide leadership for local strategies, to plan and provide high-quality services, to implement health improvement programmes and to work in partnership to improve the health of local people. People would take responsibility for their own health and make healthier choices about their lifestyle.
- *Healthy schools:* at government level high educational standards would be set; schools would give children the capacity to make the most of their lives and their future families' lives while pupils and parents would work together to share responsibility for academic achievement, healthy eating, better exercise and the development of responsible attitudes to smoking, drugs, alcohol, sex and relationships.
- *Healthy workplaces:* the government could ensure standards of health and safety as well as minimum employment rights. Employers could take measures to reduce stress at work, while employees could play their part in following health and safety rules and guidelines.
- *Healthy neighbourhood* projects could focus effort on tackling inequalities, in particular for improving the health of older people.

Our Healthier Nation (Secretary of State for Health, 1998a) was generally received well, but with caution. First, in order to make progress towards reaching the targets, effective ways of monitoring would be needed (Crail, 1998b). Secondly, no extra money had apparently been set aside to fund the new responsibilities of the health and local authorities. Thirdly, King's Fund chief executive, Julia Neuberger, welcomed the focus on disadvantaged groups at a local level but noted that, without a measure of progress in reducing inequalities, the danger was that no one would take responsibility or be held accountable (Chadda and Limb, 1998). Fourthly, a key omission was a European or wider international dimension; as a result, the importance and influence of EU directives and policy pronouncements or their critical part in shaping national policy had not been acknowledged (Hunter, 1998c).

Given the known link between poverty and ill health, Appleby (1998b) questioned whether an explicit Treasury target should not be wealth redistribution as a health target for the future. Coote and Kendall (1998) concluded that to set and attain targets to reduce health inequalities was a considerable challenge but the NHS's most significant contribution to the reduction would be through partnerships with other organizations.

The NHS Executive (1998b) followed up the government's various policies with a circular which set out an integrated programme for action. Health authorities were to take immediate steps to establish local arrangements to involve all relevant interests to plan on a partnership basis.

The Secretary of State for Scotland (1998) also published a consultative paper, amid public health consultants' concerns that insufficient doctors were available to tackle the ambitious agenda. The proposals set health outcome targets in five areas: coronary heart disease and stroke, cancer, dental and oral health, accidents, but which did include teenage pregnancy. Scottish ministers were keen to set national lifestyle targets to cover smoking, alcohol misuse, diet and exercise. Public health directors were also recommended to be co-opted onto appropriate local government committees to help to assess the impact of local policies.

The Secretary of State for Wales (1998b) similarly produced a consultation paper; a 'new approach' was unveiled to address some of the worst health problems in Europe. Life expectancy in Wales was three to four years lower than in the best European countries; the proposals focussed on the concept of health and well-being through the encouragement of sustainable communities, a healthy lifestyle and a better environment. A five-year research programme was to show the most effective ways of breaking the cycle of poor health in Wales as well as the development of indicators/targets for health inequalities and health determinants. The recommendations placed particular emphasis on joint working between local councils and health authorities which would be given new duties of collaboration.

In England, by the end of 1998, the Acheson Report (1998) on inequalities in health appeared which set out radical recommendations for the tax and benefits system, the NHS, housing, transport and education. Key priorities were for the government to target policies to reduce income inequalities, to improve health, to reduce health inequalities (especially in women of childbearing age, expectant mothers and young children) and to improve the living standards of households receiving social security benefits. The implications of the wide-ranging suggestions, from higher benefits for vulnerable groups to better fluoridation to help children's teeth, would have required substantial increases in benefits as well as major changes in government spending. Unlike the Black Report (1980) on inequalities in health, the proposals were not costed. Ministers warmly welcomed the Acheson Report (1998) and the 39 recommendations, which gave renewed emphasis to reducing inequalities in health in the UK.

Anti-smoking proposals

In April 1998, the Secretary of State for Health (1998b), together with the Secretaries of State for Scotland, Wales and Northern Ireland, brought out a White Paper on tobacco. The message was clear: smoking was killing 120 000 people a year. Those who smoked were likely to die a lingering death from tobacco-related disease in NHS hospitals which was costing the country millions. While there would not be a general ban on smoking in public places, the government pledged to protect children. Billboard advertising was to be ended by the end of 1999, while the government was to provide funds for a major anti-smoking campaign to cost £50 million. Amongst the targets set, the government wanted to see 110 000 fewer children smoking in England and 1.5 fewer million smokers overall. The *Guardian* (1998) commented that at least the government had to be given credit for making a real effort to tackle the biggest public health problem of all – for which initiatives, by June 1999, had been extended to banning most tobacco sponsorship of art and sports by 2003.

The White Paper, *Saving Lives*

Alongside the anti-smoking proposals and following on from the consultative document *Our Healthier Nation* (Secretary of State for Health, 1998a), the government continued with a £96 million crusade to help poor people to live longer. The July 1999 White Paper *Saving Lives* (Secretary of State, 1999b) called for targets to:

- reduce deaths from heart disease in those under 75 by 40%, which aimed at saving 100 000 lives;
- cut the death rate of all cancers in those under 75 by 20% within 10 years, in order to save 200 000 lives;
- cut the suicide rate by 20%, to protect 4000 lives;
- reduce death rates from accidents by one-fifth in order to save 12 000 lives;
- set up first-aid programmes for 11 and 16 year olds;
- extend the nurse-led NHS Direct telephone helpline;
- set up expert patients programmes to help people to manage their own illnesses;
- set up public health observatories in each NHS region to identify and monitor local needs and trends.

The Health Secretary, Mr Dobson, outlined the policies to be implemented nationally in schools, health centres, the workplace and even shopping centres, but most of the money made available would go to the poorest areas in England to target health inequalities. The policies were intended to improve, most of all, the health of the less healthy. A task force was to be set up by the Chief Medical Officer to design a programme for those with chronic disease (one-third of the population). The Health Education Authority was to be replaced by a new Health Development Agency to be responsible for raising standards – a public health equivalent of the National Institute for Clinical Excellence.

While the targets set out, together with the investment to be made, reflected the government's determination to address inequalities in society, David Hunter (1999) warned that the government needed to learn the lessons from the *Health of the Nation* strategy introduced by the Conservative government in 1992. That strategy had had minimal impact on the activities of trusts and primary care. Then again, although intended as a cross-sectoral initiative, the *Health of the Nation* initiative became regarded as a DoH matter in commitment and ownership, while local government felt marginalized as health authorities were given the lead agency role, which concentrated on a disease-based health strategy. Anna Coote, director of public health at the King's Fund, pointed out (Sherman, 1999) that the promotion of healthy lifestyles had to be integrated with action to tackle the underlying influences on health, such as income, environment and affordable, nourishing food (to which one would also add healthy housing).

Ann Oakley of the Social Science Research Unit at the Institute of Education argued that, as the outcomes of public health were somewhat unclear in the achievement of the aims intended, health campaigns should be subject to the same controlled trials as the rest of medicine (Watts, 1999). However, the new Health Development Agency, launched in October 1999, promised evidence-based guidelines for health programmes as well as evaluation and dissemination of research on public health (Donnelly, 1999d).

SOCIAL EXCLUSION

By September 1998, Mr Blair planned to reduce social division with an £800 million programme to address problems ranging from bad housing and health to education and crime. The government's Social Exclusion Unit (1998) identified key themes which ranged from investigating innovative approaches to getting people into work to housing improvement, while attempting to address inequality in the country's most deprived neighbourhoods. Other themes included motivating children at school, providing the poorest people with better access to services as well as developing family support to alleviate family breakdown. The Social Exclusion Unit (1998) described how the geography of poverty had changed: the poorest people had become more concentrated in small areas of acute need where some of the most deprived areas were now only a mile away from affluent areas. The centrepiece of the programme would be the initial concentration on 17 'pathfinder' districts of deprivation. The failure of previous improvement programmes had often been the result of unco-ordinated, confusing programmes. Although some felt the government's anti-poverty plans mirrored flaws that had undermined America's strategy some 35 years ago

(Kleinman, 1998), nevertheless the government wanted to bring agencies together to draw up progress reports. A new commitment was called for in which central and local government, local businesses, voluntary and statutory agencies would work together to develop policy plans for the future, to be co-ordinated overall by the Social Exclusion Unit (Hetherington, 1998).

The theme of *Partnership in Action* (DoH, 1998d) was emphasized by the government in September 1998 under the sub-heading *New Opportunities for Joint Working between Health and Social Services* which recommended integrated provision. By December 1998, integration was considered a step in the right direction by the House of Commons Health Committee (1998), which also reviewed, once again, *The Relationship between Health and Social Services*. The present situation was considered to be confused; organizations saw issues only from their own perspective. The problems of collaboration would not be properly resolved until there was an integrated health and social care system, whether in local government or as a new separate organization.

A month earlier, in launching the White Paper *Modernising Social Services* (Secretary of State for Health, 1998c), Health Secretary Frank Dobson announced the most radical overhaul of the social services in 30 years. The changes would be funded by an extra £750 million for the delivery of top-quality services, in which safeguards for vulnerable people would be increased. Above all, the proposals would ensure that local authorities, health services and other providers would work together to help people live independent and fulfilling lives. Buzz words were well in evidence, but came in pairs this time, as can be seen in the title: *Modernising Social Services: Promoting Independence; Improving Protection; Raising Standards* (Secretary of State for Health, 1998c).

By the end of the 1990s, joint working and partnerships were top of the agenda for the health and social services throughout all the new policy developments. Engagement was on but marriage was never quite achieved; in keeping with the times, the services preferred to remain in partnership.

15 Challenges for the Twenty-First Century

As the NHS headed into the new millennium, certain key issues remained, both as a legacy from the twentieth century and a challenge for the twenty-first:

- the education and training of the practitioners involved;
- the matter of NHS costs and finance, a constant factor for any age;
- the place of long-term care;
- the start of the primary care groups introduced new potential.

Training and education for health care practitioners

Doctors

By the end of the twentieth century, three key issues had emerged for the medical profession: the place of training and education, work practice and regulation.

Up until the early 1990s, little had changed with regard to the training and education of doctors. Increasingly medical bodies then began to review a range of issues for both undergraduate and postgraduate medical education, partly prompted by curriculum and work overload but also spurred on by the need to relate to European Union (EU) directives.

A spate of detailed reports appeared which provided recommendations to improve on the arrangements for medical education in general. Some of the main points are outlined below (in date order).

In April 1993, the Working Group on Specialist Medical Training (1993) for *Hospital Doctors Training for the Future* made the following recommendations:

- that opportunities should be created for a significant reduction in the duration of training without compromising standards;
- that the term 'specialist training' for the purposes of the EC (European Community) Medical Directives applied to the whole of the training period following full registration and lasted until the award of a UK CCST (Certificate of Completion of Specialist Training);
- that individuals in possession of a UK CCST could request the addition of 'CT' to the Medical Register;
- some form of EC harmonization of training, certification and standards was considered helpful, although the Department of Social Policy at the University of Bristol stated that simply co-ordinating the award of specialist status would not meet the problems of disparity in length of training nor discrimination against UK nationals.

The Working Group concluded that, despite a wide range of views in relation to career structure and registration of specialists, an overall consensus favoured the move towards a reduction in the period of time spent in training.

In December 1993, the General Medical Council (1993) looked in detail at undergraduate medical education for *Tomorrow's Doctors*. The recommendations included changes in the style of the undergraduate course to bring about a reduction in the curriculum overload. Importantly, the theme of public health was suggested to figure prominently in the education programme to encompass health promotion, illness prevention, assessment and targeting of population needs as well as awareness of environmental and social factors in disease. Even more significant was the long overdue recognition of the need for communication skills throughout the undergraduate course.

In May 1995, the Calman Report (1995) recommended that two phases of General Practitioner training should be recognized: a period of vocational training and provision for a period of higher/further training/education (to be voluntary until resources could be secured). The value of developing a coherent programme of education for general practice was acknowledged in order to address the continuum of undergraduate, postgraduate and continuing education. Further, an integrated plan for the career development of both academic and practice-based GPs should be explored for all stages of General Practitioner education.

In August 1995, the British Medical Association (BMA, 1995) pointed out that medical education had become overloaded with fact acquisition to the detriment of learning which ignored established principles of education and insights from the psychology of learning. Amongst 31 pages of recommendations, attention was drawn to:

- the need to improve the pre-registration year;
- the need for medical education to be a continuum, from entry into medical schools to retirement, in which continuing professional development encompassed all stages of the process to ensure that education should be part of doctors' contracts of employment;
- the need to develop the role of postgraduate Dean, as a purchaser of education, to ensure involvement in the control of staffing levels as well as the monitoring and assessment of educational progress.

However, the BMA drew attention to the need for change in postgraduate medical education in response to the ever-increasing base of medical knowledge, growing public awareness and demands, the NHS financial limitations which led to rationing and the effects of audit and accountability. The current system had failed to provide an adequate education because long hours of work caused fatigue, an inability to absorb information and a reduction in the desire for self-directed-learning.

The wider context of developments was, nevertheless, provided by the number of doctors and dentists in England, which had grown by 23% to 66 340 in the ten years from 1987. The sharpest increase was in the proportion of women doctors who accounted for 32% of medical staff. However, in June 1998, the BMA warned of an impending crisis if medical training was not stepped up: the NHS was set to run out of doctors by 2010 (Boseley, 1998b).

The place of interprofessional education

As government polices had encouraged ever more emphasis on joint working and collaboration in health and social care, the relevance of doctors training and working with other professions became increasingly significant. The Department of General Practice at the University of Exeter led the way in the 1980s, followed by new Masters courses at South Bank University and the Marylebone Centre Trust (later brought into the University of Westminster), in 1990 and 1993, respectively, amongst other initiatives elsewhere (Leathard, 1994). However, as Janet Storrie's (1992) survey of Masters' courses showed in the early stages, with one or two exceptions, doctors were recruited only to programmes based in medical departments, while nurses were the most heavily represented group. Storrie (1992) questioned whether the explanation indicated nurses' greater freedom from professional constraints or a trend by nurses to raise their educational and professional standards via Masters' programmes.

However, a number of impediments arose for doctors to take part in collaborative educational programmes, whether with nurses or other health care practitioners, or even with social workers. For example, levels, locations and funding arrangements for education and training significantly differed between professional groups (Leathard, 1997). Rashid et al. (1996), from GP and health visitor backgrounds, also pointed out that GPs could have difficulty with joint training when, amongst other factors, many GPs would argue that nurse practitioner training was not comparable to medical training.

Nevertheless by the mid-1990s, interprofessional developments, which involved medical students, were moving apace.

- Both the General Medical Council (1993) and the BMA (1995) had urged the 26 UK medical schools to place as much emphasis on gaining skills in clinical techniques and *teamwork experience* as on the acquisition of knowledge.
- The Schofield report (Schofield, 1996), which was largely composed of service managers, criticized professional inflexibility and, controversially, amongst various other recommendations, advocated a generic and multi-skilled workforce, flexible working among professional groups, employer-led occupational standards for training and a common core training for nurses, doctors and health workers.
- City University and St Bartholomew's School of Nursing and Midwifery had opened up an undergraduate multi-disciplinary education module for medical, dental and nursing students (Pryce, 1996).
- At Dundee University, links between medical and nursing students were being fostered to encourage multiprofessional learning (*Times Higher Educational Supplement*, 1996).
- The new Joint Faculty of Health Care Sciences at Kingston University and St George's Hospital Medical School led to the inclusion of an interprofessional module within a vocational training course in 1997. The course initially included GPs, social workers, radiographers and nurses. Subsequent

developments explored experimental courses on primary care for medical and nursing students as well as a common foundation course for medical students, students of radiography and physiotherapy which included plans to extend the course to nursing students on a BSc nursing degree.

- By November 1997, a DoH-funded fellowship, sponsored by the Royal College of General Practitioners and the Royal College of Nursing, recommended that vocational training for general practice and specialist community nursing should be part of an integrated approach to continuing development and lifelong learning. Further, interprofessional education initiatives needed to be formally developed and evaluated as the potential existed therein to transform the organizational delivery of care (Watts and Lenehan, 1997).

Despite the slowly increasing initiatives, the need to address the generic and profession-specific competencies, necessary for effective multiprofessional working, remained (Pittilo and Ross, 1998). At the St Catherine's 1998 conference at Cumberland Lodge, on *The Collaborative Imperative: Overcoming Barriers in Health and Special Care*, four main barriers were identified with regard to collaboration in health and social care: attitudinal, educational, organizational and financial. Funding streams also continued to encourage professional segregation. Furthermore, the historically based stereotypical images of the roles of doctors, nurses, other health care professionals and social workers would not be easy to break down.

While increasing interprofessional activity was taking place in Britain, no development quite matched the initiatives for medical education at the Faculty of Health Sciences in Linkoping University, Sweden, where Professor Nils Holger Areskog (1992) had pioneered multiprofessional education for six professional groups: doctors, nurses, physiotherapists, occupational therapists, laboratory technicians and community care managers. The curriculum strongly emphasized primary health care and problem-based learning, whose objectives were to meet the health care needs of the population and to provide a greater emphasis on community-based care. More recent interprofessional educational developments have taken place in Maastricht in the Netherlands and in Tromso, Norway, much influenced by the Linkoping programme.

Expansion in medical education

Following the third report of the Medical Workforce Standing Advisory Committee, chaired by Sir Colin Campbell (1998), a progressive expansion in medical student numbers, from 5000 to 6000 by 2005 (a 20% increase), with more to come, was announced in England and Wales – although how much money was to be put aside for the new medical places had yet to be resolved. By September 1998, plans for an eventual total of an additional 7000 doctors had been set out (Jinks et al., 1998). A joint DoH/Higher Education Funding Council for England implementation group was formed to recommend whether to award the additional places to existing medical schools or to look to new models for doctor training (Hinde, 1998a).

Medical schools soon moved into action. Universities started to develop innovative techniques to cash in on the increase in numbers of medical students. New medical schools, partnerships between existing schools and other universities, fast-track entry schemes, were all being considered (Goddard, 1998). The Open University was in the forefront of new thinking to set up a medical school, based at hospitals and surgeries, which would revolutionize medical training. The proposal was for medical students to be supervised by local clinical teachers but students would also benefit from the Open University's expertise in distance learning. As well as clinical training in the practice environment, virtual seminars and tutorials would take place using video-conferencing and electronic communications to provide a medical school with research and teaching facilities (Hinde, 1998b).

In June 1999, three new centres of medical education were designated to be opened as part of a drive to recruit more doctors to service poorer areas (Murray, 1999b). The new centres of medical education were to be linked with established schools: Durham (to work alongside Newcastle's medical school), Warwick (in collaboration with the medical school at Leicester) and Keele (in conjunction with Manchester University's medical school). To simplify the overall picture, figures for England only will be set out here, with the guidance of the NHS Executive in Leeds. Recruits to the new centres were to start training by September 2000 at Keele and Warwick and from the autumn of 2001 at Durham; taken together, some 248 extra places were intended. By the year 2005, the government's working target was to achieve an overall intake of 4700 medical school places per year in England. The other new places were to be spread amongst existing medical schools and consideration to be given to new initiatives. Fast-track courses for graduates who wanted to train to be doctors were also to be encouraged, such as the 35 places on a four-year course at St George's Hospital Medical School from the year 2000 (Goddard, 1999), 20 at Cambridge by 2001, 128 at Warwick by 2001 and 20 at Oxford by 2002.

The immediate outcome was one of disappointment for the University of Hull, whose bid to establish a medical school was turned down – nor were places initially allocated to the Universities of East Anglia, Plymouth and Exeter (the peninsula bid for a medical school), or to the imaginative programmes outlined by the Open University. However, the Department of Health was considering possible programmes at East Anglia and at Kings College, London, in collaboration with the University of Kent at Canterbury as well as the peninsula bid. Discussions would also be taking place with the Open University about the possibility of furnishing relevant distance learning programmes to other universities.

Medical education thus looked set to step into the twenty-first century with more places in medical schools, but just how far these new, imaginative programmes on offer would materialize remained to be seen. Meanwhile, Professor Alan Maynard (1998) gave a cautionary warning that the country did not need more doctors. Dealing with professions in isolation was no longer appropriate when most health care was delivered by teams, of which doctors were a part but who all needed good management. Plans for doctors should be seen in the light of skill-mix opportunities together with the more efficient use of nurses and pharmacists.

Work practice

In the late twentieth century, however, unrest mounted amongst junior doctors, who were not happy with the 1999 pay settlement which included 32 hours' overtime a week (Healy, 1999a). In 1998, the European Commission's proposals to cut the hours of millions of workers, including those of lorry drivers and junior doctors, brought immediate opposition from employers' organizations. The NHS claimed that the move could cause serious problems. If the regulations were agreed by the European Parliament and by national governments, the procedure would be likely to take two years to reach national statute books, followed by a further two year phasing-in-period. For junior doctors, the transition period would be much longer to allow for the training of extra staff (Bates, 1998). Meanwhile, one in six junior doctors continued to work more than 72 hours a week (Eaton, 1998).

In March 1999, leaders of 34 000 junior doctors threatened strike action over pay and conditions unless the government promised to act to stop hospitals requiring junior doctors to work excessive hours at 'derisory' wages (Brindle, 1999d).

In May 1999, the junior doctors' long campaign for a 48-hour week was rejected again. The government obtained the agreement of the 15 European Union (EU) member states to delay the reduction in junior doctors' working hours for 13 years. The news caused outrage among medical associations. The only hope of changing the plans would be if the newly elected European Parliament voted against the agreement later in 1999. The junior doctors' working hours were to remain the same under the amended regulations for four years. From then on, a graded scale of reduced hours would cover 60 hours for three years, 56 hours for three more years, 52 hours for three more years before a reduction finally to 48 hours a week, well into the next century. Although British ministers had supported the principle of the EU working hours directive, concern about the practicalities of implementation for junior doctors overruled any immediate change (Bates, 1999). In September 1999, junior doctors again threatened strike action over the length of the working week and overtime pay. Industrial unrest was eased when the government agreed to the demands for a new employment contract to reduce overtime and improve pay. The new agreement provided for a maximum average working week of 56 hours over the next three years and for the abolition of the infamous overtime rates. Different pay bands would be introduced so that doctors in busy wards would be paid more. A special conference and referendum would decide on acceptance.

The government also faced renewed calls by senior hospital doctors and consultants to be given seats on the boards of primary care groups and primary care trusts. Meanwhile, blaming inflexible and onerous working conditions, doctors at all stages of their careers were leaving the NHS. The British Medical Association pointed out that the country spent £250 000 on training a doctor but 8% of medical students left during their studies; one in five doctors had left the NHS within 10 years of qualifying (from the evidence of one study in the north-west of England), while some 1000 GP vacancies remained unfilled (Friend, 1998b). In contrast by 1999, claims were made that some 350 doctors, qualified to fill consultants post in obstetrics and gynaecology, were unable to find posts – which, argued Alan Maynard (1999a), was a reflection of poor workforce planning together with a lack of scrutiny by the royal medical colleges. The Health Secretary, Frank Dobson, had suggested that, in parallel with the phased increase in medical students, the government would seek to engage the medical profession and others in discussions about the future of the health care workforce (Crail, 1998c). Would doctors be forced to cede professional ground to nurses and other groups of staff as part of the price of a 20% expansion?

By July 1999, the doctors' annual representative meeting at the British Medical Association had swung firmly behind the junior hospital doctors campaign for shorter hours and better pay (Boseley et al., 1999).

Regulation

As the intense and exhausting lifestyle of junior doctors remained seemingly unaltered, change was blowing through GP surgeries and hospitals but which had yet to reach the royal colleges, according to Richard Horton, the editor of *The Lancet* (Boseley, 1998c). Thus reforms in the regulation of clinical practice were to become of increasing importance to primary care groups, clinical governance, the National Institute for Clinical Excellence, the Commission for Health Improvement and in the National Service Frameworks. Clinical governance was to ensure that quality assurance packages would be built into the delivery of primary health care (Davies, 1999). The Health Bill in 1999 intended to extend the jurisdiction over professional self-regulation. In February 1999, the General Medical Council also announced proposals for every doctor to be subject to regular revalidation of their skills. At the start of the new century, doctors would be facing the implementation of constant reform with the emphasis on increased regulation.

The place of dentists

The key issues for dental health were in sharp contrast to those of medical care.

First, in 1998, 80% of the cost of dental treatment by an NHS dentist was payable by the patient up to a maximum of £340, although children, pregnant women and those on low income were exempt. However, by 1999, almost half the country's dentists were not accepting NHS patients (Pratt, 1999). As a result, to reach an NHS dentist might require long-distance travel as dentists, willing to treat adults on the NHS, were in short supply. In some parts of Devon and Cornwall, there were waiting lists to get on to an NHS dentist's list. Some dentists accepted people for a check-up on the NHS but exercised their prerogative to charge private rates for some of the treatment offered (Boseley, 1998d). However, public dissatisfaction with NHS dentistry had accelerated, according to a Social Attitudes Survey, in contrast to GP services where levels of dissatisfaction had remained low (Mulligan and Judge, 1997: 128). Dickinson et al. (1998/9) showed that the two major reasons were: problems of access caused by increased charges and lack of availability of NHS dental care.

Secondly, the private sector had become buoyant for several reasons. For a start, various options now existed. Dental health schemes enabled individuals to visit the dentist privately, to have routine work done at no extra cost but paid a monthly subscription, worked out by the dentist according to the state of the individual's teeth. The schemes were effectively run by the dentist; the insurer simply collected the subscription and deducted a share for expenses. From 1994, BUPA also offered a special Dental Protector scheme, which paid for treatment of dental emergencies and accidents. However, most dentists who charged patients for private treatment (whether on a special scheme or not) worked in relatively well-off middle class areas. Furthermore, many people paid, not only because no alternative seemed available, but also because they did not think the same rights existed for publicly funded dental treatment as for GP treatment (Boseley, 1998d).

Thirdly, according to Aubrey Sheiham, a leading figure in dentistry and Professor of Dental Public Health at University College, London, public awareness of dental entitlement (such as entitlement to a second opinion on the NHS) was very low. What was needed, according to Sheiham, was consumer power – as in medicine, where the public had become much more critical of doctors' services. Paul Batchelor, Senior Clinical Research Fellow at King's College London, suggested a radical solution: that dentists should be paid for the reduction of disease progression rather than for treatment – in other words, paid by outcomes (Boseley, 1998d).

Fourthly, one key result in dental health was that, despite the government's commitment to equity in oral health, across the UK a seven-fold difference existed between the best and worst districts in the outcomes of dental health in terms of the removal of rotten teeth and multiple extractions. Socially deprived areas in the north-west of England, parts of Yorkshire, Scotland, Northern Ireland and Inner London were the most vulnerable. The public health consultation paper *Our Healthier Nation* (Secretary of State for Health, 1998a) had recognized the unacceptably large inequalities in the levels of children's tooth decay. However, while supporting the principle of water fluoridation in order to reduce tooth decay, the government stopped short of a commitment to action to ensure that water suppliers would be obliged to accede to water fluoridation (Lennon and Jones, 1998). Children's teeth in some areas without fluoride were four times worse than in treated areas. However, the matter was not straightforward: the National Pure Water Association blamed fluoride for discoloration of teeth, weakened bones, bone cancer and other health risks, although the pro-Lobby declared fluoride to be safe and effective (Moore, 1999b). Fluoridation thus remained a key issue for the year 2000 and beyond.

New Labour attributed the rundown of NHS dentistry 'by the previous government' to acute, if not long-term, problems of access to the general dental services. The problem for the twenty-first century was whether the former commitment by dentists to the NHS could be regained (Boseley, 1998d).

Nurses in the NHS

In contrast to dentists, whose earnings were increasing – dentists whose income exceeded £200 000 had risen from 20 in 1991 to 500 in 1998 (while most dentists earned around £45 000 a year after deductions of 55% for running costs and expenses (*Health Service Journal*, 1999b)) – most nurses considered themselves badly paid. Nurses' pay therefore represented one key issue; nurse education had also become a second matter of importance.

Nurses' pay

Nurses' pay was linked to the sheer numbers involved and the attrition rate. Even at the start of the NHS in 1948, in England and Wales, the NHS employed 137 000 nurses, but there was an alleged shortage of 30 000 nurses. By 1999, the figure for whole-time equivalent nurses employed by the NHS for England exceeded 300 000, with a reported shortage of between 8000 and 12 000. Although the number of GPs had increased by 50% in the last 50 years, the number of nurses appeared to have more than doubled (Ainsworth, 1999).

In a strong bid to reward nurses as well as to encourage new recruits, in the 1999 NHS pay settlement the Health Secretary, Frank Dobson, awarded a 12% pay rise for junior nurses, which would take a newly qualified nurse to £14 400. While welcomed by the Royal College of Nursing (RCN), concern remained for the average 4.7% increase which, according to the RCN, would not keep older nurses in the NHS. Mr Dobson said the above-inflation pay award was the best award, in real terms, for nurses and professionals allied to medicine in the last 10 years; £100 million was to be found from the NHS modernization fund to support the full implementation (Healy, 1999b). Christine Hancock, RCN general secretary, reflected the nurses' grudging acceptance of the pay award with the comment that improvements in patient care depended on a pay boost, not just for the newly qualified, but for all nurses (Healy, 1999c); nor should NHS trusts try to save money by employing fewer senior nurses.

In July 1999, a further government initiative attempted to halt the nursing exodus to the private sector. Top pay for nurses on the ward was to rise by a third to £40 000 a year – a carrot to keep 'super nurses' in the NHS. Announcing the creation of a new grade, Tony Blair and Frank Dobson said the initiative was part of the most comprehensive strategy ever produced to improve the status, training, pay and job opportunities for nurses, based on plans for a new four tier structure: health care assistants, qualified nurses, qualified staff with advanced qualifications and skills and a fourth ('super nurse') grade of consultant practitioner (DoH, 1999d). NHS trusts were expected to fund the new posts from general allocations, although more money would be made available to finance nurse education and training proposals (Healy, 1999e). At the start, only a few new 'super nurses' would be appointed, but the new approach would be piloted at ten sites from September 1999, jointly run by the RCN and the Department of Health. Eventually, some 5000 super nurses would be needed, each in charge of 50 nurses (DoH, 1999d). The government claimed that 1200 nurses had already rejoined the NHS since the beginning of the recruitment drive in February 1999. However, Mr Dobson also hinted at further pay improvements to come for the middle grades who were disappointed with the 1999 settlement. The RCN welcomed the breakthrough initiative with the call for greater emphasis on the acquisition of practical skills linked to more effective clinical placements for students (Murray, 1999c).

Various factors, as well as pay, influenced the recruitment, retention and service delivery by nurses. For example, the Audit Commission (1999) found that the district nursing services had been misused; one in ten referrals to district nursing services could be inappropriate. District nurses treated 2.75 million patients a year at a cost of £660 million; the demand was likely to increase as the ageing population was likely to incur more home care for terminally ill people. However, the Audit Commission (1999) argued that few NHS trusts had considered the strategic purpose of district nursing; the result was demand-led care, duplication and gaps in patient services.

Next was the wide variation in nurses and their skills. At one end came health care assistants (HCAs: introduced in 1990), who were not trained nurses but a new grade of staff who were also known as support workers. Up to 80% of NHS trusts employed HCAs, who averaged 8% of the workforce: by September 1996, 20 220 HCAs were employed by the NHS. After an intended six-month training period, HCA salaries ranged from £6000 to nearly £12 000. Some HCAs became engaged in various activities such as administering drugs, counselling, venepuncture; some could be in charge of a shift. The RCN remained concerned that regulation was left to individual employers (Snell, 1998).

Increasingly, boundaries between what HCAs and nursing staff were expected to do (Thornley, 1997) became blurred, leading to the government's 1999 promise to look into whether HCAs should be brought into some system of regulation.

By the winter of 1999, as the 'NHS crisis' deepened, families of patients at two Portsmouth hospitals were even asked to help wash, feed and shave relatives (Hope, 1999). Equally problematical was the role of health visitors who, in 1998, fought a bitter battle in Cambridge, but conceded defeat when health visiting was merged with school nursing into Lifespan Healthcare Trust's child and family nursing service. In an attempt to retain identity and position, the Health Visitors' Association (with 17 000 members), added the words 'community practitioner' to the title, in 1998, to become the CPHVA. Debates remained as to whether health visitors should continue to be registered separately from nurses and midwives; some health visitors wanted to become 'specialist community practitioners', others wanted to retain the title of health visitor. Most agreed that health visitors should continue to have a first-level nursing qualification, although others argued that to be placed with nursing in general prevented the profession from developing into the particular field of health visiting (Hempel, 1998).

The variation in nursing continued on to the highest levels of nurse practitioners. Nurse prescribing had also been increasingly encouraged, after eight pilot sites had undertaken trial runs, in the light of the Crown Report's (1989) recommendations together with positive evaluations from an official evaluation team from the Universities of Liverpool and York (Luker et al., 1997). Although health visitors and district nurses were included in the nurse prescribing programme, the position of other groups, such as practice nurses, had yet to be resolved. By April 2000, all nurses, health visitors and district nurses employed by NHS trusts or GP practices should be trained in nurse prescribing, according to the Nurse Prescribers' Formulary (NHS Executive, 1998c).

The developments of nursing into an upwardly mobile profession with an increasing graduate entry inevitably led to demands for higher pay to match new skills and responsibilities commented Ainsworth (1999). For example, by the end of 1999, an anticipated 60% of the population was to be covered by the nurse-led telephone helpline, even though doubts remained as to whether the service actually helped cut visits to doctors or accident and emergency departments (Snell, 1999). Training and skill mix could therefore also influence nurses' choices as much as pay. Nevertheless, as the 7 January leader in *The Times* (1999) pointed out, however many more nurses were recruited, more hospitals built and wards opened, the public's expectations would always exceed the NHS's capacity.

Nurse training and education

The basic programme to train and educate nurses, the Project 2000 diploma which was introduced in the early 1990s (see Chapter 6) was, according to Maynard (1999b), over-ambitious in trying to turn nursing into an academic profession. The Council of Deans and Heads of Universities' Faculties of Nursing, Midwifery and Health Visiting (1998) called for a re-think on nursing and health professional training, proper clinical career paths for nurses and nurse academics and a clear code of conduct between the NHS purchasers' consortia and university provision. The Council also demanded better workforce planning together with moves to stop pre-registration nurses leaving: one in seven did not seek registration. Poor pay and career prospects were partly blamed. Nursing needed to be an all-graduate profession. The RCN also agreed that nurses should be at the same level as other health care professionals if patients were to benefit from multidisciplinary learning (Brindle, 1998d).

A new, smaller Nursing, Midwifery and Health Visiting Council was to replace the four national boards that had governed nurse education. However, the debate over the future of the Project 2000 diploma raged on. Dr Anne Marie Rafferty (1999), from the Centre for Policy in Nursing Research, London School of Hygiene and Tropical Medicine, argued that, without university trained staff, the ambitious and much-needed NHS reforms would not work. Certainly, most would acknowledge that the Project 2000 diploma needed a radical overhaul to enable an effective combination of practice and academic learning. As RCN General Secretary, Christine Hancock's (1998) vision of the future foresaw the skills of caring, communication and disease prevention (skills traditionally the domain of the nurse) as becoming increasingly important for all health profes-sionals. Meanwhile, the growing debate on nurse education had been fuelled in part by concern over high drop-out rates, insufficient time spent on learning practical skills and the need to widen the entry gates into nursing (Thompson,

1999). For the twenty-first century, the Department of Health's strategy was spelt out by Tony Blair and Frank Dobson in *Making a Difference* (DoH, 1999d) (see page 266). The second initiative, in September 1999, was the report of the commission into nurse education, set up by nursing's regulatory body, the UKCC (United Kingdom Central Council), which opened up further debate.

Complementary medicine

Alongside the main professions in health care were the developments in alternative medicine. By the mid-1990s, data from *Social Trends* (CSO, 1994) provided evidence, for the first time, on the use of various therapies.

Table 15.1   Use of alternative medicine, 1989.

	Seriously consider (%)	Personally used (%)
Homoeopathy	37	11
Osteopathy	32	10
Faith or spiritual healing	12	5
Acupuncture	33	4
Hypnosis	19	3
Chiropractice	13	3

Source: CSO (Central Statistical Office) (1994: 108).
Reproduced by kind permission of the Office for National Statistics.

Other treatments could be added to the list by 1997 – such as reflexology, aromatherapy and herbal medicine. Changing attitudes were reflected in the British Medical Association's report *Complementary Medicine: New Approaches to Good Practice* (BMA, 1993) and the General Medical Council's (1993) report *Tomorrow's Doctors*. By 1997, some complementary therapies were available within the NHS, while almost 40% of GP partnerships in England provided access to complementary medicine, either by treating the patients within their own practice or by delegation to a complementary therapist. Furthermore, standard setting and education progressed as an increasing number of accredited university courses for students who wished to study for a career in a number of different complementary medical professions had become available – for example, at the University of Westminster's Centre for Community and Primary Health Care. Moreover, chiropractice and osteopathy, under the 1993 *Osteopathy Act*, had become regulated by an Act of Parliament.

By 1999, nearly 100 000 NHS staff had become members of the professions supplementary to medicine through completing approved training – often to degree level – and were state registered with the Council for Professions Supplementary to Medicine, set up by statute in 1960 to regulate the professions. Clause 47 of the 1999 Health Bill sought to regulate the professions allied to medicine far more closely which was intended to benefit both patients and *bona fide* practitioners (Harris, 1999).

In 1997, with a long-held interest in complementary medicine and holistic health care, the Prince of Wales called for an integrated approach to medicine and was instrumental in setting up four working groups from different scientific and educational backgrounds. The Foundation for Integrated Medicine (1997) published the results in a report. Recommendations were made for the introduction of effective systems of self-regulation for complementary medical professions and therapies in order to protect the public, for educational developments and for good practice in the delivery for integrated health care. The overall intention was to stimulate a wider public and professional debate about the possible role of complementary medicine within the changing pattern of health care in Britain.

By November 1998, from the Research Council for Complementary Medicine, Rebecca Rees (1998) had brought together a summary, from papers held on the CISCOM database, on the use of complementary medicine in the UK. Of interest was the gender of users (women only slightly outnumbered men by 55 to 45); most users were between 35 and 64 years old, mostly with problems linked to musculoskeletal conditions. However, no study had looked at the effect of income on use. Meanwhile, physicians perceived complementary medicine as 'moderately effective'.

Meanwhile, the scope and definition of alternative medicine remained problematical. Cant and Sharma (1999: 5) in analysing *A New Medical Pluralism*, considered that alternative medicine referred to forms of healing that depended on knowledge bases distinct from that of biomedicine nor shared by the special legitimisation conferred by the state upon biomedicine. Interestingly, the shift in terms also became clearer in their publication; 'alternative' medicine was predominately used up to the end of the 1980s but implied associations with alternative lifestyles. As greater acceptance became apparent by the medical profession, so the term 'complementary' came to be more widespread which signified the possibility of a more co-operative relationship with biomedicine. As Cant and Sharma (1999) went on to investigate, four key players had interests, at times conflicting, in complementary therapy: users, alternative practitioners, doctors and governments. In answer to the question 'why had alternative medicine achieved popularity in recent years?' Cant and Sharma (1999: 21) suggested that a significant change in the behaviour of users of health care had taken place: patients, with higher incomes and expectations, had become more discerning and discontented.

New trends for the twenty-first century were also reflected in the work of Dr Craig Brown, a GP in Sussex and President of the National Federation of Spiritual Healers. Dr Brown (1998) had set out to achieve *Optimum Healing* by integrating healing and spirituality into general medical care. In Dr Brown's view (1998: 7), the main thrust of conventional modern medicine was to eliminate symptoms, but health was more than being free of illness. The optimum healing approach was therefore one of integrating healing with modern medicine.

FINANCING HEALTH CARE IN THE TWENTY-FIRST CENTURY

The government had set out on an ambitious and impressive path of change in the NHS which was supported by a comprehensive spending review to result in generous allocation of resources to the NHS for the next three years. However, warned Barry Elliott (1999), chair-elect of the Healthcare Financial Management Association, the government's NHS reforms were in danger without a stable financial baseline. To avoid financial instability at the turn of the century, urgent steps were needed to manage the transition from the current to the new NHS funding regime.

New financial initiatives were also likely to make an impact on the twenty-first century. For example:

- the Road Traffic (NHS Charges) Bill would enable the NHS to claim back treatment costs for crash victims; the new system would be introduced in England, Scotland and Wales from April 1999;
- sweeping powers to curb the cost of drugs were included in the 1999 Health Bill;
- lottery money became part of mainstream NHS funding in the March 1999 budget, when £100 million was to be invested in cancer care.

Risk management and long-term care presented two further major financial challenges for the future.

Risk management

Risk management for the next century was likely to incur rising costs. Soaring litigation bills, together with the introduction of clinical governance, had led NHS trusts to appoint risk managers – which also increased financial outlay. Although training in the management of non-clinical risk had become well established, clinical risk management was a relatively new concept. The money that had been put aside for the eventual settlements of the 1998 cases had virtually doubled to £145 million on the previous year. The extra £120 million (£430 million over three years), which Chancellor Gordon Brown had found in the March 1999 budget for the NHS from the previously announced capital modernization fund, mainly for accident and emergency improvements, put the mounting costs of medical litigation into perspective.

The case at Newham Healthcare Trust reflected the rising financial outlay when a Trust had no risk strategy. Following the death of an 83-year old patient, who fell from an open window in 1998, the Trust was fined nearly £16 500 for breaching the *Health and Safety at Work Act*, at a time when the Trust was also operating a £4 million deficit. The new chief executive quickly installed a risk co-ordination group and relevant staff training (*Health Service Journal*, 1999c).

Overall, as White (1999a) commented, risk management reflected the law of unintended consequences. As procedures had been made more open and doctors had become more accountable, so patients started to sue more.

The Royal Commission on Long-Term Care

A far bigger financial legacy for the twenty-first century was the decision to be made by the government on long-term care. Appointed by the New Labour government in December 1997, the Royal Commission was asked to examine the short and long-term options for a substantial system of funding of long-term care for elderly people, both in their own homes and in other settings (Sutherland, 1999). Under the chairmanship of Sir Stewart Sutherland (1999: xvii) the Royal Commission began from the point of view that: 'old age should not be seen as a problem, but a time of life with fulfilment of its own'.

The Royal Commission's main recommendations (Sutherland, 1999) were for:

- a new contract between the individual and the state;
- bringing health, social care and housing services into a cohesive approach for rehabilitation, assessment of needs and commissioning;
- establishing a national care commission to bring together the different income strands of health and social services in a 'single pot of money'; the national care commission would ensure accountability;
- safeguarding the value of an elderly person's home for the first three months in residential care;
- changing the cut-off point for receiving state help from £16 000 in assets, including property, to £60 000;
- taking Department of Health proposals on pooled health and social services budgets further, with clear timetables and responsibility devolved to care managers;
- joint assessment of care needs by health and social services to provide a single entry point;
- a national carer support package to be introduced, with £229 million a year set aside to help carers which would need to rise to £700 million by 2050;
- the central recommendation was to split the costs of care between living costs, housing costs and personal care. People would contribute to living and housing costs, but all personal and nursing care would be available according to need and paid for from general taxation.

The Royal Commission claimed that there was no time-bomb as far as long-term care was concerned, as a result the costs of care would be affordable (Sutherland, 1999: xviii). Set out clearly were the unacceptable variations in standards across the country, the unequal charging systems between free hospital nursing care and means-tested care in nursing and residential homes in the community, the lack of clear lines of responsibility between the individual and the state and too little security for those approaching old age (Sutherland, 1999). Normal living and housing costs would remain the responsibility of care home residents under the Royal Commission's proposals which would cost £1.2 billion to implement in the first year. The nation currently paid £11.1 billion a year on long-term care for elderly people, which included contributions from individuals; the overall costs would rise to £45 billion by the middle of the twenty-first century. If the Royal Commission's proposals were implemented, the state's share of costs would increase from £8.2 billion at current levels to £33 billion by 2050 (Frean, 1999).

The *Guardian* (1999a) perceived a third way forward between the universal and redistribution approaches: a compulsory social insurance system (rejected by the Royal Commission) which could provide collective cover for those needing long-term care. However, such a move would be perceived as a tax rise.

By early March 1999, Health Secretary Frank Dobson told the House of Commons that he supported the Royal Commission's call for an 'informed debate' on the proposals, but that the government's response had to await the outcome of the discussions (Healy and McIntosh, 1999). However, as months went by without a decision on the Royal Commission's proposals, ministers were accused of shelving the report while older people were still forced to sell their homes to fund essential care in local authority nursing homes. The charities Age Concern, Help the Aged and Council and Care, as well as private insurers, complained that older people were being left in limbo (Inman, 1999).

As the twenty-first century approached the issues sharpened up; decisions were needed. By July 1999, research from Leeds University and Liverpool University had shown that, despite the recognition of the importance of seamless health and social care, to enable elderly peopel to live independently, there was little evidence that continuing health care policies were achieving these objectives. The transition between hospital and home or residential care needed to be improved by better co-operation between staff in the different sectors; the links between most GPs and social workers were especially weak (Johnson and Abbott, 1999). However, the introduction of an interprofessional care co-ordinator at St Bartholomew's and the London Trust had helped hospital discharge. Nevertheless, tensions over professional boundaries between nursing and social work remained (Bridges et al., 1999).

Matters were brought into legal contention when the Court of Appeal ruled on Pamela Coughlan's case in July 1999. Miss Coughlan had been paralysed in a road accident in 1971. Subsequently North and East Devon Health Authority decided to close Mardon House, an NHS rehabilitation centre, whereupon Pamela Coughlan and other long-term disabled residents were moved into a local authority nursing home where means-tested nursing care was operational. The Appeal Court ruling proved significant in that the three judges stated that the health authority had acted unlawfully as Miss Coughlan had been told that NHS-funded nursing care and a home for life would be provided at Mardon House. Miss Coughlan won her case as well as the legal costs (Shaw, 1999).

The critical issue in the appeal case was whether nursing care for a chronically ill patient could be provided by a local authority as a social service – in which case the patient paid according to means – or whether the NHS should be required to provide nursing care, free at the point of use, by law. The three appeal judges did not accept the previous High Court judge's conclusion that all nursing care should be the sole responsibility of the NHS, therefore to be provided by the health authority. The Appeal Court judges stated that the NHS did not have sole responsibility for all nursing care. Nursing care for a chronically sick patient might be provided by a local authority; the patient could then be liable to meet the cost of nursing care according to financial means. However, the Appeal Court ruled that where a person's need for accommodation and support was primarily to meet health needs, as in the case of Pamela Coughlan, care should be free; but social service departments as well as the health service might be the providers (Dyer and Gibbs, 1999).

More than 150 000 elderly people who receive long-term nursing care could be affected by the Coughlan case. During the 1990s, numerous long-stay hospitals closed; health authorities nation-wide then transferred patients needing indefinite care to local authority nursing homes. However, the Appeal Court upheld the government's 1995 guidelines, which stated that the NHS could shift responsibility for some long-term nursing care to local authorities, who could pass on the costs of care to patients if individuals had the means to pay (DoH, 1995b). Nevertheless, the 1999 Appeal Court ruling meant that the NHS would have to pay the care bill for some nursing home residents with needs for extensive care that were currently met by local authority social services or by the patient's mean-tested resources. The upshot of the case was that where the line was exactly drawn was not clear.

As a result of the Coughlan case, the government had to review the Department of Health guidelines (DoH, 1995b). Health authorities were also likely to receive a round of further legal challenges to fees charged for local authority nursing care. Health Secretary, Frank Dobson was delighted with the outcome, which went against the High Court's ruling that all nursing care was the sole responsibility of the NHS, acting through health authorities and that financial burden could not be transferred to local authority social services departments – a judgment which could have landed the NHS with an annual bill of £220 million. However, according to the RCN's understanding, the Appeal Court ruling could herald the end of means-testing for long-term nursing care, as anyone in a nursing home was there primarily for health needs. In the view of Stephen Thornton, chief executive of the NHS Confederation, had the Appeal Court judges come to the conclusion that the NHS should carry the financial burden of all nursing care provided in nursing homes, the NHS could have been bankrupted (Hall, 1999a).

The structural division between local authority means-tested community care and NHS health care, free at the point of use, therefore continued as a legacy across the twentieth centry and into the twenty-first century. Whatever the outcome of the Royal Commission's proposals (Sutherland, 1999) and the Department of Health's review of continuing care guidelines (DoH, 1995b) in the light of the Coughlan judgement, the issue for the next century was to face up to some difficult decisions at a cost.

A primary care-led NHS

On 1 April 1999, the GP fundholding scheme effectively came to an end. In place of the fundholding arrangements, which covered just over half of all patients, a more unified system of 481 Primary Care Groups, with some 50 GPs per PCG to cover roughly 100 000 patients, took over. For the PCGs of the future lessons could be learnt from the Department of Health's research, by the health service management centre at Birmingham University, into the GP commissioning pilot programmes. Forty pilot programmes in the English regions were started in April 1998, all of which became PCGs in April 1999. Prefiguring an important aspect of PCGs, each programme held a group cash-limited prescribing budget. Key points to emerge from the evaluation included:

- the importance of high-quality dedicated management support;
- the health authority–PCG dynamic was of particular importance to the effective development and functioning of PCGs;
- service user and public involvement were likely to remain problematic unless clear guidance and support for PCGs about models of good practice were forthcoming (Smith et al., 1999b).

The time commitment of clinical staff had also been considerable which had deterred some GPs from taking part in PCGs (Brindle, 1999e).

PCGs were intended to develop into trusts over time, to include former community health trusts and to be responsible not only for commissioning care but also for providing health services. As a result the purchaser/provider split would become less clear cut. However, the government had decided not to extend GP control to the arrangements for Primary Care Trusts. Doctors would not necessarily retain a majority on trust executives. Of the 11 members of a PCT, six members (including the chair) would be appointed by the Secretary of State for Health. According to the newly appointed Health Minister, John Denham, PCG boards would be responsible for overall performance, but the membership would be formed by a lay majority with a strong professional presence (Brindle, 1999e).

First-wave PCTs were to go live in April 2000 to provide community and primary health care as well as commissioning acute hospital services. John Denham stated that health authorities must begin to 'let go' to enable primary care groups to become primary care trusts. Peterborough and Hertfordshire were commended as good examples of areas where progress had been made towards PCT developments. Meanwhile, local experience had shown that Community Health Care Trusts needed to work effectively with PCGs and PCTs to prevent becoming 'dysfunctional' organizations in times of local health economy change (McIntosh, 1999c).

The challenge for the future was whether the reforms could lead to a radical primary care-led health service – a vision which, according to official NHS historian Charles Webster (1998/9), was held by the planners of the NHS over 50 years ago who were drawn to the original blueprint, set out by the Dawson Committee (1920) of primary care centres (Brindle, 1999e).

However, by July 1999, GPs were becoming increasingly concerned over the loss of their gatekeeper role as NHS Direct spread nation-wide, while high street drop-in centres offered another point of access to health care. The government's capital modernization fund had set aside £280 million for fast-access NHS walk-in centres, to be run by primary care groups, but GPs doubted whether any benefits would be provided by such centres (Crail, 1999b). Furthermore, the rise of the Medicentre chain of private GP clinics, such as the clinic at a Sainsbury's branch in Sheffield, had also been met with alarm by NHS family doctors (McIntosh, 1999d).

Only in the twenty-first century would patients be able to judge whether all the changes had been worth while.

16 INTO THE TWENTY-FIRST CENTURY: RETROSPECT AND PROSPECTS

In retrospect, the NHS principles, strengths and weaknesses will now be reviewed and a wider assessment of health care provision discussed, set within four models for analysis. Finally, prospects for the twenty-first century will be considered in the light of new possibilities for health care in the future, while some final questions are considered for the NHS in the new century.

INTO THE TWENTY-FIRST CENTURY: RETROSPECT

After over 50 years from the start of the NHS, any form of evaluation has become problematical. First, the original principles of the NHS were somewhat ambiguous; secondly, monitoring techniques have emerged only in recent years and often for different purposes; thirdly, the NHS has evolved over time, so outcomes could not necessarily be compared as systems have moved through different stages. The NHS could not therefore be evaluated in terms of a single currency, which led Powell (1997) to construct a formula for temporal (over time), intrinsic (meeting objectives) and extrinsic (comparing systems abroad) evaluation. At a more simplistic level, the next section concentrates on certain key factors that have emerged and which could point the way forward into the twenty-first century.

The Ministry of Health's (1944: 5) White Paper established the broad aims and principles of the NHS:

> *The government want to ensure that in the future every man and woman and child can rely on getting ... the best medical and other facilities available, that their getting them shall not depend on whether they can pay or any other factor irrelevant to real need.*

From this somewhat entangled statement, various key concepts emerged: need, adequacy, comprehensiveness, universality, services free at the point of use, equality and equity. Given the intended NHS agenda, in retrospect the pre-war services looked gravely deficient with a track record of inadequacy, inefficiency, barriers to access as well as geographical and social inequalities. However, as Powell (1997: 36) has pointed out, the criticism of inequality would be relevant only to an NHS system of provision not to a collection of pre-war individual hospital providers. Further, local authorities were responsible for health care in their locality which, despite diversity in provision, did offer local democracy. Throughout the history of the NHS, the organizational barriers between the NHS and local authority social services left a continuing legacy which only New Labour had, by the end of the century, attempted to address more fundamentally through a policy of integrated care based on partnership (DoH, 1998d). A remaining question for the twenty-first century was whether joint working would be sufficient to overcome the twentieth-century tensions.

Need

Need was never defined, although the concept of need, embodied in the principles, was interpreted as an ability to benefit from the use of the NHS (Birch, 1986). The nature of health care demand was not recognized, nor was consideration given as to how the scarce resources of the NHS were to be rationed in the absence of the traditional price mechanism. The medical profession was largely left to resolve the issue of need, where the severity of the condition or urgency of treatment tended to be given higher priority. By the mid-1980s, management and resource imperatives began to assume greater predominance in determining need. By the 1990s, the internal market had introduced priced treatments based on assessed need in which the purchasing of health care was separated from the provision. However, the concept of need stood the test of time as New Labour, by 1997, placed meeting need at the centre of health care policy but, in keeping with an era of neat buzz terms, under the caption 'A modern and dependable NHS there when you need it' (Secretary of State for Health, 1997c: 4). The concept of need is likely to remain into the twenty-first century.

Adequacy and the best

As Minister of Health, Aneurin Bevan's vision in 1946 of an optimum service proved an unrealizable ideal. The reason soon became manifest as 'the best' assumed unlimited resources which was incompatible with the financial basis of the NHS as the system became an instrument for rationing scarce resources. Furthermore, health care needs and demands have always proved infinite and in tension with finite resources. The 'best' became watered down to the notion of adequacy. What the NHS did, in effect, achieve was universalization of the adequate: the delivery of health care was rationalized to assure a minimum of service provision for all (Klein, 1983). As Klein (1995: 235) commented: Bevan's original aim of 'universalizing the best', an objective reaffirmed by *Working for Patients* (DoH, 1989a), had not been realistic. Universalizing adequacy was probably the most that could be achieved. By 1997, the Secretary of State for Health (1997c: 4) also offered a vision of a government committed 'to giving the people of this country the very best system in the world'. By 1997, 'best' for the NHS meant prompt high quality treatment and care when and where needed, regulated and accountable, alongside working with others to improve health and to reduce inequalities. The agenda for 'best' in the twenty-first century was certainly ambitious, but the problem could well be in the implementation.

Comprehensive services for all

Providing appropriate care for most conditions on a universal basis has been generally assumed. However, to the extent that the NHS has offered inadequate facilities or none at all, then such fundamental principles have been eroded. Nevertheless, although the NHS set out to become a universal service, people did not have automatic and enforceable entitlements to treatment. Although GPs might see all registered patients on request, some patients might not move beyond the GP gatekeeper, assessed on the basis of clinical need rather than by patient demand (Powell, 1997: 123). Increasingly, the notion of comprehensiveness has become diluted. Differing views over access to abortion facilities on the NHS, for example, has led to wide variations across the country. In 1996, a national average of 72% of abortions were undertaken in NHS hospitals; the remainder were performed in the private sector under contract from the NHS on behalf of NHS patients (Office for National Statistics: 1996).

Rationing (as set out in Chapter 11) also lowered the level of comprehensive provision so that limited targets for specific treatments became increasingly likely (such as for *in vitro* fertilization). Viagra for male impotence raised another issue: a new form of treatment which could raise costs astronomically if issued on a universal, comprehensive basis. Viagra sparked a long overdue debate about rationing in the NHS. In May 1999, the High Court ruled that the government's interim guidance, which restricted Viagra's availability, was unlawful (Murray, 1999d). The then Health Secretary, Frank Dobson, had been striving to restrain spending to ensure that money was spent on NHS priorities. By 1999, the NHS was funded by £42 billion of taxpayers' money which meant that care had to be rationed. The NHS could only provide a fixed sum for Viagra, which the Health Secretary had hoped to cap at around £15 million. However, Mr Dobson had to bow to pressure from doctors and patients to announce that Viagra could be prescribed on the NHS for men with a wider range of medical conditions than previously planned, although the Health Secretary stuck to his resolve not to allow unlimited NHS funds to be spent on the expensive drug. Mr Dobson's announcement was a landmark in that a minister was prepared to make a difficult decision on rationing NHS resources. In the past, health authorities were left to find money for treatments or turn patients away (Boseley, 1999c). However, drugs that made life seemingly better for patients without actually helping to cure individuals then immediately raised the issue of rationing in the NHS.

A further factor was the developments in medical technology which could offer hip, knee and other joint replacements as well as cancer screening services, to cite two widely used present-day forms of treatment and illness prevention. Into the twenty-first century, comprehensive services for all were likely to be trimmed by rationing and cost availability.

Services free at the point of use

A basic principle of the NHS established that health care was to be available to all citizens, free at the point of delivery, financed largely by general taxation. Charges for certain services were, however, introduced early in the life of the NHS (1951). Prescription charges went up continuously: by 1 April 1999 the charge for a single prescription was £5.90.

A fundamental question then remained as to whether charges were important as a deviation from basic principles in their own right or only if charges deterred use (Walshe, 1995). As Powell (1997: 120) has pointed out, many people were exempt from charges which, in theory, were then only paid by those who could afford charges. Nevertheless, the effects of regular and frequent increases in NHS charges led to a significant reduction in patient utilization (Birch, 1986; Ryan and Birch, 1988). However, the principle of free health care, at the point of use, was to remain a key feature of the New NHS, under Prime Minister Tony Blair's signature: to deliver dependable, high-quality care based on need not ability to pay (Secretary of State for Health, 1997c: 2). The basic principle looked firmly secured by political commitment for the start of the twenty-first century. A key question for the future remained as to how far public financial resources could be made available to uphold the principle of services free at the point of use in the light of rising needs and demands.

Equality and equity

Embedded in the notion of 'real need' were the concepts of equality of access (aiming to provide equal services for equal need irrespective of income) and equity (seeking to offer fair, just and impartial health care services according to need). In theory, the principles of equality and equity remained intact, but the NHS had to contend with regional, social class, race and gender inequalities, in both health care access and in outcome (Black Report, 1980; Whitehead, 1987; McNaught, 1988; Benzeval et al., 1995; Acheson Report, 1998).

Initially aggravated by the legacy of uneven health care facilities across the country, geographical equality of access to NHS services remained unattainable. The mid-1970s Resource Allocation Working Party solution went some way to eradicate regional inequalities, but the subsequent policy of marked public expenditure restraint impeded progress, compounded by differences in local policies, clinical practices and professional attitudes. A decade later, Smith and Jacobson (1988) charted mounting inequalities which showed that, while the country's health as a whole had improved, the gap between north and south, as well as between rich and poor, had widened.

The NHS had been even less successful in achieving equity, in terms of the quality and care provided, once individuals had access to the system (equity had largely been achieved regarding service access) (Klein, 1989: 148). Again, surveys (Black Report, 1980; Whitehead, 1987; Benzeval et al., 1995) had consistently shown that higher income, white people had benefited most from the NHS in terms of the quality received, through their knowledge of how to work the system to their advantage – but also as the NHS was structured according to the values, assumptions and preferences of the sophisticated middle-class consumer (Black Report, 1980; Klein, 1989). On the other hand, Klein (1995: 235) considered that the internal market model of 1991 would not necessarily discriminate against equity as, potentially, the model offered an opportunity to 'manipulate incentives in such a way as to enhance equity'.

However, as Benzeval et al. (1995: 119) had pointed out, health care provision was not the most important way to tackle inequalities in health, but the NHS had a contribution to make through ensuring greater equity of access to care by distributing resources in relation to need and by removing barriers to effective use of services. In looking forward to the new century, New Labour had shown a determined effort to address the issues through the consultation paper *Our Healthier Nation* (Secretary of State for Health, 1998a), the Social Exclusion Unit and through Health Action Zones in socially deprived areas, amongst other initiatives. The challenge for the future was to surmount the twentieth century's seeming neglect.

Overall, due to the problematical nature of the exercise, Powell (1997: 190) concluded that no definitive evaluation of the NHS could be effectively mounted. Earlier government attempts to evaluate the NHS had identified efficiency with economy which led to concern over controlling costs rather than measuring outcomes. For the twenty-first century, Powell (1998) called for a broader NHS remit to look at evidence-based health: the evaluation of environmental interventions as well as evidence-based policy making.

NHS STRENGTHS AND WEAKNESSES BY 1999

The positive views of patients and users

Although the founding principles of the NHS in 1948 were not fully satisfied over the subsequent 50 years, features such as equality of access, equity, comprehensiveness and services free at the point of delivery were highly valued by the general public. One major NHS achievement had been the continuous public acclaim which, in 1995, was reflected in the 77% support for extra public spending on health – as always, to feature above all other public expenditure outlays, according to the *British Social Attitudes* survey (Brook et al., 1996). Mulligan and Judge (1997: 128) also pointed out that, as people became more demanding, dissatisfaction with the state of the NHS had increased, although favourable attitudes had always been expressed about the services provided by the professionals.

NHS shortcomings from the consumer perspective

- Paternalism in the health service.
- Rationing by queuing (waiting lists).
- The need to rebuild confidence in public services over time.
- The perennial problem of hospital bed shortages. The Ministry of Defence (MoD) offered a novel solution in the use, by the NHS or private companies, of two new hospital ships (with 200 hospital beds each) to be set up under the private finance initiative, whenever the MoD did not need the ships (Gow, 1999).
- Low level of consumer choice together with the information needed to exercise choice (Leavey et al., 1989).
- Lack of individual involvement and community participation in decision-making and in health care provision more generally (Barnes and Evans, 1998).
- Lack of local democracy.

Health status: some strengths

- Infant mortality had fallen dramatically from 36 to 9.1 deaths for every 1000 live births between 1948 and 1987 (Smith and Jacobsen, 1988).
- Younger people had far better teeth than in previous generations: better diet,

- better hygiene and fluoride in water or toothpaste had all combined to reduce teeth fillings and dental decay (Boseley, 1998d).
- UK life expectancy had risen to over 74 years for men and 79 years for women in 1996; life expectancy had increased every decade by about two years for men and 1.5 years for women (Office for National Statistics, 1999: 120).
- Deaths from diphtheria, polio and whooping cough had fallen from 1468 in 1948 to 33 in 1974 (Abel-Smith, 1978). By 1988 diseases such as tuberculosis had shrunk from being recurrent killers to clinical rarities, although where vaccination programmes lapsed, dangers still lurked. However, by 1999, globalization had increased international transmission and as a result the incidence of multi-drug resistant tuberculosis was rising significantly in London (Boseley, 1999d).

Health status: some continuing weaknesses

- The death rate for coronary heart disease was virtually the highest in the world.
- The significant health gap between professional and unskilled classes continued (Smith and Jacobsen, 1988; Office for National Statistics, 1999: 120).
- Up to 25 000 deaths from cancer could be avoided every year if Britain was as effective at treating the disease as the best countries in Europe. Britain was below average in Europe for the number of cancer sufferers who survived longer than five years, while the standard of care patients received varied radically around Britain (Boseley, 1999e).

The NHS delivery system: the drawbacks

- The backlog of demand and accumulated pre-First World War deficiencies represented some of the greatest problems in the early NHS whose financing, as Charles Webster (1988) recorded, made little allowance for the correction of inherited maldistribution and general inadequacies in standards.
- The initial absence of symmetry and lack of co-ordination between the three arms of the NHS (hospitals, general practice, community health) obstructed continuity of treatment and planning overall (Webster, 1988; Kings Fund, 1988).
- Lack of patient choice was a constant feature, except for the 10% of the population (by 1999) with access to private health insurance (MacAskill, 1999a).
- Gaps persisted between the intention of policy makers and what happened in practice which resulted in the failure to develop adequate community-based services for mentally ill, mentally handicapped and elderly people (Ham, 1982; IHSM, 1988).
- One notably neglected area was the place of the public health tradition whose decay stood in contrast to the relatively high watermark of concern and activity in the nineteenth century. The NHS had traditionally encouraged other bodies to tackle social inequalities (Hawker, 1999), despite Ashton and Seymour's (1988) call for *The New Public Health*, as well as important recommendations from both Acheson Reports (1988, 1998) on the future

development of the public health function. However, even New Labour's much-heralded *Our Healthier Nation* (Secretary of State for Health, 1998a) might founder, warned Steve Peckham (1998), on 'hidden icebergs left floating in an NHS structure that was set up to focus on ill health'.

- Overall, too little systematic attention had been given to the quality of the services (IHSM, 1988) until the 1990s.
- However, the major drawback throughout the history of the NHS was the lack of public funds to meet the demands. Even when private sector initiatives were brought into the spectrum during the 1990s to help boost NHS monies, demand still outstripped supply. By 1999, even the principle of the government's private funding initiative (PFI) had come under attack. Under the PFI, a private sector consortium was intended to design, build, finance and operate a new hospital. The NHS hospital trust would then make a single annual payment to the consortium for the use of the building and provision of basic services. Although six hospitals had been given the go-ahead since 1997, together with plans for a further six PFI hospitals announced in July 1999, concerns lingered amongst the trade unions as well as the *British Medical Journal*, influenced by work from a number of university academics (Brown, 1999). Nor did the purchaser/provider split, across the 1990s, which had set out to assess needs in order to curb unlimited demands, provide the intended solution to cut costs. By 1999, the NHS was running into ever more financial problems. Two thirds of hospital trusts were heading into the red despite an injection of £21 billion into the NHS before 2002. The extra cash had been absorbed by pay deals, above-inflation increases in capital charges, the cost of blood products, the impact of the European working time directives and a steep rise in NHS pension costs (which alone would cost an additional £500 million a year by 2001). Mr Blair's vision of modernization for the NHS had therefore been 'hit by doubts' (Brindle, 1999f) for the start of the new century.

The NHS delivery system: the strengths

The NHS was an immense advance on the inadequate, uncoordinated pre-war health care facilities which were out of financial reach for many.

- Following the Griffiths Report (1983), those who considered the NHS had suffered from inadequate management welcomed the introduction of general management; however, the outcome did vary according to whose perception was invoked (Petchey, 1986; Strong and Robinson, 1988).
- By international standards, a relative strength of the NHS had been the family-oriented General Practitioner service; although geographically patchy, especially in the inner cities, the personalized primary care doctor system had been able, on the whole, to deal with the vast majority of ill health economically (Maxwell, 1988; Timmins, 1988).

In retrospect the outcome of the internal market from 1991 would have to be seen as disadvantageous, in the outcome of service fragmentation and in the failure to curb costs but, given that New Labour intended to continue with the purchaser/provider split, the outcome could be seen as advantageous where purchaser contracts, based on assessed needs serviced by health care providers, were concerned. By the turn of the century the architect of the internal market, Professor Alain Enthoven, commented that, while still an advocate of the internal market (although developments had needed more time and political space to develop in Britain), there was general agreement that the purchaser/ provider split was a good idea (Crail, 1999a).

Despite uncertainty about funding, the general direction of policy was positive with New Labour's emphasis on collaboration and co-operation both within the NHS and between the NHS and social services. Further, a new attempt had been made to highlight health promotion in the widest sense (Klein et al., 1998).

Overall, curious outcomes could be seen retrospectively in the NHS delivery system: increasingly, a near obsession to reorganize the structure of the NHS gripped all incoming administrations. No consideration was given to effective management until the 1980s but not until the 1990s under quality assurance programmes, and more particularly with the arrival of New Labour in 1997, was any serious detailed programme set out to address the important element of regulated quality services, to be extended to private sector hospitals under government proposals for the year 2000 (MacAskill, 1999a).

HEALTH CARE PROVISION SET WITHIN SOCIAL POLICY MODELS

An overview of past, present and future health care provision could only be usefully assessed on a broader basis when applied to a set of social policy models. The models explored in *Not Just for the Poor* (Bayley et al., 1986) have always been particularly relevant for the developments in the NHS. Five basic social policy models were outlined to illustrate the possible alternative approaches to providing health and welfare services. The three models most appropriate to the delivery of health care in twentieth century Britain will be discussed here. The models of the state, acting as an exclusive provider, or where only private and voluntary agencies were available, have been omitted. However, an extended model has been added to reflect The Third Way in New Labour's outlook for the new century.

Model 1: the state as a safety net

This approach has been especially relevant to the post-war social security system in Britain. The model aimed to restrict the role of the state to that of providing a safety net to prevent those unable to fend for themselves from falling into deprivation and poverty. This route to social welfare also corresponded to the pre-war model of health care where first the Poor Law, then local authorities provided a municipal safety net. Thus the state offered a minimal back-up service for those who could not afford any other kind of health care or welfare. For the rest, provision was by private or voluntary means, through insurance schemes and specialist private agencies. Individuals were therefore largely responsible for their own provision; public action was restricted to providing services for those who were likely to fall below the minimum standard considered necessary for survival. Nevertheless, the state also had a role in setting and enforcing minimum standards.

Reluctant collectivists favoured such an approach as individuals had the freedom to take responsibility for their own welfare but were protected against serious hardship, ill health and deprivation. The state also recognized that society had a duty to poor and sick people. However, the snags of the safety net model reflected the drawbacks of the pre-war health services: the stigmatizing effect of residual provision, the perpetuation of inequalities, the inadequacy of facilities, the lack of co-ordination and planning, services directed to poor people invariably became poor services, while individuals unable to make provision by private means therefore received second-class treatment. As the NHS replaced the pre-war health care system the state became the main provider.

Model 2: the state as primary provider

The second model accepted and valued the place of voluntary and private agencies but contended that comprehensive care could be guaranteed only when state services were provided on a community-wide basis through collective action, financed largely by taxation. Both the education and health services in Britain adhered to the primary provider model from the mid-1940s onwards.

The advantages of this approach were essentially two-fold. First, taxation was an effective funding mechanism which represented a cheap method of raising funds but which could control the level of public expenditure. Secondly, collective action and state responsibility could aim for comprehensive, egalitarian, co-ordinated and planned public services. The snags in the primary provider model were precisely those criticized by Mrs Thatcher's government throughout the 1980s: growth of large-scale paternalistic, cumbersome bureaucracies, lack of consumer choice, fostering of dependence on the 'nanny state' and organizational resistance to change.

The government's subsequent proposals for change in the NHS for the 1990s, outlined in *Working for Patients* (DoH, 1989a), essentially moved the state provision of health care over to Model 3, along with other aspects of the social services.

Model 3: the state as primary funder

Model 3 accepted the need for some services to be provided for the whole community irrespective of their circumstances. However, under Model 3 the state primarily planned a leading role in financing services for all. The actual provision of services was made by a variety of statutory, voluntary and private institutions.

The advantages of the primary funder model, in theory, offered greater consumer choice and flexibility in provision. The model was also strong on responding to changing needs. Nevertheless, where the state became a primary funder, rather than a provider, it needed to take on a regulatory and monitoring role.

As the services moved into the 1990s, so provision in housing (through voluntary and private housing trusts and associations), in education (through the private schools-assisted places scheme and the local business-led youth training programme), in welfare (via private and voluntary residential homes) and in health (through aspects of the internal market such as private hospital provision) was significantly moving over to Model 3, where public resources were increasingly destined to finance private and voluntary provision. So what were the drawbacks of the state acting as a primary funder rather than a provider?

1 The means of ensuring universal availability of services and protecting poorer and weaker members of society were uncertain, when wealthier people could gain relatively more from the effective deployment of choice.
2 The possible duplication of services and unhelpful competition between agencies were likely to escalate.
3 Questions remained about the effective co-ordination of provision as well as the guarantee and maintenance of standards.
4 The need to secure some agreement about what should be expected of private and voluntary bodies, in relation to the responsibility of the public services, remained a matter of importance.
5 Dilemmas continued as to how the system would actually function in a deeply divided and unequal society.

So far, all models have been shown to have advantages and disadvantages. So would the incoming New Labour government in 1997 choose a former model or continue with the primary funder model, or construct a new approach?

Model 4: The Third Way

In keeping with the main theme, that evolution has been the key factor in healthcare provision in Britain, The Third Way was supremely evolutionary. New Labour did not construct a new model but selected elements from all previous models. Social security continued to be based on a safety net approach but with an emphasis on welfare to work, although the prime intent was to curb expenditure on state social security. However, education and health were to be held in high esteem, in which the state would be both a primary provider and funder. The private and voluntary sectors were also to play a key part in funding (as with the private finance initiative for new hospital buildings) and provision. Private organizations were to take over badly run state schools, for example Nord Anglia was contracted to improve failing parts of the educational services in the London borough of Hackney (*The Guardian*, 1999b), together with the ongoing role of the private and voluntary sectors for the provision of residential and nursing homes. Housing was to remain largely within the private sector. Nevertheless, Tony Blair had set a 20-year deadline to end child poverty, with a high profile attempt to show that the government meant business on welfare reform (White, 1999b). The whole was to be financed on a slightly decreasing personal taxation basis, using complex (thus almost disguised) measures of indirect taxation together with the use of lottery funds.

The model for The Third Way represented all things to all people, for health as for all other aspects of the social services. The political advantage was that any opposition or criticism could be absorbed within such a wide remit. The disadvantage, as the Opposition leader, Mr Hague, had found, was that short of moving rapidly to the right or left of any issue, the difficulty was to pin anything down. The NHS had the political advantage of a highly committed Secretary of State for Health in Frank Dobson. However, only developments in the twenty-first century would reveal just how successfully the NHS was to fare along The Third Way.

INTO THE TWENTY-FIRST CENTURY: PROSPECTS

While the NHS went into the new century with a certain level of goodwill on the part of the public, whatever else was to occur, new medical developments were likely to transform lives. How far the NHS would be able to finance the potential breakthroughs in medical technology would remain to be seen. The innovations were likely to include the following:

- An artificial heart, being pioneered by Dr Michael Debakey in Britain: whereby a thumb-sized electronic pump could be planted into or next to a patient's heart as a permanent replacement or as treatment for chronic conditions (*Horizon*, BBC2, 18 February 1999).
- Missing and damaged teeth could one day be regrown with a gel being developed by Paul Sharpe, Professor of craniofacial development at Guy's Hospital, London, to contain the genetic information to order a particular type of tooth to grow (Prigg, 1999).
- Cancer research laboratories were working on a new generation of drugs to kill cancer cells (Weinberg, 1999).
- A tongue transplant to restore speech, planned by a team led by Dr Bruce Haughey at the University of Washington, which would use a revolutionary technique to give back some cancer sufferers the ability to eat and speak (Farrar and Gadher, 1999).
- A cervical cancer vaccine could be available within 10 years, which would make smear tests all but obsolete. The aim would be to give the vaccine to all children, male and female, at the age of 12, to provide immunization for life against the sexually transmitted germ responsible for 99% of this type of cancer (Murray, 1999e).
- American scientists had announced a marrow cell find that could allow crippled immune systems to become functional again which would herald the end of bone marrow transplants for people with advanced leukaemia (Dodd, 1999).
- Surgeons at the Queen's Medical Centre in Nottingham had evolved a groundbreaking technique to grow eye transplant material, which could revolutionize the lives of people with damaged corneas (Wilson, 1999).
- Scientists at the Institute of Ophthalmology had developed a pioneering transplant technique for rebuilding damaged eyes that could help thousands of blind and partially sighted people to recover their vision. The technique involved taking nerve cells from other parts of the body (such as the leg), and injecting the cells into the eye to replace cells damaged by disease (Macaskill, 1999b).

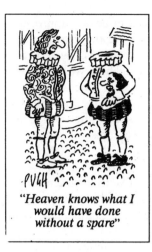

"*Heaven knows what I would have done without a spare*"

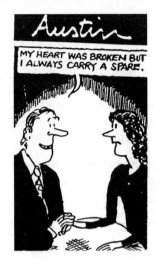

Source: Pugh, The Times, 8 December 1998.
Reproduced by kind permission of The Times and Pugh.

Source: Austin, The Guardian, 6 November 1998.
Reproduced by kind permission of The Guardian and Austin.

- Children born in 1999 could expect to live to 130 years of age due to medical breakthroughs in human genetics, organ cloning and the biology of ageing (Farrar, 1999a). A more fundamental question might be whether people would actually *want* to live to 130 years.

Such a range of developments brought up the whole perspective of ethics. If the ethical principles of autonomy, beneficence, non-maleficence and justice (Seedhouse, 1988; Singleton and McLaren, 1995) were to be applied to future decisions about genetically modified food, for example (to be addressed by the proposed Food Standards Agency under the draft 1999 Food Standards Bill, which would report to health ministers with a UK wide remit (Crail, 1999c)), the issues would become increasingly complex. The development in human cloning also raised more ethically questionable matters. In 1998, American scientists announced a discovery that could revolutionize medicine – a way had been found to grow any kind of human tissue in a laboratory. The breakthrough, the most dramatic since the cloning of Dolly the sheep, came with the cultivation of human embryonic cells which contained the potential to become blood, muscle, skin or other organic tissue in the growing human body (Radford, 1998).

Nevertheless, one danger for the twenty-first century was that millennium man might become a 14-stone sloth as almost all physical activities could be replaced or augmented by computers and machinery within 50 years (Farrar, 1999b). However, medical ethics had not, so far, been engaged in such a prospective.

A more immediate problem for the NHS at the end of the twentieth century was just how the new primary care groups were going to work out what the outcome would be for health care professionals and patients. In reviewing the NHS, both present and future, with a group of postgraduate health care practitioner students at South Bank University in March 1999, we also looked at the arrangements in Scandinavia, at the European social insurance approach and the private insurance model in the USA. Which system did the group most favour? 'The NHS in Britain' came the answer from all, except two nurse practitioners who felt that the relatively low pay was a drawback. Then, with the approval of all, one student said that the NHS represented a moral commitment which the country supported. Regardless of financial means, everyone had entitlement to health care, free at the point of use. Over 50 years after the start of the NHS, one felt Aneuran Bevan would have liked to have been present.

The moral consensus and future options

The big question for the future of the NHS in the twenty-first century was: just how long would the moral consensus last? How long would nurses, despite potentially significant pay rises for a few, be prepared to act as moral agents when often required to work in severely under-resourced conditions? At the British Medical Associations annual meeting in July 1999, doctors claimed that a climate of alienation and stress had been created within the medical profession by the government, as a result of endless reforms without consultation. Doctors considered that shortages of money, beds and doctors' time jeopardised the health of patients (Boseley, 1999f). The Prime Minister, Mr Blair, responded that the BMA was out of touch with doctors who had been working with the government on the new projects such as NHS Direct and walk-in clinics (Boseley, 1999g). Indeed, details of the new scheme for walk-in clinics were announced by the Health Secretary, Mr Dobson, a week after the BMA conference. Some 20 pilot schemes would include centres at Manchester airport and Birmingham New Street station. The walk-in clinics would be open 7am–10pm on weekdays and at times during weekends to provide free information and minor treatment from doctors and nurses in a programme worth £10 million. Ministers perceived the walk-in clinics as a key part of a strategy to modernize the NHS; many doctors saw the clinics as a threat to GP practices (Brindle, 1999g, 1999h).

The number of complaints to the NHS Ombudsman had risen by 8% in 1998–99 to 2869, of which 62% were upheld. Patients were also becoming increasingly critical of an 'impersonal' NHS. Developments that ministers and managers perceived as progress, which included primary care groups, high-tech. medicine and computerization, had alienated patients according to four focus groups set up by the Institute for Public Policy Research (Lenaghan, 1999).

Toynbee (1999) argued that, although complaints from doctors added to the public's anxiety about the NHS, the facts showed a gradual improvement (waiting times down; £21 billion of new money). Outcomes were not outstanding but the NHS was doing well enough for the seriously ill, although less well for others. The question for the future was whether 'muddling through' was good enough. Should the NHS settle for less in the twenty-first century or raise taxation to pay for more?

A rather different perspective for the future came from Cardiff Community Healthcare Trust chair, David Crosby (1999), who argued that one or more of the NHS's founding principles were likely to be relinquished in the light of the resources available to meet the needs and demands. Although many advocated an increase in the percentage of the gross domestic product accorded to the NHS – 6.7% in the UK (5.7% for the public sector, 1% from the private sector) – almost the lowest in the global league of affluent nations (based on OECD figures for 1998): France 9.9%; Germany 10.4%; Sweden 8.6%; USA 14%), this view often overlooked that the higher percentage abroad was the result of private health care contributions. Chapters 7 and 11 have also shown that different health care systems provided no easy solutions. Crosby (1999) then suggested that, while continued fudging was likely to be the way forward in Britain, 'thinking the unthinkable' was another option for the next century: the introduction of extra charges could not be postponed much longer.

The *Sunday Times* (1999) contended that Britain's population was changing, as medical technology and new drugs enabled people to live longer; the nation was also three times more prosperous than in 1948 when the NHS was founded. Should not the NHS of the future face up to the challenge of adapting to fit the needs of a society that was very different from when the NHS was founded? As health insurance schemes abroad had a tendency to exclude high-risk applicants, charges therefore looked a better option for funding the NHS without raising taxation.

Another set of views came from the Social Market Foundation (Morgan, 1999), who suggested that ways should be found to incorporate private insurance or co-operative payments into health care funding. The ideas echoed the more extreme thinking of John Spiers, a former health authority chairman, who argued that everyone should have guaranteed access to the moral minimum which the NHS currently delivered. Hospitals should be released from central government control to be turned into charities directly accountable to community representatives or institutions. Financial control of health care could then be removed from the government, to be delivered into the 'hands of the people'. The government would transfer money into vouchers weighted in favour of poor people, while everyone would invest in mutual institutions which would buy health services for subscribers, but individuals would be required to insure against 'catastrophic care' (Phillips, 1999b). Such proposals completely overlooked the relatively low NHS administrative costs in comparison with the complexity of health insurance schemes abroad. Furthermore, pre-war health care provision in Britain had already revealed the snags of decentralization and provision by charities.

At the other end of the spectrum, the NHS had increasingly, but not entirely, lost sight of altruism which had been overtaken by managerialism and the market economy. Ann Oakley and John Ashton's (1997) publication *Richard Titmuss: The Gift Relationship: From Human Blood to Social Policy*, reminded everyone once again of the central argument that markets in blood were wasteful, exploitative and supplied an inferior product – such a market had largely been avoided in Britain as blood has been given freely by donors throughout the history of the NHS. Professor Richard Titmuss was one of the great intellectual theorists behind the Welfare State, for whom the central achievement of the NHS was to set out to provide health care, free at the point of use, but where the costs were shared through a progressive taxation system, in order to meet need on the basis of equality, equity and comprehensive services. The vision turned out to be altruistic but increasingly unattainable.

Meanwhile, users could only express a national view at each general election. In 1997, New Labour had been elected on the pledge to save and modernize the NHS by cutting back on costly bureaucracy in order to spend the money where it was most needed: on frontline care.

The pace of modernization was expected to be stepped up when, in October 1999, Alan Milburn, former Health Minister then Chief Secretary to the Treasury, returned to the Department of Health as Secretary of State for Health, when Frank Dobson set off to fight for the Labour candidature in the race to become Mayor of London. After two years in the post of Health Secretary, Mr Dobson left office with his reputation enhanced, respected for his personal integrity and a willingness to take the right decisions even if they were unpopular at the time.

For the twenty-first century, the October reshuffle led to a modification in the ministerial arrangements at the Department of Health. As Parliamentary Under-secretary for Health, Gisela Stuart was responsible for NHS Direct; the millennium winter planning and information technology alongside other arenas. Yvette Cooper, a former economic journalist, succeeded Tessa Jowell as Parliamentary Under-secretary for Public Health. John Denham continued in office as Minister of State for Health with a remit to cover human resources, primary care, medical training and waiting lists amongst other functions. Former Junior Health Minister John Hutton was promoted to Minister of State with a responsibility for social services and mental health; while Lord Hunt replaced Baroness Hayman to concentrate on pharmaceuticals, dental and optical services, nursing strategy, as well as the professions allied to medicine.

The arrival of Alan Milburn at the Department of Health was greeted with almost universal welcome: as the author of *The New NHS, Modern and Dependable* (Secretary of State for Health, 1997c), much was expected of the incoming secretary. Within a week of entering office, Alan Milburn had warned doctors that the pace of change in the NHS was going to accelerate. At the start of the second week, he outlined a shift in focus from waiting list targets to the three biggest challenges which faced the NHS: heart disease, cancer and mental health, for which extra resources were to be found from the Health Secretary's budget. In the third week, the professor of cancer medicine at Guy's and St Thomas's hospitals, Mike Richards, was appointed Britain's first 'cancer tsar' to ensure that patients received the same level of treatment throughout the country. Further, in order to modernize and improve access to services, the speed of reform was to be quickened; NHS Direct and walk-in centres would be expanded; while the numbers of doctors and nurses would also be increased.

Modernization was therefore the key word for the future. However, the major issue remained the question of resources. At the start of the new millennium, the NHS would inherit a mounting deficit of £200 million from 1999 (*The Guardian*, 1999c), staff shortages and waiting lists. A further challenge for the twenty-first century was how far the NHS would respond to or could absorb major new scientific developments. By October 1999, Propecia had received a British Medicines Controls Agency licence, as a safe and effective treatment against male-pattern baldness which affected 50% of men. However, the government and the manufacturers decided that hair loss was not a health priority so the baldness pill was to be available only on private prescription. Then again, would Celera Genomics, which claimed to have unravelled 1.2 billion of the estimated 3 billion building blocks that determined the human genetic code in the design of the human body, cause long-term implications for the NHS through genetically based cures? In the light of ever-expanding developments, public expectations were continuously rising, which created demands on the NHS. 'Patients' were increasingly being perceived as 'consumers' who expected wider access to and choice of quality services.

Only the future could tell how long the basic principles of the National Health Service would be upheld or modified – or how long the twentieth-century resource system could adequately meet the needs and demands of health care in the twenty-first century.

THE NHS PLAN

To address the needs of the new century, subsequent government action was swift. By July 2000, the Department of Health (DoH) had published a plan for NHS reform with far-reaching changes: a health service designed around the patient, and a plan for investment in the NHS with sustained increases in funding. The emphasis was four-fold. First on quality and raising standards: a Modernisation Agency was to be introduced to spread best practice; national standards were to be set by the DoH, but local health bodies were to be inspected by the Commission for Health Improvement. A national inequalities target was to be established, to bring health improvements for patients; national standards for elderly care aimed at combatting ageism. Secondly, joint working between social services and the NHS was to be rewarded with financial incentives and further agreements to pool resources. New care trusts were to commission health and social care in a single organisation (a new level of primary care trust) to enable closer integration. One-stop health and social care services were also to provide a single local care network where GPs and social workers would work together with primary and community health teams as part of a single care network. By 2004, a £900m package of new intermediate care services was intended to enable older people to lead more independent lives through rapid response teams of GPs, nurses, care workers, social workers and therapists. Thirdly, a significant staffing increase was envisaged to include 7500 more consultants, 2000 more GPs, 20 000 extra nurses, 6500 extra therapists, 1000 more medical school places and 100 new hospitals by 2010. Fourthly, a concordat with the private health care providers would enable the NHS to make better use of facilities in private hospitals.

Although sympathetic to the broad thrust of the plan, the medical profession was adamantly opposed to a ban on private practice for the first seven years of the appointment of new consultants. Next, although nursing care was now to be free in nursing homes for all users, the government continued to oppose the Royal Commission's (Sutherland, 1999) recommendation for free personal care, but where the dividing line was remained unclear. The proposed wider role for community pharmacists was largely welcomed, but doubts were expressed about treating more NHS patients in private hospitals as more NHS staff might then move to the private sector. However, the intended abolition of the Community Health Councils, to be replaced by patients' representatives on various bodies, raised fundamental questions about the place of users in the NHS. Overall, the NHS plan certainly presented an ambitious vision for the future, but the reality had yet to be achieved.

APPENDIX 1
GENERAL ELECTIONS, PRIME MINISTERS AND HEALTH MINISTERS FROM 1945

A	B	C	D	E
General elections	**Prime Ministers**	**Changed in**	**Health Ministers**	**Replaced in**
26 July 1945	Clement Attlee		Aneurin Bevan	
23 February 1950	Clement Attlee		Aneurin Bevan	
			Hilary Marquand	January 1951
25 October 1951	Winston Churchill		Harry Crookshank	
			Ian Macleod	May 1952
26 May 1955	Anthony Eden		Ian Macleod	
			Robert Turton	December 1955
	Harold Macmillan	January 1957	Dennis Vosper	
			Derek Walker-Smith	September 1957
8 October 1959	Harold Macmillan		Derek Walker-Smith	
			Enoch Powell	July 1960
	Alec Douglas-Home	October 1963	Anthony Barber	
15 October 1964	Harold Wilson		Kenneth Robinson	
31 March 1966	Harold Wilson		Kenneth Robinson	November 1968
			Richard Crossman*	and onwards
18 June 1970	Edward Heath		Sir Keith Joseph*	
28 February 1974	Harold Wilson		Barbara Castle	
10 October 1974	Harold Wilson		Barbara Castle	
	James Callaghan	April 1976	David Ennals	
3 May 1979	Margaret Thatcher		Patrick Jenkin	
			Norman Fowler	September 1981
9 June 1983	Margaret Thatcher		Norman Fowler	
11 June 1987	Margaret Thatcher		John Moore	
			Kenneth Clarke†	July 1988
				and onwards
	John Major	28 November 1990	William Waldegrave†	
9 April 1992	John Major		Virginia Bottomley	
			Stephen Dorrell	July 1995
1 May 1997	Tony Blair		Frank Dobson	October 1999
			Alan Milburn	

* as Secretary of State for Social Services at the newly combined Department of Health and Social Security.
† as Secretary of State for Health.

In Scotland health functions were exercised by the Secretary of State for Scotland. Following New Labour's devolution proposals, certain central government powers were devolved to the newly elected Scottish Parliament in May 1999, when Susan Deacon was appointed Minister for Health and Community Care.

In Wales, since 1969, the health functions have been exercised by the Secretary of State for Wales. Following devolution, the election of the Welsh Assembly in May 1999 brought about a transfer of powers. In July 1999, Jane Hutt was appointed as Assembly Secretary of Health and Social Services.

The earlier part of the chart has been tabulated from Webster (1998: 220–221) with the kind permission of Dr Charles Webster and Oxford University Press.

Appendix 2
NHS organizational developments in Scotland and Northern Ireland: the background in brief

General principles

- The general principles governing the NHS have been the same throughout the United Kingdom in England, Wales, Scotland and Northern Ireland.
- The Secretaries of State for Wales, Scotland and Northern Ireland have been responsible for the health services in their respective parts of the UK but accountable to Parliament.

Scotland

The National Health Service Act 1947 established the Scottish Health Service. The organization was based on the same tripartite principle as in England and Wales. The Secretary of State for Scotland was responsible for the whole of the NHS in Scotland under whom the Scottish Home and Health Department ran the central administration.

The hospital and specialist services were administered by five regional hospital boards and 65 boards of management. Family practitioner services were administered by 25 executive councils. A total of 55 local health authorities provided community and environmental health services.

Under the *National Health Service (Scotland) Act 1972*, 15 health boards were created for each area of Scotland, each to act as the single authority for administering the three branches of the former tripartite structure, underpinned by a district organization. The Scottish Health Service Planning Council (to establish policy) and the Common Services Agency (to provide support services to the health boards to prevent uneconomic duplication of work) were created. These developments were not mirrored in England, where the equivalent functions were shared by the Department of Health and Social Security and the regional health authorities.

No specific bodies were established to pursue collaboration between local authorities and health authorities, such as the joint consultative committees created in England and Wales. Local health councils were set up to represent the views of the users of health services. The 1972 legislation also established the Health Service Commissioner for Scotland, who was the equivalent of the Commissioner for England and Wales and Parliamentary Ombudsman. The *Local Government (Scotland) Act 1973* created new local authorities in Scotland from May 1975, the boundaries of which closely followed the health board boundaries.

Scotland differed from England and Wales in that the integrated administration of the contracts for family practitioners, dentists, pharmacists and opticians was held directly with the 15 health boards, who were responsible to the Secretary of State for Scotland for the planning and provision of integrated services in their respective areas.

NORTHERN IRELAND

From 1948, under the Ministry of Health and Local Government, a tripartite structure prevailed. The Northern Ireland Hospitals Authority, supported by 29 hospital management committees, were responsible for the hospital services. General Practitioner contracts came under the Northern Ireland General Health Services Board; local authorities were responsible for community health and social services. A significant change took place from 1973 when, under the Health and Personal Social Services (HI) Order 1972, the Province was organized into four health and social services boards, although still accountable to the Secretary of State for Northern Ireland. Health and social services were then run by one administration. The Central Services Agency undertook the work of the Family Practitioners Committees in England.

The health and social services boards, with subordinate districts, were responsible for administering, planning and co-ordinating health and social services in their area. District committees represented consumer interests. Following proposals confirmed in the circular HSS (P) 1/81, *The Structure and Management of Health and Personal Social Services Northern Ireland*, issued in 1981, the four health and social services boards remained. Below the boards, units supported by unit management groups, replaced the districts.

The key differences between Northern Ireland and England were:

- absence of a regional tier;
- joint appointment of academic posts in hospitals and universities;
- inclusion of social services.

The Griffiths management inquiry in 1983 (see Chapter 5) did not cover Scotland, Wales or Northern Ireland, but the major recommendations were gradually applied to these parts of the UK. For example, in Northern Ireland general management was established at board level in 1985 but not in districts until 1990. Chapter 8 briefly takes up the relevance of the White Paper *Working for Patients* (DoH, 1989a) for Scotland and Northern Ireland. Chapter 14 details the implications of New Labour's 1997 proposals and outcomes. Further reading overleaf provides a list of useful references for more information.

FURTHER READING

For those who would like further reading on particular aspects of health care provision in Britain and abroad this is a select bibliography arranged under specific headings. These publications have mostly not featured in the references.

HISTORICAL BACKGROUND

Abel-Smith. B. (1964) *The Hospitals 1800–1948*, London: Heinemann.
Abel-Smith, B. (1960) *A History of the Nursing Profession*, London: Heinemann.
Dingwall, R., Rafferty, A. and Webster, C. (1988) *An Introduction to the Social History of Nursing*, London: Routledge.
Frazer, W. (1950) *A History of English Public Health 1838–1939*, London: Baillière, Tindall and Fox.
Honigsbaum, F. (1979) *The Division in British Medicine: A history of the separation of general practice from hospital care 1911–1968*, London: Kogan Page.
Jones, K. (1960) *Mental Health and Social Policy 1845–1959*, London: Routledge & Kegan Paul.

DEVELOPMENTS UNDER THE BRITISH NHS

Allsop, J. (1984) *Health Policy and the National Health Service*, London: Longman.
Atkinson, P., Dingwall, R. and Murcott, A. (1979) *Prospects for the National Health*, London: Croom Helm.
Beck, E., Lonsdale, S., Newman, S. and Patterson, D. (1992) *In the Best of Health? The status and future of health care in the UK*, London: Chapman & Hall.
Carrier, J. and Kendall, I. (1998) *Health and the National Health Service*, London: The Athlone Press.
Eckstein, H. (1964) *The English Health Service*, Oxford: Oxford University Press.
Ham, C. (1982) *Health Policy in Britain*, London: Macmillan.
Klein, R. (1983) *The Politics of the National Health Service*, London: Longman.
Illife, S. and Munro, J. (eds) (1997) *Healthy Choices: Future Options for the NHS*, London: Lawrence & Wishart.
Lindsey, A. (1962) *The National Health Service 1948–1961: Socialised Medicine in England and Wales*, Chapel-Hill: University of North Carolina Press.

PRIVATE HEALTH CARE IN BRITAIN

Audit Commission (1987) *Competitive Tendering for Support Services in the NHS*, London: HMSO.
Higgins, J. (1988) *The Business of Medicine: Private Health Care in Britain*, London: Macmillan.
Jackson, P. and Price, C. (1994) *Privatisation and Regulation: A Review of the Issues*, London: Longman.
Laing, W. (1987) *Laing's Review of Private Health Care 1987*, London: Laing and Buisson. (An annual publication.)

Le Grand, J. and Robinson, R. (1984) *Privatisation and the Welfare State*, London: Allen & Unwin.

THE OUTCOME OF THE 1983 GRIFFITHS REPORT AND THE NHS MANAGEMENT INQUIRY

Carrier, J. and Kendall, I. (1986) 'NHS management and the 'Griffiths Report', in Brenton, M. and Ungerson, C. (eds) *The Year Book of Social Policy in Britain 1985–6*, London: Routledge & Kegan Paul.

Cox, D. (1991) 'Health Service Management – A Sociological View: Griffiths and the Non-Negotiated Order of the Hospital', in Gabe, J., Calnan, M. and Bury, M. (eds), *The Sociology of the Health Service*, London: Routledge.

Glennerster, H., Owens., Gatiss, S. and Kimberley, A. (1988) *The Nursing Management Function after Griffiths: A study in the North West Thames region*, London: The London School of Economics and North West Thames Regional Health Authority.

Ham, C. and Hunter, D. (1988) *Managing Clinical Activity in the NHS*, London: Kings Fund Institute.

Harrison, S., Hunter, D. Marnoch, G. and Pollit, C. (1989) *The Impact of General Management in the National Health Service*, University of Leeds and the Open University, Milton Keynes: Nuffield Institute for Health Studies.

Robinson, J., Strong, P. and Elkan, R. (1989) *Griffiths and the Nurses: A National Survey of CNAs*, University of Warwick: Nursing Policy Studies Centre.

Strong, P. and Robinson J. (1988) *New Model Management Griffiths and the NHS*, University of Warwick: Nursing Policy Studies Centre.

THE 1989 NHS REVIEW AND THE INTERNAL MARKET

Department of Health (1989) *National Health Service Review Working Papers*, London: HMSO.

Harrison, S., Hunter, D., Johnston, I. and Wistow, G. (1989) *Competing for Health: A commentary on the NHS Review*. Leeds University: Nuffield Institute for Health Service Studies.

Harrison, S., Hunter, D., Marnoch, G. and Pollitt, C. (1989) *General Management in the National Health Service: Before and After the White Paper*, Report No. 2, Leeds University: Nuffield Institute for Health Service Studies.

Harrison, S. and Wistow, G. (1992) 'The Purchaser/Provider Split in English Health Care: towards explicit rationing', *Policy and Politics*, **20** (2), 123–30.

Holliday, I. (1992) *The NHS Transformed*, Manchester: Baseline Books.

Judge, K. (1989) *Managed Competition: A new approach to health care in Britain*, London: King's Fund Institute.

Ovretveit, J. (1995) *Purchasing for Health*, Buckingham: Open University Press.

Maynard, A. and Holland, W. (1989) *Reforming UK Health Care to Improve Health: The case for research and experiment*, York University: Centre for Health Economics.

Paton, C. (1998) *Competition and Planning in the NHS*, second edition, Cheltenham: Stanley Thornes.

Rafferty, J., Mulligan, J. Forrest, S. and Robinson, R. (1994) *Third Review of Contracting*, Leeds: NHS Executive.

Walshe, D. (1995) 'The internal market in health: sham or saviour?', *British Journal of Health Care Management*, **1**, 352–355.

Williams, A. (1989) *Creating a Health Care Market*, York University: Centre for Health Economics.

THE NEW NHS 1997

Dixon, J. and May, N. (1997) 'New Labour, New NHS?', *British Medical Journal* 315, 1639–40.

Klein, R. (ed.) (1998) *Implementing the White Paper: Pitfalls and Opportunities*, London: King's Fund.

Lugon, M. and Secker-Walker, J. (1999) *Clinical Governance – making it happen*, London: Royal Society of Medicine.

Sussex, J. (1998) *Controlling NHS Expenditure: The Impact of Labour's NHS White Papers*, London: Office of Health Economics.

PUBLIC HEALTH

Griffiths, S. and Hunter, D. (eds) (1999) *Perspectives in public health*, Abingdon: Radcliffe Medical Press.

Vetter, N. (1998) *The Public Health and the NHS*, Oxford: Oxford Radcliffe Medical Press.

HEALTH CARE SYSTEMS ABROAD

Abel-Smith, B. (1976) *Value for Money in Health Services*, London: Heinemann.

Abel-Smith, B. (1984) *Cost Containment in Health Care*, London: Bedford Square Press.

Elling, R. (1980) *Cross-National Study of Health Systems*, London: Transaction Books.

Greenberg, W. (1999) *The healthcare marketplace*, New York: Springer.

Johnson, N. (ed.) (1995) *Private Markets in Health and Welfare: an International Perspective*, Oxford/Providence, USA: Berg.

Leichter, H. (1979) *A Comparative Approach to Policy Analysis: Health care policy in four nations*, Cambridge: Cambridge University Press.

Light, D. (1998) *Effective Commissioning: Lessons from purchasing in American managed care*, London: Office of Health Economics.

Maxwell, R. (1981) *Health and Wealth: An international study of health care spending*, Toronto: Lexington Books.

Maynard, A. (1982) *Health Care in the European Community*, fourth edition, London: Croom Helm.

OECD (1987) *Financing and Developing Health Care: A comparative analysis of OECD countries*, Social Policy Studies No. 4, Paris: OECD.

Robinson, R. (1990) *Competition and Health Care: A Comparative Analysis of UK Plans and US Experience*, London: King's Fund Institute.

Roemer, M. (1986) *An Introduction to the US Health Care System*, 2nd edition, New York: Springer.

Seedhouse, D. (ed.) (1995) *Reforming Health Care: The Philosophy and Practice of International Health Reform*, Chichester: Wiley.

Timmins, N. (1988) *Cash, Crisis and Cure: The Independent guide to the NHS debate*, London: Newspaper Publishing PLC.

Wood, R. (ed.) *Eurohealth*, quarterly journal, London: LSE Health. (London School of Economics, Houghton Street, London WC2 2AE).

WALES, SCOTLAND AND NORTHERN IRELAND

Birch, S. and Maynard, A. (1986) *The RAWP review: RAWPing primary care: RAWPing the United Kingdom*, York University: Centre for Health Economics.

Chaplin, N. (ed.) (1982) *Health Care in the United Kingdom: Its organisation and management*, London: Institute of Health Service Administrators and Kluwer Medical.

Cohen, D. (1997) *NHS Wales: Business or Public Service?* Cardiff: Institute of Welsh Affairs.

Connah, B. and Lancaster, S. (eds) (1989) *NHS Handbook: NAHA, The National Association of Health Authorities*, 4th edition, London: Macmillan.

Department of Health for Northern Ireland (1998) *Fit for the Future*, Belfast: Department of Health.

Hayward, D. (1986) *Nursing Care in the Community: An initial study*, Joint Management Study of the Community Nursing Services in Northern Ireland, Belfast: Department of Health and Social Services.

McLachlan, G. (ed.) (1987) *Improving the Common Weal: Aspects of Scottish health services, 1900–1984*, Edinburgh: Edinburgh University Press.

Northern Ireland Department of Health and Social Services (1988) *Primary Care Review*, Belfast: DHSS.

Secretary of State for Scotland (1997) *The Scottish Health Service: Ready for the Future*, Cm. 3614, Edinburgh: The Stationery Office.

Scottish Home and Health Department (1989) *Implications for Primary Health Care*, *National Health Service Review*, Scottish Working Paper No. 1, Edinburgh: HMSO.

The Scottish Office: Department of Health (1997) *Working together for a healthier Scotland: a consultation paper*, January, Cm. 3584, Edinburgh: The Stationery Office.

The Scottish Office (1997) *Scotland's Parliament*, Cm. 3658, July, Edinburgh: The Stationery Office.

The Welsh Office (1998) *Putting Patients First*, Cm 3841, Cardiff: The Stationery Office.

The Welsh Office (1997) *A Voice for Wales*, Cm. 3718, Cardiff: The Stationery Office.

SOCIAL POLICY DEVELOPMENTS

Blakemore, K. (1998) *Social Policy: An Introduction*, Buckingham: Open University Press.

Ellison, N. and Pierson, C. (eds) (1998) *Developments in British Social Policy*, London: Macmillan.

Glennerster, H. (1995) *British Social Policy since 1945*, Oxford: Blackwell.

Hill, M. (1993) *The Welfare State in Britain: A Political History since 1945*, Aldershot: Edward Elgar.

Hills, J. (1993) *The future of welfare: A guide to the debate*, York: Joseph Rowntree Foundation.

Hutton, W. (1995) *The State We're In*, London: Jonathan Cape.

Lowe, R. (1999) *The Welfare State in Britain since 1945*, second edition, London: Macmillan.

THE THIRD WAY

Giddens, A. (1998) *The Third Way: The Renewal of Social Democracy*, Cambridge: Polity Press.

Green, D. (1998) 'Mutuality and Voluntarism: A Third Way', in *Social Policy Review 10*, Brunsdon, E., Dean, H. and Woods, R. (eds), London: Social Policy Association.

Powell, M. (1999) *New Labour, New Welfare State?* Bristol: Policy Press.

JOINT WORKING, TEAMWORK AND COLLABORATIVE CARE

Barr, H. (General Editor) *Journal of Interprofessional Care*. (Quarterly journal, Centre for Community Care and Primary Health, University of Westminster, 115 New Cavendish St. London W1M 8JS.)

Hornby, S. (1993) *Collaborative Care: Interprofessional, Interagency and Interpersonal*, Oxford: Blackwell Scientific Publications.

Gorman, P. (1998) *Managing Multi-disciplinary Teams in the NHS*, London: Kogan Page.

Loxley, A. (1997) *Collaboration in Health and Welfare: Working with Difference*, London: Jessica Kingsley.

Owens, P. Carrier, J. and Horder, J. (1995) *Interprofessional Issues in community and primary health care*, London: Macmillan.

Ovretveit, J., Mathias, P. and Thompson, T. (1997) *Interprofessional Working for Health and Social Care*, London: Macmillan.

Pearson, P. and Spencer, J. (1997) *Promoting Teamwork in Primary Care: A research based approach*, London: Arnold.

Soothill, K., Mackay, L. and Webb, C. (1995) *Interprofessional Relations in Health Care*, London: Edward Arnold.

REFERENCES

Abel-Smith, B. (1960) *A History of the Nursing Profession*, London: Heinemann.

Abel-Smith, B. (1964) *The Hospitals 1800–1948*, London: Heinemann.

Abel-Smith, B. (1976) *Value for Money in Health Services*, London: Heinemann.

Abel-Smith, B. (1978) *National Health Service: The first thirty years*, London: HMSO.

Abel-Smith, B. (1988) 'A New Regime', *New Society*, 24 April, 16–18.

Abel-Smith, B. (1995) 'Health Reform: Old Wine in New Bottles', *Eurohealth*, 1 (1) 7–9.

Abel-Smith, B. (1996) 'Health care costs: An International Dilemma', *LES Magazine*, Summer, 7–9.

Abel-Smith, B. and Titmuss, R. (1956) *The Cost of the National Health Service in England and Wales*, Cambridge: Cambridge University Press.

Abel-Smith, B., Mossialos, E., McKee, M. and Holland, W. (1995) *Choices in Health Policy: An Agenda for the European Union*, Aldershot: Dartmouth Publishing Company.

ACHCEW (Association of Community Health Councils for England and Wales) (1988) *The Impact of General Management on the National Health Service: The views of Community Health Councils*, London: ACHCEW.

Acheson Report (1988) *Public Health in England. The Report of the Committee of Inquiry into the Future Development of the Public Health Function*, London: HMSO.

Acheson Report (1998) *Independent Inquiry into Inequalities in Health*, London: The Stationery Office.

Age Concern (1994) *Community Care and Older People: Mapping the Change. The Next Steps: Lessons for the Future of Community Care*, London: Age Concern.

Ainsworth, S. (1999) 'A fatal outbreak of ambition', *Health Service Journal*, 109 (5642) 18–19.

Allan, P. and Jolley, M. (1982) *Nursing, Midwifery and Health Visiting since 1900*, London: Faber and Faber.

Allen, I. (1981) *Family Planning, Sterilisation and Abortion Facilities*, London: Policy Studies Institute.

Allen, I. (1988) *Any Room at the Top: A Study of Doctors and their Careers*, London: Policy Studies Institute.

Alleway, L. (1985) 'No rush of new blood into the NHS', *Health and Social Service Journal*, 12 September, 1120–1.

Alleway, L. (1987) 'Back on the outside looking in', *Health Service Journal*, 97 (5059) 818–19.

Alibhai, Y. (1988) 'Black nightingales', *New Statesman and Society*, October, 26–7.

Allsop, J. (1995) *Health Policy and the NHS: Towards 2000*, Second Edition, London: Longman.

AMA (Association of Metropolitan Authorities) (1994) *Local Authorities and Health Services: the Future Role of Local Authorities in the Provision of Health Services*, Birmingham: AMA.

Appleby, J. (1994a) 'Fundholding', *Health Service Journal*, 104 (5415) 32–3.

Appleby. J. (1994b) 'Evaluating the NHS Reforms', *Health Service Journal*, 104 (5390) 32–3.

Appleby, J. (1995) 'Managers in the Ascendancy', *Health Service Journal*, 105 (5471) 32–3.

Appleby, J. (1996a) 'PFI: RIP?', *Health Service Journal*, **106** (5515) 32–3.

Appleby, J. (1996b) 'Factfile', *Budget Special Health Service Journal*, **106** (5531) 5.

Appleby, J. (1998a) 'Population Projections', *Health Service Journal*, **108** (5603) 38–9.

Appleby, J. (1998b) 'Our growing inequalities', *Health Service Journal*, **108** (5594) 40–1.

Areskog, N. (1992) 'The New Medical Education at the Faculty of Health Sciences, Linkoping University – A Challenge for both students and teachers', *Scandinavian Journal of Social Medicine*, **20** (1) (no page number recorded).

Arora, S., Davies, A. and Thompson, S. (1999) *Developing Health Improvement Programmes: Lessons from the First Year*, London: King's Fund.

Ashton, J. (1992) 'The Origins of Healthy Cities, in *Healthy Cities*, Ashton, J. (ed.) Buckingham: Open University Press.

Ashton, J. and Seymour, H. (1988) *The New Public Health*, Milton Keynes: Open University Press.

Audit Commission (1985) *Managing Services for the Elderly more Effectively*, London: HMSO.

Audit Commission (1986) *Making a Reality of Community Care*, London: HMSO.

Audit Commission (1987) *Competitive Tendering for Support Services in the NHS*, London: HMSO

Audit Commission (1992a) *Homeward Bound: A New Course for Community Health*, NHS Report No. 7, London: HMSO.

Audit Commission (1992b) *Community Care: Managing the Cascade of Change*, London: HMSO.

Audit Commission (1992c) *The Community Revolution: Personal Social Services and Community Care*, London: HMSO.

Audit Commission (1993a) *Their Health, Your Business: The New Role of the District Health Authority*, London: HMSO.

Audit Commission (1993b) *Practices Make Perfect: The Role of the Family Health Services Authority*, London: HMSO.

Audit Commission (1993c) *What Seems to be the Matter: communications between hospitals and patients*, London: HMSO.

Audit Commission (1994a) *Taking Stock: Progress with Community Care*, London: HMSO.

Audit Commission (1994b) *Finding a Place. A Review of Mental Health Services for Adults*, London: HMSO.

Audit Commission (1995) *Briefing on GP Fundholding*, London: HMSO.

Audit Commission (1996a) *What the Doctor ordered: A Study of GP Fundholders in England and Wales*, London: HMSO.

Audit Commission (1996b) *Balancing the Care Equation: Progress with Community Care*, London: HMSO.

Audit Commission (1997a) *Higher Purchase: Commissioning Specialized Services in the NHS*, London: Audit Commission.

Audit Commission (1997b) *The Coming of Age: improving care services for older people*, London: Audit Commission

Audit Commission (1999) *First Assessment: A review of district nursing services in England and Wales*, London: Audit Commission.

Baggott, R. (1994) *Health and Health Care in Britain*, London: Macmillan.

Bailey, S. and Bruce, A. (1994) 'Funding the National Health Service: the Continuing Search for Alternatives', *Journal of Social Policy*, **23** (4) 459–542.

Baker, M. (1998) *Making sense of the new NHS White Paper*, Abingdon: Radcliffe Medical Press.

Ballantyne, A. (1989) 'GPs may face dilemma of cash limits versus a suitable case for treatment', The Guardian, 1 February.

Banyard, R. (1988) 'How do UGMs perform?', Health Service Journal, 98 (5110) 824–5.

Barnes, J., Parsley, K. and Walshe, K. (1994) 'Star Quality', Health Service Journal, 104 (5427) 20–2.

Barnes, M. and Evans, M. (1998) 'Who wants a say in the NHS?', Health Matters, Issue 34, Summer/Autumn, 6–7.

Bartlett, W. and Harrison, L. (1993) 'Quasi-markets and the National Health Service Reforms', in Quasi-Markets and Social Policy, Le Grand, J., Bartlett, W. (eds) London: Macmillan.

Bartlett, W. and Le Grand, J. (1993) 'The Performance of Trusts', in Evaluating the NHS Reforms, Robinson, R., Le Grand, J. (eds) London: King's Fund Institute.

Bates, S. (1998) 'EC plans to cut hours of doctors and drivers', The Guardian, 19 November.

Bates, S. (1999) 'Doctors' long wait for 48 hour week', The Guardian, 26 May.

Baxter, C. (1988) Black Nurses: An endangered species, Cambridge: National Extension College.

Bayley, M., Bessell, R., Preston, R., Wicks, M. and Wilding, P. (1986) Not Just for the Poor: Christian perspectives of the Welfare State, Report of the Social Policy Committee of the Board for Social Responsibility, London: Church House Publishing.

Beattie, A. (1994) 'Going Inter-Professional: Working together for health and wealth' in Leathard, A. (ed.) Healthy alliances or dangerous liasions? The challenge of working together in health promotion, London: Routledge.

Benzeval, M., Judge, K. and Whitehead, M. (1995) 'Tackling Inequalities in Health. An agenda for action', London: King's Fund.

Berliner, H. (1996) 'Forlorn in the USA', Health Service Journal, 106 (5498) 19.

Best, G. (1985) 'Secrets of success for happy families', Health and Social Service Journal, 26 September, 1194–5.

Best, G. (1988) 'NHS's Unhappy Returns', Marxism Today, July, 20–3.

Best, G. (1989) 'Exciting journey into the unknown', Health Service Journal, 99 (5137) 166.

Beveridge Report (1942) Interdepartmental Committee on Social Insurance and Allied Services, Cmd 6404, London: HMSO.

Birch, S. (1986) 'Increasing patient charges in the National Health Service: a method of privatizing primary care', Journal of Social Policy, 15 (2) 163–84.

Black, D. (1993) 'Poverty will always make you ill', Guardian, 9 September.

Black Report (1980) Inequalities in Health, London: DHSS.

Blair, T. (1996) 'My vision of a one nation Britain', The Sunday Times, 14 January.

Blair, T. (1998) The Third Way. New Politics for the New Century, London: Fabian Society.

BMA (British Medical Association) (1929; revised 1938) A General Medical Service for the Nation, London: BMA.

BMA (1993) Complementary Medicine: New Approaches to Good Practice, London: BMA.

BMA (1986) Cervical Cancer and Screening in Great Britain, London: BMA.

BMA (1987) Deprivation and Ill Health, London: BMA.

BMA (1995) Report of the Working Party on Medical Education, London: BMA.

Booth, C. (1903) Life and Labour of the People in London, London: Macmillan.

Bosanquet, N. (1989) 'A framework with much potential', *Health Service Journal*, **99** (5137) 167–8.

Bosanquet, N. (1993) 'Two cheers for the internal market', *Journal of Interprofessional Care*, **7** (2) 125–30.

Bosanquet, N. (1994) 'Improving health', in *British Social Attitudes the 11th Report*, Jowell, R., Curtice, J., Brook, L., Ahrendt, D. and Park, A. (eds) Aldershot: Dartmouth Publishing Company.

Bosanquet, N. (1995) 'Reviving the sleeping beauty', *Health Service Journal*, **105** (5448) 20–2.

Boseley, S. (1998a) 'Viagra maker defiant on price' *The Guardian*, 16 September.

Boseley, S. (1998b) 'NHS set to run out of doctors by 2010', *The Guardian*, 18 June.

Boseley, S. (1998c) 'Colleges hinder reform of NHS', *The Guardian*, 29 June.

Boseley, S. (1998d) 'Teeth and smiles?', *The Guardian*, 2 July.

Boseley, S. (1999a) 'Outrage at breast screening doubts', *The Guardian*, 12 March.

Boseley, S. (1999b) 'Not-so-nice dilemma', *The Guardian*, 10 February.

Boseley, S. (1999c) 'Dobson gives way on Viagra prescriptions', *The Guardian*, 8 May.

Boseley, S. (1999d) 'Killer disease out of control', *The Guardian*, 24 March.

Boseley, S. (1999e) 'Cancer 'killing too many' in UK', *The Guardian*, 10 March.

Boseley, S. (1999f) 'Angry doctors say NHS is failing', *The Guardian*, 6 July.

Boseley, S. (1999g) ' "BMA out of touch with doctors", says Blair', *The Guardian*, 8 July.

Boseley, S., Watt, N., White, M. (1999) 'BMA backs juniors on hours and pay', *The Guardian*, 7 July.

Bottomley, V. (1993) 'My new year resolution for the NHS, *Health Service Journal*, **103** (5334) 13.

Bridges, J., Meyer, J., Davidson, D., Harris, J. and Glynn, M. (1999) 'Hospital discharge: Smooth passage', *Health Service Journal*, **109** (5659) 24–25.

Briggs, A. (1978a) 'Making health every citizen's birthright: the road to 1946', *New Society*, 16 November, 383–6.

Briggs, A. (1978b) 'The achievements, failures and aspirations of the NHS', *New Society*, 23 November, 448–51.

Briggs Committee (1972) *Report of the Committee on Nursing*, Cmnd 5115, London: HMSO.

Brindle, D. (1996a) 'Health chief seeks yearly contract end', *The Guardian*, 16 May.

Brindle, D. (1996b) 'The end of the welfare state', *The Guardian*, 8 May, front page.

Brindle, D. (1996c) 'Plan to give away cottage hospitals', *The Guardian*, 8 June.

Brindle, D. (1996d) 'NHS tops list of private health care providers', *The Guardian*, 30 September.

Brindle, D. (1996e) 'US firms buy into private care homes', *The Guardian*, 26 January.

Brindle, D. (1996f) 'Unemployment kills, survey reveals', *The Guardian*, 25 January.

Brindle, D. (1997) 'Why parties must face the real problems', *The Guardian*, 18 April.

Brindle, D. (1998a) 'Doctors urge NHS scoring system for waiting lists', *The Guardian*, 30 December.

Brindle, D. (1998b) 'Sleight of hand' in waiting list fall', *The Guardian*, 27 August.

Brindle, D. (1998c) 'Depth charge', *The Guardian*, 11 March.

Brindle, D. (1998d) 'Nursing 'needs to be all-graduate', *The Guardian*, 31 March.

Brindle, D. (1999a) 'Children to assist in crusade to save lives', *The Guardian*, 7 July.

Brindle, D. (1999b) 'Dobson waiting list claim attacked', *The Guardian*, 5 June.

Brindle, D. (1999c) 'GPs demand slowdown on NHS reform', *The Guardian*, 25 June.

Brindle, D. (1999d) 'Junior doctors consider strike', *The Guardian*, 20 March.

Brindle, D. (1999e) 'Up for grabs', *The Guardian*, Society section, 31 March.

Brindle, D. (1999f) 'Blair NHS vision hit by doubts', *The Guardian*, 27 May.

Brindle, D. (1999g) 'Airport and station get walk-in NHS centres', *The Guardian*, 16 July.

Brindle, D. (1999h) 'Walk-in clinics "pose a threat" to GP practices', *The Guardian*, 14 April.

Brindle, D. and Johnson, A. (1988) 'Gambling chiefs question validity of lottery for NHS', *The Guardian*, 22 April.

British Diabetic Association. (1996) *Counting the Cost: the real impact of non-insulin dependent diabetes*, London: British Diabetic Association.

Brook, L., Hall, J. and Preston, I. (1996) 'Public Spending and Taxation' in *British Social Attitudes 13th report*, Jowell, R., Curtice, R., Park, A., Brook, L. and Thomson, K., (eds) Aldershot: Dartmouth.

Brotherton, P. and Jenkins, J. (1989) 'Primary lessons', *New Statesman and Society*, 20 January, 15.

Brown, C. (1990) 'MPs back continued embryo research: Huge majority ends six-year battle after emotional debate', The *Independent*, 24 April.

Brown, C. (1998) *Optimum Healing: A life-changing new approach to achieving good health*, London: Rider.

Brown, H. and Smith, H. (1992) *Normalisation: A reader for the 90s*, London: Routledge.

Brown, R. (1979) *Reorganising the National Health Service*, Oxford: Blackwell & Robertson.

Brown, S. (1999) 'Fresh Initiative', *The Guardian*, Society Finance, 21 July.

BUPA (British United Provident Association) (1998) *Your BUPACare Membership Guide*, London: BUPA

Burkitt, B. and Baimbridge, M. (1994/5) 'The Maastricht Treaty's impact on the welfare state', *Critical Social Policy*, 42, Winter, 100–11.

Butler, J. (1992) *Patients, Policies and Politics: Before and after Working for Patients*, Milton Keynes: Open University Press.

Butler, P. (1996a) 'Hundreds of HA jobs to go as government targets bite', *Health Service Journal*, **106** (5489) 3.

Butler, P. (1996b) 'Beggars can't be choosers', *Health Service Journal*, **106** (5501) 10.

Butler, P. (1998) Together again?, *Health Service Journal*, **108** (5621) 10–11.

Butler, E. and Pirie, M. (1988) *The Health of Nations*, London: Adam Smith Institute.

Calman Report (1995) *Hospital Doctors: Training for the Future: The Report of the Working Group on Specialist Medical Training*, Leeds: NHS Executive.

Calman-Hine Report (1995) *A Policy Framework for Commissioning Cancer Services*, London: Department of Health.

Campbell, C. (1998) *Planning the Medical Work Force – The Third Report of the Medical Manpower Standing Advisory Committee on long-term demand for doctors*, London: Department of Health.

Campbell, D. (1988) 'The amazing AIDS scramble', *New Statesman and Society*, 24 June, 10–13.

Campbell, D. (1989) 'AIDS: the race against time', *New Statesman and Society*, 6 January, 9–14.

Cant, S. and Sharma, U. (1999) *A New Medical Pluralism?* London: UCL Press.

Carrier, J. and Kendall, I. (1986) 'NHS management and the Griffiths Report', in *The Year Book of Social Policy in Britain*, Brenton, M. and Ungerson, C. London: Routledge & Kegan Paul.

Carson, J. and Sharma, T. (1994) 'In-patient psychiatric care. What helps? Staff and patient perspectives'. *Journal of Mental Health*, 3 99–104.

Cervi, B. (1996) 'Government set to bail out troubled trust PFI schemes', *Health Service Journal*, 106 (5533) 8.

Chadda, D. (1993) 'Trust leaders call for help as mergers get set to soar', *Health Service Journal*, 103 (5367) 8.

Chadda, D. (1996a) 'Welsh Chorus', *Health Service Journal*, 106 (5518), 8.

Chadda, D. (1996b) 'Dorrell condemns blanket ban on types of treatment', *Health Service Journal*, 106 (5485) 6.

Chadda, D. (1997) 'Private league table of trusts shows vast range in clinical performance', *Health Service Journal*, 107 (5580) 5.

Chadda, D. (1998) 'Only a quarter of bids for HAZ status will get approval', *Health Service Journal*, 108 (5587) 3.

Chadda, D. and Limb, M. (1998) 'Anger as green paper falls short on inequalities and funding pledges, *Health Service Journal*, 108 (5591) 9.

Challis, L., Klein, R. and Webb, A. (1988) *Joint Approaches to Social Policy: Rationality and Practice*, Cambridge: Cambridge University Press.

Chambaud, L. (1993) 'A La Carte', *Health Service Journal*, 103 (5344) 24–7.

Clarke, K. (1989) 'Clarke on the Review', *Nursing Times*, 85 (6) 20.

Clay, T. (1987) *Nurses: Power and Politics*, London: Heinemann.

Clay, T. (1989) 'Clay on the Review', *Nursing Times*, 85 (6) 21.

CNA (Carers National Association) (1995a) *Better Tomorrow*, London: Carers National Association.

CNA (1995b) *Working for a Fair Deal for Carers, Annual Report*, London: Carers National Association.

Cohen, N. (1989) 'Unworkable plans for a hard pressed surgery', The *Independent*, 31 January.

Cole, A. (1995) 'Should complaints be treasured?', *Health Service Journal* 105 (5472) 24–6.

Collins, R. (1988) 'Lessons in compassion for student doctors', The *Sunday Times*, 7 August.

Commons Public Accounts Committee (1986) *Preventive Medicine*, London: HMSO, London.

Conroy, S. and Mohammed, S. (1989) 'Rooting out NHS racism', *Health Service Journal*, 99 (5132) 19.

Cook, R. (1989) 'A private hospital by any other name', *The Guardian*, 30 January.

Coote, A. (1999) 'Divisions no longer add up', *Health Service Journal*, 109 (5662) 18–19.

Coote, A. and Kendall, L. (1998) 'Evening all', *Health Service Journal*, 108 (5632) 30–31.

Corea, G. et al. (1985) *Man-Made Woman: How new reproductive technologies affect women*, London: Hutchinson.

Corea, G. (1988) *The Mother Machine: Reproductive technologies from artificial insemination to artificial wombs*, London: The Women's Press.

Council of Deans and Heads of Universities' Faculties of Nursing, Midwifery and Health Visiting (1998) *Breaking the Boundaries: Educating Nurses, Midwives and Health Visitors*, Manchester: Manchester University.

Court Report (1976) *Report of the Committee on Child Health Services: Fit for the future*, Cmnd 6684, London: HMSO.

Cousins, C. (1987) *Controlling Social Welfare*, Brighton: Wheatsheaf.

Cox, B. et al. (1987) *The Health and Lifestyle Survey*, London: Health Promotion Trust.

Cox, D. (1986) 'Implementing Griffiths at District Level', Unpublished Paper given to the BSA Medical Sociology Group, University of York, September.

Cox, D. (1988) *Short-term prediction of HIV Indications and AIDS in England and Wales. Report of a Working Group*, London: HMSO.

Craig, G. and Manthorpe, J. (1996) *Wiped off the Map? – Local government reorganization and community care*, School of Policy Studies, Papers in Social Research No. 5, Kingston upon Hull: University of Lincolnshire and Humberside.

Crail, M. (1995) 'Rational judgements', *Health Service Journal*, 105 (5478) 12.

Crail, M. (1997) 'Dobbo: Time to Talk Frankly', *Health Service Journal*, 107 (5565) 10–13.

Crail, M. (1998a) 'Homa truths', *Health Service Journal*, 108 (5622) 12–13.

Crail, M. (1998b) 'Moving targets', *Health Service Journal*, 108 (5588) 12–13.

Crail, M. (1998c) 'Price of new doctors may be changed in role', *Health Service Journal*, 108 (5615) 8.

Crail, M. (1999a) 'All Right now', *Health Service Journal*, 109 (5653) 8–9.

Crail, M. (1999b) 'Brothers grim', *Health Service Journal*, 109 (5661) 12–13.

Crail, M. (1999c) 'Once bitten', *Health Service Journal*, 109 (5646) 13.

Cranbrook Committee (1959) *Report of the Committee on the Maternity Services*, London: HMSO.

CRE (Commission for Racial Equality) (1986) *Overseas Doctors*, London: CRE.

CRE (1987) *Ethnic Origins of Nurses Applying for In-Training*, London: CRE.

CRE (1988) Medical School Admissions: Report of a formal investigation into St. George's Hospital Medical School, London: CRE.

Crosby, D. (1999) 'Archie's enemies', *Health Service Journal*, 109 (5649) 24.

Cross, M. (1995) 'Will the NHS get wired?', *Health Service Journal*, 105 (5470) 24–7.

Cross, M. (1996) 'Time to byte back', *Health Service Journal*, 106 (5494) 16.

Crown Report (1989) *Report of the Advisory Group on Nurse Prescribing*, Department of Health, London: HMSO.

CSO (Central Statistical Office) (1989) *Social Trends 19*, London: HMSO.

CSO (1993) *Social Trends 23*, London: HMSO.

CSO (1994) *Social Trends 24*, London: HMSO.

Cumberlege Report (1986) *Neighbourhood Nursing: A focus for care; report of the Community Nursing Review*, London: HMSO.

Culyer, A. (1976) *Need and the National Health Service: Economics and social choice*, London: Martin Robertson.

Daily Telegraph (1989) 'Voters concern over NHS cuts Tory lead to 1.5 pc', 16 February.

Davies, M. (1999) 'The servician vision', *Health Service Journal*, 109 (5646) 24.

Davies, P. (1988) 'The public speaks out on the NHS', *Health Service Journal*, 98 (5101) 556–7.

Davies, P. (1989a) 'Flexing muscle on flexible pay', *Health Service Journal*, 99 (5134) 69.

Davies, P. (1989b) 'White Paper show – with no support act', *Health Service Journal*, 99 (5139) 223.

Davies, P., Hunter, H., Limb, M. and Lyall, L. (1996) 'Beds not bureaucracy, says Blair', *Health Service Journal*, 106 (5509) 12–13.

Dawson Committee (1920) *Interim Report on the Future Provision of Medical and Allied Services*, Cmnd 7468, London: HMSO.

Day, P. Klein, R. and Redmayne, S. (1996) *Why regulate? Regulating residential care for elderly people*, Bristol: Policy Press.

Deffenbaugh, J. (1996) 'Playing by different rules', *Health Service Journal*, 106 (5507) 25.

Department of Health for Northern Ireland (1998) *Fit for the Future*, Belfast: Department of Health.

Dewar, S. (1999) *Clinical Governance Under Construction*, London: King's Fund.

DHSS (Department of Health and Social Security) (1970) *National Health Service: The Future Structure of the National Health Service*, London: HMSO.

DHSS (1971a) *Better Services for the Mentally Handicapped*, Cmnd 4683, London: HMSO.

DHSS (1971b) *National Health Service reorganisation consultative document*, London: HMSO.

DHSS (1972a) *National Health Service reorganisation: England*, London: HMSO.

DHSS (1972b) *National Health Service: England*, London: HMSO.

DHSS (1975) *Better Services for the Mentally Ill*, Cmnd 6223, London: HMSO.

DHSS (1976) *Priorities for Health and Personal Social Services in England*, London: HMSO.

DHSS (1977a) *The Way Forward*, London: HMSO.

DHSS (1977b) *Prevention and Health Everybody's Business*, London: HMSO.

DHSS (1978a) *A Happier Old Age*, London: HMSO.

DHSS (1978b) *Review of the Mental Health Act 1959*, Cmnd 7320, London: HMSO.

DHSS (1979) *Patients First*, London: HMSO.

DHSS (1980a) *Mental Handicap: Progress, Problems and Priorities, a review of mental handicap services in England since the 1971 White Paper 'Better Services for the Mentally Handicapped'*, London: DHSS.

DHSS (1980b) *Health Service Development, Structure and Management*, Health Circular (80) 8, London: DHSS.

DHSS (1981a) *Care in Action*, London: HMSO.

DHSS (1981b) *Report of a Study on Community Care*, London: DHSS.

DHSS (1981c) *Care in the Community*, London: DHSS.

DHSS (1983a) *Competitive Tendering in the Provision of Domestic Catering and Laundry Services*, HC (83) 18, London: DHSS.

DHSS (1983b) *Health Care and its Costs*, London: HMSO.

DHSS (1984a) *Health Service Management: Implementation of the Management Inquiry Report*, HC (84)13, London: DHSS.

DHSS (1984b) *The Next Steps: Management in the Health Services*, London: HMSO.

DHSS (1986a) *General Managers Arrangements for the Introduction of Performance Related Pay*, PM (86) 11 September, London: DHSS.

DHSS (1986b) *Primary Health Care: An agenda for discussion*, Cmnd 9771, London: HMSO.

DHSS (1987a) *Promoting Better Health: The Government's programme for improving primary health care*, Cm 248, London: HMSO.

DHSS (1987b) *Human Fertilisation and Embryology: A framework for legislation*, Cm 259, London: HMSO.

Dickson, R. Fullerton, D. and Sheldon, T. (1997) 'Birth control', *Health Service Journal*, **107** (5541) 40–1.

Dickinson, M., Calnan, M. and Manley, G. (1998/9) 'Why are some dentists a pain?', *Health Matters*, Issue 35, Winter, 12–13.

Dingwall, R. and Hughes, D. (1990) 'What's in a name', *Health Service Journal*, **100** (5229), 1770–1.

Dobson, R. (1994) 'Bones of Contention' *Health Service Journal*, **104** (5392) 11.

Dodd, V. (1999) 'Marrow cell find may end transplants', *The Guardian*, 10 July.

DoH (Department of Health) (1989a) *Working for Patients: The Health Service, Caring for the 1990s*, Cm. 555, London: HMSO.

DoH (1989b) *National Health Service Review Working Papers*, London: HMSO.

DoH (1989c) *Caring for People: Community Care in the Next Decade and Beyond. Caring for the 1990s*, London: HMSO.

DoH (1990) *Caring for People: Community Care in the Next Decade and Beyond. Policy Guidance*, London: HMSO.

DoH (1991a) *Medical Audit in the Hospital and Community Health Services*, Health Circular HC(91)2, London: Department of Health.

DoH (1991b) *The Patient's Charter*, London: Department of Health.

DoH (1991c) *The Health of the Nation, A Consultative Document for Health in England*, London: HMSO.

DoH (1992a) *Memorandum on the Financing of Community Care*, 2 October, London: Department of Health.

DoH (1992b) *Health of the Nation*, Cmnd. 1986, London: HMSO.

DoH (1993a) *Managing the New NHS*, London: Department of Health.

DoH (1993b) *Clinical Audit: Meeting and Improving Standards in Healthcare*, London: Department of Health.

DoH (1993c) *Working Together for Better Health*, London: Department of Health.

DoH (1994) *Working in Partnership: A collaborative approach to care*. Report of the Mental Heath Nursing Review Team, London: Department of Health.

DoH (1995a) *Acting on Complaints: the government's proposals in response to Being Heard*, London: HMSO.

DoH (1995b) *NHS Responsibilities for Meeting Continuing Health Care Needs*, London: Department of Health.

DoH (1995c) *The Health of the Nation. A Strategy for People with Learning Disabilities*, London: Department of Health.

DoH (1996a) *Primary Care: The Future*, June, London: Department of Health.

DoH (1996b) *Choice and Opportunity: Primary Care: The Future*, October, London: The Stationery Office.

DoH (1996c) *Primary Care: Delivering the Future*, December, London: The Stationery Office.

DoH (1997) *Departmental Report*, Cm. 3612, Annexe E, London: The Stationery Office.

DoH (1998a) *A First Class Service Quality in the New NHS*, London: Department of Health.

DoH (1998b) *Modernising Mental Health Services: Safe, sound and supportive*, London: Department of Health.

DoH (1998c) *The New NHS, Modern and Dependable: A National Framework for Assessing Performance*, Consultation document, London: Department of Health.

DoH (1998d) *Partnerships in Action; New Opportunities for Joint Working Between Health and Social Services*, London: Department of Health.

DoH (1999a) 'Dobson hails biggest waiting list fall yet as NHS delivers even more than promised', *Press Release* 1999/0278, 10th May, Leeds: NHS Executive.

DoH (1999b) *NHS Direct: Summary of Findings from the First Nine Months*, Leeds: NHS Executive.

DoH (1999c) *High Level Performance Indicators*, London: Department of Health.

DoH (1999d) *Making a Difference: Strengthening the Nursing, Midwifery and Health Visiting Contribution to Health and Health Care*, London: Department of Health.

Donabedian, A. (1966) 'Evaluating the quality of medical care', *Millbank Memorial Fund Quarterly*, **44** (3, Section 2) 166–207.

Donaldson, L. (1995) 'The listening blank', *Health Service Journal*, **105** (5471) 22–4.

Donnelly, L. (1999a) 'Ready sorted', *Health Service Journal*, **109** (5637) 14.

Donnelly, L. (1999b) 'Clinical governance needs 'extra powers', *Health Service Journal*, **109** (5679) 7.

Donnelly, L. (1999c) 'Sound post', *Health Service Journal*, **109** (5460) 10–11.

Donnelly, L. (1999d) 'Head of HEA resigns as new era dawns', *Health Service Journal*, **109** (5659). 5.

Donovan, J. (1986) *We Don't Buy Sickness, It Just Comes*, Aldershot: Gower.

Douglas Home, M. (1988) 'Doctors propose world revolution in training', *Independent*, 13 August.

Dudman, J. (1999) 'Software bidding war hots up for NHS Direct roll-out', *Health Service Journal*, **109** (5662) 5.

Dunford, H. and Smith, C. (1992) 'Family Planning and Audit: Anyone for Audit?' *British Journal of Family Planning*, **18** (2) 56–8.

Durham, V. (1993) 'Tomlinson: what it means for the Black community', *Share*. Issue 5, April, 4.

Dyer, C. and Gibbs, G. (1999) 'How law student won landmark ruling', *The Guardian*, 17 July.

Earwicker, S. (1998) *GP Commissioning Groups – The Nottingham Experience*, OHE Briefing No. 38, London: Office of Health Economics.

Eaton, L. (1998) 'Guidance brings 48-hour week as exempt junior doctors fight on', *Health Service Journal*, **108** (5632) 8.

Elkeles, R. (1989) 'The cash register may drown out the sound of the ambulance', *Independent*, 24 January.

Ellis, R. (1988) 'Quality Assurance: The Professional's Role', *Public Money and Management*, Spring/Summer, 37–40.

Elliott, B. (1999) 'Ready, steady?', *Health Service Journal*, **109** (5644) 23.

Elliott, L. (1996) 'Learn the hard lesson and freeze the health budget', *The Guardian*, 17 June.

Ely Report (1969) *Report of the Committee of Enquiry into Allegations of Ill-Treatment of Patients and Other Irregularities at the Ely Hospital, Cardiff*, Cmnd 3975, London: HMSO.

Enthoven, A. (1985) *Reflections on the Management of the NHS*, London: Nuffield Provincial Hospitals Trust.

EOC (Equal Opportunities Commission)(1982) *Who Cares for the Carers?*, Manchester: EOC.

Ewles, L. (1999) 'Avon calling', *Health Service Journal*, **109** (5660) 24–5.

Exworthy, M. and Moon, G. (1998) 'The shape of things to come', *Health Service Journal*, **108** (5615) 20–2.

Farrar, S. (1999a) 'Today's babies can expect to live to 130', *The Sunday Times*, 14 February.

Farrar, S. (1999b) 'Millennium man will be 14-stone sloth', *The Sunday Times*, 21 February.

Farrar, S. and Gadher, D. (1999) 'First tongue transplant will restore speech', *The Sunday Times*, 24 January.

Feldman, R. (1987) 'The politics of the new reproductive technologies', *Critical Social Policy*, Issue 19, Summer, 21–40.

Field, F. (1989) 'Time bomb set to blow apart NHS', *The Sunday Times*, 19 February.

Field, F., Deacon, A., Alcock, P., Green, D. and Phillips, M. (1996) *Stakeholder Welfare*, Choice in Welfare Series No. 32, London: The Institute of Economic Affairs.

Finch, J. (1999) 'Boots lays out its battle plan', *The Guardian*, 4 June.

Finch, J. and Groves, D. (1983) *A Labour of Love: Women, work and caring*, London: Routledge & Kegan Paul.

Flynn, R., Pickard, S. and Williams, G. (1995) 'Contracts and the Quasi-market in Community Health Services', *Journal of Social Policy*, **24**, Part 4, October, 529–50.

FPSC (Family Policy Studies Centre) (1988) *An Ageing Population*, Fact Sheet 2, London: FPSC.

Forrest Report (1987) *Breast Cancer Screening*, London: HMSO.

Foundation for Integrated Medicine (1997) *Integrated Healthcare: A Way Forward for the Next Five Years?*, London: Foundation for Integrated Medicine.

Frazer, W. (1950) *A History of English Public Health 1838–1939*, London: Baillière, Tindall and Fox.

Frean, A. (1999) 'Elderly may not have to sell up to afford care', *The Times*, Long-Term Care Report, 2 March.

Friend, B. (1998a) 'The cost of living', *Health Service Journal*, **108** (5614) 22–4.

Friend, B. (1998b) 'Quick march', *Health Service Journal*, **108** (5633) 26–8.

Gardner, P. (1988) *Health Care in Britain: Progress, problems and options for reform*, London: Conservative Central Office.

General Medical Council (1993) *Tomorrow's Doctors: Recommendations on Undergraduate Medical Education*, London: General Medical Council.

Gibbs, G. (1997) 'Policy decision on prescription charges 'ducked'', *The Guardian*, 8 January.

Gillam, S. (1998) 'Clinical governance', in *Implementing the White Paper Pitfalls and opportunities, A King's Fund Policy Paper*, Klein, R. (ed.) London: King's Fund.

Gillie, O. (1988a) 'Obstacle course for Alton Bill', *The Independent*, 6 May.

Gillie, O. (1988b) 'AIDS death toll passes "sombre" 1,000 milestone', *The Independent*, 9 November.

Gillie Report (1963) *The Field of Work of the Family Doctor*, Central Health Services Council, Standing Medical Advisory Committee, London: HMSO.

Ginsberg, N. (1992) *Division of Welfare: A Critical Introduction to Comparative Social Policy*, London: Sage.

Glassman, D. (1997) 'Those magical zones', *Health Matters*, Issue 31, Autumn, 6–7.

GLARE (Greater London Action for Racial Equality) (1987) *No Alibi No Excuses*, London: GLARE.

Glendinning, C. (1998) 'From General Practice to Primary Care: Developments in Primary Health Services 1990–1998', *Social Policy Review 10*. Brundson, E., Dean, H., and Woods, R. (eds) London: Social Policy Association.

Glennerster, H. (1995) *British Social Policy since 1945*, Oxford: Blackwell.

Glennerster, H. (1998) 'Substance or Rhetoric? The New NHS White Paper', *Eurohealth*, 4 (4) Autumn, 38–9.

Glennerster, H., Korman, N. and Marsden-Wilson, F. (1983) *Planning for Priority Groups*, Oxford: Martin Robertson.

Glennerster, H., Owens, P. and Kimberley, A. (1986) *The Nursing Management Function after Griffiths: A Study in the North West Thames Region*, London: The London School of Economics and North West Thames Regional Health Authority.

Glennerster, H., Owens, P., Gatiss, S. and Kimberley, A., (1988) *The Nursing Management Function after Griffiths: A Study in the North West Thames Region: A second interim report*, London: London School of Economics and North West Thames Regional Health Authority.

Glennerster, H., Matsaganis, M., Owens, P. and Hancock, S. (1993) 'GP Fundholding: Wild Card or Winning Hand?', in *Evaluating the NHS Reforms*, Robinson, R. and Le Grand, J. (eds) London: King's Fund Institute.

Glennerster, H., Matsaganis, M., Owens, P. and Hancock, S. (1994) *Implementing GP Fundholding: Wild Card or Winning Hand?* Buckingham: Open University Press.

Goddard, A. (1998) 'Medics to rise by 1,000', *The Times Higher*, 31 July.

Goddard, A. (1999) 'Medical schools win go-ahead' *The Times Higher*, 25 June.

Goodwin, N. (1996) 'GP fundholding: a review of the evidence', in *Health Care UK 1995/96: an annual review of health care policy*, Harrison A. (ed.) London: King's Fund.

Gow, D. (1995) 'Pharmacist fights NHS drugs fee', *The Guardian*, 21 June.

Gow, D. (1999) 'Hospital ship plan floated for NHS', *The Guardian*, 21 July.

Graham, H. (1988) 'The limits to health promotion: unfiltered tips from women who smoke'. Paper given to the Social Policy Association's Annual Conference, Edinburgh University, 14 July.

Green, D. (1986) *Challenge to the NHS: A study of competition in American health care and the lessons for Britain*, London: Institute of Economic Affairs.

Green, D. (1988) *Everyone a Private Patient: An analysis of the structural flaws in the NHS and how they could be remedied*, London: Institute of Economic Affairs.

Green, D. (1989) 'A step in the right direction', *Health Service Journal*, 99 (5137) 168.

Green, H. (1988) *General Household Survey 1985: Series GHS No. 15 Supplement A: Informal Carers*, London: HMSO.

Grice, E. (1987) 'Queueing for a cure', *The Sunday Times*, 29 November.

Griffiths Report (1983) *NHS Management Inquiry*, London: DHSS.

Griffiths Report (1988) *Community Care: An agenda for action*, London: HMSO.

Griffiths, J. (1991a) 'Promoting gain to end pain', *Health Service Journal*, 101 (5265) 20–1.

Griffiths, J. (1991b) 'Lessons in Class', *Health Service Journal*, 101 (5266) 20–1.

Guillebaud Committee (1956) *Report of the Committee of Enquiry into the Cost of the National Health Service*, Cmnd 9663, London: HMSO.

Gunn, S. (1989) 'Drug-users most at risk from AIDS'. *The Times*, 14 January.

Hall, C. (1999a) 'Free care ruling 'may led to chaos', *The Daily Telegraph*, 17 July.

Hall, S. (1999b) 'Men missing out on health care cash', *The Guardian*, 25 May.

Halpern, S. (1985) 'How should the Centre be spread?', *Health and Social Service Journal*, 28 February, 248–50.

Ham, C. (1982) *Health Policy in Britain*, London: Macmillan.

Ham, C. (ed.) (1997) *Health Care Reform: Learning from International Experience*, Buckingham: Open University Press.

Ham, C. (1998) 'Mix and match', *The Guardian*, (Society: Health Administration) 18 February.

Ham, C. and Calltorp, J. (1992) 'Money Money Money', *Health Service Journal*, 102 (5295) 22–5.

Ham, C. and Heginbotham, C. (1991) *Purchasing Together*, London: King's Fund College.

Ham, C. and Hunter, D. (1988) *Managing Clinical Activity in the NHS*, London: King's Fund Institute.

Ham, C. and Robinson, R. (1988) 'National Health Service PLC', *New Society*, 19 February, 11–12.

Ham, C., Robinson, R. and Benzeval, M. (1990) *Health Check: Health care reforms in an international context*, London: King's Fund Institute.

Hancock, C. (1994) 'Two into one won't go', *Health Service Journal*, **104** (5416) 19.

Hancock, C. (1998) 'Party to a vision of the future', *Health Service Journal*, **108** (5585) 20.

Hansard (1986) *House of Commons: Parliamentary Debates*, **105**, No. 8, 21 November, Cols. 801–866, London: HMSO.

Hansard (1989a) *House of Commons: Parliamentary Debates*, **144**, No. 27, 13 January, Col. 1100–1162, London: HMSO.

Hansard (1989b) *House of Commons: Parliamentary Debates*, **147**, No. 5, 21 February, Col. 820, London: HMSO.

Harman, H. (1988) *Cervical Cancer Screening: The risk remains*, London: Transport and General Workers Union.

Harris, C. (1999) 'Toeing the line', *Health Service Journal*, **109** (5650) 24–25.

Harrison, A. (ed.) (1992) *Health Care UK 1991*, London: King's Fund Institute.

Harrison, A. and New, B. (1996) *Health Care UK 1995/6: An annual review of health care policy*, London: King's Fund.

Harrison, L. and Neve, H. (1996) *A Review of Innovations in Primary Health Care*, University of Bristol: Policy Press.

Harrison, S., Hunter, D., Marnoch, G. and Pollitt, C. (1989) *The Impact of General Management in the National Health Service*, Milton Keynes: Nuffield Institute for Health Studies, University of Leeds and the Open University.

Hastings, G. and Scott, A. (1987) 'AIDS publicity: pointers to development', *Health Educational Journal*, **46** (2) 58–9.

Hawker, J. (1999) 'Parity begins at home', *Health Service Journal*, **109** (5636) 18–20.

Hayes, A. (1998) 'The EU and Public Health beyond the Year 2000', *LSE Health*, **4** (4) Autumn, 2–4.

Haywood, S. (1985) 'Making the most of the HA members', *Health and Social Service Journal*, 16 May, 612.

Hazell, R. and Jervis, P. (1998) *Devolution and Health*, Nuffield Trust Series No. 3, London: The Nuffield Trust; London: The Constitution Unit.

Healthcare 2000 (1995) *UK Health and Healthcare Services, Challenges and Policy Options*, London: Healthcare 2000.:

Health Care Information Services (1988) *The Fitzhugh Directory*, London: Euston House.

Health Quality Service (1999) *Feeling the Pulse: quality improvement and assurance in the NHS*, London: King's Fund.

Health Service Journal (1989) 'Flawed by the fanatics', **99** (5136) 131.

Health Service Journal (1998) 'Social services chiefs oppose integration', **108** (5595) 6.

Health Service Journal (1999a) 'GPs stand firm on board boycott', **109** (5640) 7.

Health Service Journal (1999b) 'Steep rise in NHS dentists earning more than £200 000', **109** (5639) 8.

Health Service Journal (1999c) 'Death-plunge trust had no risk strategy', **109** (5659) 4.

Healy, P. (1998a) 'Unfinished business', *Health Service Journal*, **108** (5603) 11.

Healy, P. (1998b) 'A poor fit', *Health Service Journal*, **108** (5626) 15.

Healy, P. (1998c) 'Mayor 'should be strong on health', *Health Service Journal*, **108** (5635) 9.

Healy, P. (1999a) 'Splitting the difference', *Health Service Journal'*, **109** (5461) 9–10.

Healy, P. (1999b) 'Broad welcome for pay awards – if fully funded', *Health Service Journal*, **109** (5460) 2–3.

Healy, P. (1999c) 'Damning with faint praise', *Health Service Journal*, **109** (5646) 10–11.

Healy, P. (1999d) 'Equal to the task', *Health Service Journal*, **109** (5649) 6–7.

Healy, P. (1999e) 'No extra cash to fund Blair's nurse posts', *Health Service Journal*, **109** (5563), 2–3.

Healy, P. and McIntosh, K. (1999) 'Dobson stalls on proposal for free long-term care', *Health Service Journal*, **109** (5644) 2–3.

Heginbotham, C. (1990) *Return to Community: The Voluntary Ethic and Community Care*, London: Bedford Square Press.

Hempel, S. (1998) 'Title fight', *The Guardian*, 12 August.

Hencke, D. (1984) 'Fowler names health service manager', *The Guardian*, 14 December.

Hencke, D. (1995) 'NHS unable to account for £422m', *The Guardian*, 4 December.

Hetherington, P. (1998) 'Social Exclusion', *The Guardian*, 16 September.

Hetherington, P. (1999) 'Scottish MPs may be cut, admits Reid', *The Guardian*, 20 July.

Higgins, J. (1988) *The Business of Medicine: private health care in Britain*, London: Macmillan.

Higgins, J. (1998) 'HAZs warning', *Health Service Journal*, **108** (5600) 24–5.

Hinde, J. (1998a) 'Committee starts work on extra medic places', *The Times Higher*, 30 September.

Hinde, J. (1998b) 'OU revolution for doctor training', *The Times Higher*, 6 February.

Hodges, R. (1993) 'In the pink?', *Health Service Journal*, **103** (5361) 24–6.

Holland, P. (1996) 'How should primary care be developed?', in *Health Care UK1995/96: An annual review of health care policy'*, Harrison, A. (ed.) London: King's Fund.

Hoggart, S. (1998) 'Blair bons mots prove a palpable hit', *The Guardian*, 25 March.

Hooper, J., Edwards, N. and Ujah, S. (1997) 'How to get started' in *Needs to Know: A guide to needs assessment for primary care*, Harris, A. (ed.) London: Churchill Livingstone.

Hope, J. (1999) 'Nurse your own patient', The *Daily Mail*, 8 January.

Hopton, J., Leahy, G. (1997) 'Locality needs assessment', in *Needs to Know: A guide to needs assessment for primary care*, Harris, A. (ed.) London: Churchill Livingstone.

House of Commons Health Committee (1996) *Long-term Care: Future Provision and Funding*. Session 1995–6. Third Report, Volume I, London: HMSO.

House of Commons Health Committee (1998) *The Relationship between Health and Social Services*, First Report, Volume 1, London: The Stationery Office.

House of Commons Social Services Committee (1988) *The future of the National Health Service*, Fifth Report, Session 1987–88, HCP 613, London: HMSO.

House of Commons Treasury Committee (1996) *The Private Finance Initiative: sixth report*, Session 1995–6, HoC paper 146, London: HMSO.

Hudson, B. (1998a) 'Take your partners', *Health Service Journal*, **108** (5590) 30–1.

Hudson, B. (1998b) 'Prospects of partnership', *Health Service Journal*, **108** (5600) 26–7.

Hughes, D. (1990) 'Same story; different words', *Health Service Journal*, **100** (5193) 432–3.

Hughes, D. (1991) 'A question of judgement', *Health Service Journal*, **101** (5256) 22–4.

Hughes, D. and Dingwall, R., (1990) 'What's in a name?', *Health Service Journal*, **100** (5229) 170–1.

Human Fertilisation and Embryology Authority (1995) *The Patient's Guide to DI and IVF clinics*, London: Human Fertilisation and Embryology Authority.

Hunter, D. (1988) 'They who shout loudest', *Health Service Journal* 98 (5082) 18.

Hunter, D. (1993) *Rationing Dilemmas in Health Care*, Research Paper no. 8, Birmingham: NAHAT.

Hunter, D. (1996a) 'New line on age-old problems', *Health Service Journal*, **106** (5508) 21.

Hunter, H. (1996b) 'Treasury gives go-ahead for private hospital plan', *Health Service Journal*, **106** (5498) 6.

Hunter D. (1998a) Which way lies The Third Way? *Health Service Journal*, **108** (5615) 16–17.

Hunter, D. (1998b) I re-think therefore I am, *Health Service Journal*, **108** (5603) 20.

Hunter, D. (1998c) Cruel illusions of progress, *Health Service Journal*, **108** (5598) 22.

Hunter, D. (1999) 'Horizontally challenged', *The Guardian*, 12 May.

Hunter, D. and O'Toole, S. (1995) 'Rosy Outlook', *Health Service Journal*, **105** (5451) 20–1.

Hunter, H. and Shamash, J. (1996) 'Leeds cash crisis part of wider financial 'meltdown', *Health Service Journal*, **106** (5502) 3.

Hutton, W. (1995) 'Technology leaps to wrong diagnosis', *The Guardian*, 20 September.

Inman, P (1999) 'Fury at new care delay', *The Guardian*, 22 May.

Institute of Health Services Management (IHSM) (1988) *Alternative Delivery and Funding of Health Services, Final Report*, London: IHSM.

IPPF (International Planned Parenthood Federation) (1988) Open File, 15 March, London: IPPF.

Jack, B. and Oldham, J. (1997) 'Taking steps towards evidence based practice', *Nurse Researcher*, **5** (1) 65–71.

Jameson Committee (1956) *An Inquiry into Health Visiting*, London: HMSO.

Jay Report (1979) *Report of the Committee of Enquiry into Mental Handicap, Nursing and Care*, Cmnd 7468, London: HMSO.

Jenkins, L. (1988) 'No more PIs in the sky', *Health Service Journal*, **98** (5097) 450–1.

Jenkins, P. (1989a) 'Notice to quit vested interests', *The Independent*, 1 February.

Jenkins, P. (1989b) 'Doctors draw the political battle lines', *The Independent*, 21 March.

Jervis, P. and Hazell, R. (1998) 'Separate ways', *Health Service Journal*, **108** (5632) 26–7.

Jinks, C., Nio Ong, B. and Paton, C. (1998) 'Catching the drift', *Health Service Journal*, **108** (5622) 24–5.

Jofre, S. (1988) 'Humanising health', *New Statesman and Society*, 19 August, 29.

Johnson, L. and Abbott, S. (1999) 'Long-term care: Wait 'til your dad gets home', *Health Service Journal*, **109** (5661) 24–25.

Johnson, S. et al. (1997) *London's Mental Health*, London: King's Fund.

Jones, A. and Duncan, A. (1995) *Hypothecated Health Taxes: an evaluation of recent proposals*, London: Office of Health Economics.

Jones Elwyn, G., Rapport, F. and Kinnersley, P. (1998) 'Primary health care teams re-engineered', *Journal of Interprofessional Care*, **12** (2) 189–98.

Jones, K. (1960) *Mental Health and Social Policy 1845–1959*, London: Routledge & Kegan Paul.

Joss, R., Henkel, M. and Kogan, M. (1994) *An evaluation of total quality management in the National Health Service, Final Report to the Department of Health*, Uxbridge: Brunel University.

Joss, R. and Kogan, M. (1995) *Advancing Quality: Total Quality Management in the National Health Service*, Buckingham: Open University Press.

Jowell, R., Witherspoon, S. and Brook, L. (1986) *British Social Attitudes: The 1986 Report*, Aldershot: Gower.

Jowell, R., Witherspoon, S. and Brook, L. (1988) *British Social Attitudes: The 5th Report*, Aldershot: Gower.

Judge, K. (1999) 'National Evaluation of Health Action Zones', in *PSSRU Bulletin*, Bebbington, A. and Judge K. (eds). Canterbury: Personal Social Services Research Unit.

Kerrison, S., Packwood, T. and Buxton, M. (1993) 'Monitoring Medical Audit', in *Evaluating the NHS Reforms*, Robinson, R. and Le Grand, J. (eds) London: King's Fund Institute.

Kaletsky, A. (1998) 'Field guide points to 'third way', *The Times*, Analysis, 27 March.

King's Fund (1988) *Health and Health Services in Britain, 1948–88*, London: King's Fund Institute.

King's Fund (1992) *London Health 2010 – the report of the King's Fund London Initiative*, London: King's Fund.

Kingston, W. and Rowbottom, R. (1989) *Making General Management Work in the NHS*, Uxbridge: Brunel University.

Kirkman-Liff, B. (1997) 'The United States', in *Health Care Reform: Learning from International Experience*, Ham. C. (ed.) Buckingham: Open University Press.

Klein, R. (1982) 'Performance, evaluation and the NHS', *Public Administration*, 60, 385–407.

Klein, R. (1983) *The Politics of the National Health Service*, London: Longman.

Klein, R. (1989) *The Politics of the NHS*, second edition, London: Longman.

Klein, R. (1995) *The New Politics of the NHS*, third edition, London: Longman.

Klein, R. (1996) 'Who's to decide the NHS menu?', *The Guardian* (Society section) 25 September.

Klein, R. (1999) 'Reviews', *Journal of Social Policy*, 28, Part 1, January, 165.

Klein, R. and Day, P. (1989) 'NHS review: the broad picture', *British Medical Journal*, 298, 11 February, 339–40.

Klein, R., Perry, J. and Travers, T. (1998) 'Clinical depression', *The Guardian*, Society section, 29 April.

Kleinman, M. (1998) 'New deal, old barriers', *The Guardian*, 30 September.

Korner Steering Group (1982) *Health Services Information*, London: HMSO.

Labour Party (1943) *National Service for Health: The Labour Party's post-war policy*, London: Labour Party.

Labour Party (1996) *New Labour: New Life for Britain*, London: Labour Party.

Laetz, T. (1996) 'An American View: Health Care Policy Comparisons between the European Union and the United States', *EuroHealth* 2 (1) March, 35–6.

Laing, W. (1987) *Laing's Review of Private Health Care 1987*, London: Laing and Buisson.

Laing, W. (1995) *Laing's Review of Private Healthcare 1995*, London: Laing and Buisson.

Laing, W. (1997) *Laing's Review of Private Healthcare 1997*, London: Laing and Buisson.

Lalonde Report (1974) *A New Perspective on the Health of the Canadians*, Ottowa: Government of Canada.

Lamb, J. (1994) 'Beaten by the system', *The Guardian*, 16 February.

Lancet (1989) 'Curtains up on the NHS review', 1 (8632) 247–9.

Lane Committee (1974) *Report of the Committee on the Working of the Abortion Act*, Cmnd 5579, London: HMSO.

Larbie, J. (1985) *Black Women and the Maternity Services*, London: Health Education Council.

Laurance, J. (1982) 'Solid for health workers', *New Society*, 10 June, 424–5.

Laurance, J. (1983) 'The collapse of the BUPA boom', *New Society*, 24 February, 295–6.

Laurance, J. (1986a) 'The rising cost of prescriptions is deterring patients', *New Society*, 14 March, 460.

Laurance, J. (1986b) 'Unemployment health hazards', *New Society*, 21 March, 492–3.

Laurance, J. (1987a) 'NHS: How spending has fallen', *New Society*, 2 January, 5.

Laurance, J. (1987b) 'The patient factory', *New Society*, 8 May, 21.

Laurance, J. (1988a) 'Silencing the NHS', *New Statesman and Society*, 10 June, 14–15.

Laurance, J. (1988b) 'AIDS: the politics of panic', *New Society*, 22 January, 22.

Laurance, J. (1989a) 'Doctors prepare for a showdown on NHS reforms', *The Sunday Times*, 12 March.

Laurance, J. (1989b) 'Pioneering GPs cut drugs bill', *The Sunday Times*, 19 March.

Laurance, J. (1996) 'Positive results vary five-fold in tests for cervical cancer', *The Times*, 21 February.

Law Commission (1996) *Damages for Personal Injury: Medical, Nursing and other Expenses – the Cost of Care*, London: HMSO.

Layzell, A. (1994) 'Perspectives on Purchasing: Local and Vocal', *Health Service Journal*, 104 (5395) 28–30.

Leathard, A. (1980) *The Fight for Family Planning*, London: Macmillan.

Leathard, A. (1985) *District Health Authority Family Planning Services*, London: Family Planning Association.

Leathard, A. (1987) *Consumer Views and Family Planning Perspectives*, London: Family Planning Association.

Leathard, A. (ed.) (1994) *Going Inter-Professional: Working Together for Health and Welfare*, London: Routledge.

Leathard, A. (1997) 'Interprofessional Education and the Medical Profession: The Changing Context in Britain', *Education for Health*, 10, (3) 359–370.

Leathard, A. (1998) 'Collaborative care for health and welfare', in *Fifty years of the National Health Service: continuities and discontinuities in health policy'*, Skelton, R. and Williamson, V. (eds) Brighton: University of Brighton.

Leavey, R., Wilkin, D. and Metcalfe, D. (1989) 'Consumerism and general practice', *British Medical Journal*, 298 737–9.

Le Grand, J. (1993) 'Evaluating the NHS Reforms', in *Evaluating the NHS Reforms*, Robinson, D. and Le Grand, J. (eds) London: King's Fund Institute.

Le Grand, J. and Bartlett, W. (eds) (1993) *Quasi-markets and Social Policy*, London: Macmillan.

Le Grand, J., Mays, N. and Mulligan, J. (1998) *Learning from the NHS Internal Market: A Review of the Evidence*, London: King's Fund.

Le Grand, J. and Robinson, R. (eds) (1984) *Privatisation and the Welfare State*, London: Allen & Unwin.

Leiba, T. (1994) 'Inter-professional approaches to mental health care', in *Going Inter-Professional: Working Together for Health and Welfare*, Leathard, A. (ed.) London: Routledge.

Lenaghan, J. (1999) *Rights and Responsibilities*, London: Institute for Public Policy Research.

Lennon, K. and Jones, S. (1998) 'Give health authorities some teeth', *Health Matters*, Issue 33, Spring, 11.

Lewis, J. (1993) 'Community care policy imperatives, joint planning and enabling authorities', *Journal of Interprofessional Care*, 7 (1) Spring, 6–14.

Lewis, J. and Glennerster, H. (1996) *Implementing the New Community Care*, Buckingham: Open University Press.

Lilley, R. (1997) 'Why health will not be 'free' for all', *Health Service Journal*, 107 (5536) 20.

Limb, M. (1992) 'The poverty of theory', *Health Service Journal*, 102 (5311) 13.

Lindsey, A. (1962) *The National Health Service 1948–1961: Socialised medicine in England and Wales*, Chapel Hill: University of North Carolina Press.

Ling, K. (1993) 'Grasping the nettle of NHS staff equality', *Share*, Issue 5, April, 5.

Linstead, D. and McMahon, L. (1987) 'Clinicians in management: in transit: back-up required', *Health Service Journal*, **97** (5056) 730.

Longfield, J. (1984) *Ask the Family: shattering the myths about family life*, London: NCVO.

Lorbiecki, A. (1995) 'Clinicians as managers: Convergence or collision?', in *Inter-professional Relations in Health Care*, Soothill, K., Mackay, L. and Webb, C. (eds) London: Edward Arnold.

Luker, K. et al. (1997) *Evaluation of Nurse Prescribing*, Final Report, Liverpool: University of Liverpool and University of York.

MacAskill, E. (1999a) 'Dobson private care threat, *The Guardian*, 18 March.

Macaskill, M. (1999b) 'Surgeons rebuild eyes with cell transplants', *The Sunday Times*, 6 June.

Macpherson, G. (1989) 'BMA's measured response', *British Medical Journal*, **298** 340–1.

Maddock, S. and Morgan, G. (1999) 'Identifying conditions for partnership', *CAIPE Bulletin*, Spring, No. 16, 15.

Mahon, A., Wilkin, D. and Whitehouse, C. (1993) 'Choice of Hospital for Elective Surgery Referral: GPs' and Patients' Views', in *Evaluating the NHS Reforms*, Robinson, R. and Le Grand, J. (eds) London: King's Fund Institute.

Mandelson, P. and Liddle, R. (1995) *The Blair Revolution – can New Labour deliver?* London: Faber and Faber.

Marks, L. (1988) *Promoting Better Health? An Analysis of the Government's Programme for Primary Health Care*, London: King's Fund Institute.

Marsh, D. and Chambers, J. (1981) *Abortion Politics*, London: Junction Books.

Maxwell, R. (1984) 'Quality assessment in health', *British Medical Journal*, **288** 1470–2.

Maxwell, R. (1988) 'Life begins at 40? The NHS in 1988', *Health Services Management*, **84** (3) 10–13.

Maxwell, R. (1992) *Purchasing and Poverty: a guide to commissioning health services for homeless people*. London: King's Fund.

May, A, (1995) 'Doing the Continental', *Health Service Journal*, **105** (5461) 14–15.

Maynard, A. (1987) 'Making the health technology revolution more cost effective' *Health Service Journal*, **97** (5051) 587.

Maynard, A. (1989a) 'Budget holding and how it will affect GPs' usual work practices', *Pulse*, **498**, No. 8, 25 February, 65.

Maynard, A. (1989b) 'Carrots to blend with choice cuts', *The Guardian*, 30 January.

Maynard, A. (1995a) 'Dispensing with the paradoxes', *Health Service Journal*, **105** (5466) 17.

Maynard, A. (1995b) 'Are they barking mad?', *Health Service Journal*, **105** (5472) 21.

Maynard, A. (1996) 'Lean, mean rationing machine', *Health Service Journal*, **106** (5488) 21.

Maynard, A. (1998), 'We don't need more doctors', *The Times Higher*, 3 July.

Maynard, A. (1999a) 'Troubles down below', *Health Service Journal*, **109** (5645) 15–16.

Maynard, A. (1999b) 'Loot is not the only route', *Health Service Journal*, **109** (5639) 16–17.

Maynard, A. and Holland, W. (1988) *Reforming UK Health Care to improve Health: The case for research and experiment*, York University: Centre for Health Economics.

Mays, N. and Dixon, J. (1996) *Purchaser Plurality in UK Health Care: Is a consensus emerging and is it the right one?* London: Kings Fund.

Mayston Report (1969) *Report of the Working Party on Management Structure in the Local Authority Nursing Service*, DHSS, London: HMSO.

McClenahan, J., Flux, R., Ijebor, L. and Mumford, P. (1986) 'Korner preparing for the pay off', *Health Service Journal*, 96 (5018) 1258–9.

McGlone, F. (1993) 'A million new carers – but how many more to come?', *Family Policy Bulletin*, (Family Policy Studies Centre), June.

McGrath, M. (1991) *Multi-disciplinary Teamwork. Community Mental Handicap Teams*, Aldershot: Avebury.

McIntosh, K. (1999a) 'Only two PCG chairs to be held by nurses', *Health Service Journal*, 109 (5643) 7.

McIntosh, K. (1999b) 'Virtual reality', *Health Service Journal*, 109 (5650) 11–12.

McIntosh, K. (1999c) 'Community trusts win praise for PCT moves', *Health Service Journal*, 109 (5629) 8.

McIntosh, K. (1999d) 'A word in private', *Health Service Journal*, 109 (5652) 9–11.

McKie, D. (1989) 'Health tops poll on Budget', *The Guardian*, 17 February.

McKeown, T. (1976) *The Role of Medicine – Dream, Mirage or Nemesis*, London: Nuffield Provincial Hospitals Trust.

McNaught, A. (1988) *Race and Health Policy*, London: Croom Helm.

Medical Research Council (1994) *The Health of the UK's Elderly People*. London: Medical Research Council.

Merrison Report (1979) *Report of the Royal Commission on the National Health Service*, Cmnd 7615, London: HMSO.

Mihill, C. (1995) 'Top surgeon quits over waiting list', *The Guardian*, 8 December.

Mihill, C. (1996a) 'Cash limits pushing NHS 'to brink', 'Hospitals head for 'meltdown', *The Guardian*, 17 May, front page.

Mihill, C. (1996b) 'Privatising NHS could destroy it', *The Guardian*, 23 April.

Mihill, C. (1996c) 'Cervical tests rules tightened', *The Guardian*, 19 March.

Milburn, A. (1996) 'Breaking the tension', *The Guardian*, 14 February.

Milburn, A. (1998) 'The chance we've been waiting for', *Health Service Journal*, 108 (5597) 20.

Millar, B. (1988) 'Public Health served the Canadian way', *Health Service Journal*, 98 (5120) 1116.

Millar, B. (1989a) 'Christine Hancock ... a manager joins the union', *Health Service Journal*, 99 (5133) 39.

Millar, B. (1989b) 'Bigwigs, worthies and gentlemen', *Health Service Journal*, 99 (5138) 192.

Millar, B. (1996) 'The facts of life', *Health Service Journal*, 106 (5488) 16.

Millar, B. (1997) 'Gym'll fix it', *Health Service Journal*, 107 (5569) 12.

Millar, B. (1999a) 'Standard bearer', *Health Service Journal*, 109 (5644) 12–13.

Millar, B. (1999b) 'Whole new ball game', *Health Service Journal*, 109 (5643) 12–13.

Mind (1987) *Mental Health Services in a Multi-Racial Society*, London: Mind.

Ministry of Health (1944) *A National Health Service*, White Paper, Cmnd 6502, London: HMSO.

Ministry of Health (1962) *Hospital Plan for England and Wales*, Cmnd 1604, London: HMSO.

Ministry of Health (1963) *Health and Welfare: The Development of Community Care*, Cmnd 1973, London: HMSO.

Ministry of Health (1968) *National Health Service: The Administrative Structure of the Medical and Related Services in England and Wales*, London: HMSO.

Mohammed, S. (1991) 'Improving health services for Black populations', *Share*, Issue 1, November, 1–3.

Moks, D. (1996) 'From high and dry to PFI', *Health Service Journal*, **106** (5494) IT update, 15–16.

Moore, J. (1988) Letter to Miss Audrey Emerton, chairman UKCC. (Unpublished.) 20 May, London: DHSS.

Moore, W. (1995) 'Power of the People', *The Guardian*, Society section, 12 April.

Moore, W. (1999a) 'Final check-up', *The Guardian*, Society section, 17 February.

Moore, W. (1999b) 'The gap widens', *The Guardian*, Society section, 19 May.

Moran, M. (1992) 'Between the Lines', *Health Service Journal*, **102** (5299) 20–3.

Morgan, O. (1999) *A Cue for Change: Global Comparisons in Health Care*, London: Social Market Foundation.

Mossialos, E. and McKee, M. (1997) 'The European Union and health: past, present and future', in *Health Care UK 1996/7*, Harrison. A. and New, B. (eds) London: King's Fund.

Mulcahy, L. (1995) *Redress in the Public Sector*, London: National Consumer Council.

Mulcahy, L. and Tritter, J. (1994) 'Hidden depths', *Health Service Journal*, **104** (5411) 24–6.

Mullen, P. (1995) *'Is Health Service Rationing Really Necessary?'*, Discussion Paper No. 36, Birmingham University: Health Services Management Centre.

Mulligan, J. and Judge, K. (1997) 'Public Opinion and the NHS', *Health Care UK 1996/7*, London: King's Fund.

Munro, J. (1997/98) 'NHS trusts increasingly turn to private earnings', *Health Matters*, Issue 32, Winter, 2.

Murray, I. (1997) 'Hospital waiting lists are growing by 1,000 a week', *The Times*, 19 November.

Murray, I. (1999a) 'Flu crisis at hospitals dents Dobson's waiting list hopes', *The Times*, 7 January.

Murray, I. (1999b) 'New medical schools will serve poor areas', *The Times*, 23 June.

Murray, I. (1999c) '£40,000 carrot to keep super-nurses in NHS', *The Times*, 10 July.

Murray, I. (1999d) 'NHS curb on Viagra supply is ruled illegal', *The Times*, 27 May.

Murray, I. (1999e) 'Cervical cancer vaccine 'ready within ten years', *The Times*, 23 June.

NAHA (National Association of Health Authorities) (1988a) *Action Not Words: A Strategy to improve Health Services for Black and Ethnic Minority Users*, Birmingham: NAHA.

NAHA (1988b) *The Nation's Health: A Way Forward*, Birmingham: NAHA.

NAHAT (National Association of Health Authorities and Trusts) (1994) *Priority Setting: purchasing*, Birmingham: NAHAT.

NAHAT (1996) *The 1996/7 Contracting Round: NAHAT's Survey of NHS Purchasers and Providers*, Birmingham: NAHAT.

National Consumer Council (1988) *Funding the NHS*, London: National Consumer Council.

National Health Service Advisory Service (1997) *Services for People who are Elderly*, London: The Stationery Office.

National Infertility Awareness Campaign (1999) *The Sixth National Survey of the Funding and Provision of Infertility Services*, London: NAC.

Nattrass, H., Jarrold, K., Knowles, D. and Spry, C. (1985) 'Keeping the district family happy', *Health and Social Service Journal*, 19 September, 1158–61.

Neuberger, J. (1989) 'Putting the patient last', *The Times*, 3 February.

New, B. and Le Grand, J. (1996a) *Rationing in the NHS: Principles and Pragmatism*, London: King's Fund.

New, B. and Le Grand, J. (1996b) 'A la carte? No, choose from what's on the menu', *The Guardian*, Society section, 24 July.

New, B., Mays, N. (1997) 'Age, renal replacement therapy and rationing', in *Health Care UK 1996/97: The King's Fund annual review of health policy*', Harrison, A. (ed.) London: King's Fund.

NHS Advisory Service (1997) *Services for People who are Elderly. Addressing the balance: the multidisciplinary assessment of elderly people and the delivery of high quality continuing care*, London: The Stationery Office.

NHS Executive (1995) *Developing NHS Purchasing and GP Fundholding: Towards a Primary Care-led NHS*, Leeds: Department of Health.

NHS Executive (1997) *Health Action Zones – Invitation to Bid*, EL(97)65, Leeds: Department of Health.

NHS Executive (1998a) *The new NHS – Modern and Dependable. Developing Primary Care Groups*, HSC 1988/139, Leeds: Department of Health.

NHS Executive (1998b) *Better Health and Better Health Care: Implementing the new NHS and Our Healthier Nation*, HSC 1998/021 Leeds: Department of Health.

NHS Executive (1998c) *Nurse Prescribing*, Leeds: Department of Health.

NHSME (National Health Service Management Executive) (1992) *Local Voices: The views of local people in purchasing for health*, EL(92)1 January, Leeds: NHSME

Nissel, M. and Bonnerjea, L. (1982) *Family Care of the Handicapped Elderly: Who Pays?*, London: Policy Studies Institute.

Norman, I. and Redfern, S. (1995) 'What is Audit?', in *Making Use of Clinical Audit: A guide to practice in the health professions*, Kogan, M. and Redfern, S. (eds) Buckingham: Open University Press.

North, C., Moore, H. and Owens, C. (1996) *Go Home and Rest? The Use of an Accident and Emergency Department by Homeless People*, London: Shelter.

Nundy, J. (1993) 'France increases health tax in austerity package', *The Independent*, 11 May, 8.

Oakley, A. and Ashton, J. (1997) *Richard Titmuss: The Gift Relationship: From Human Blood to Social Policy*', Original edition with new chapters edited by Ann Oakley and John Ashton, London: LSE Books.

OECD (Organization for Economic Cooperation and Development) (1987) *Financing and Developing Health Care: A Comparative Analysis of OECD Countries*, Social Policy Studies No. 4, Paris: OECD.

OECD (1996) *Health Data 96*, Paris: OECD.

Office for National Statistics (1989) *Social Trends 19*, London: HMSO.

Office for National Statistics (1996) *ONS Monitor AB 97/5, Legal Abortions*, London: Office for National Statistics.

Office for National Statistics (1997) *Social Trends 27*, London: The Stationery Office.

Office for National Statistics (1998) *Social Trends 28*, London: The Stationery Office

Office for National Statistics (1999) *Social Trends 29*, London: The Stationery Office.

OHE (Office of Health Economics) (1987) *Compendium of Statistics*, London: OHE.

OHE (1988) *Briefing: Health Services in Europe: 1988*, No. 24, London: OHE.

OHE (1989) *People as Patients and Patients as People*, London: OHE.

OHE (1993) *The Impact of Unemployment on Health*, London: OHE.

Old, P. (1993) 'HA Law', *Health Service Journal*, 103 (5334) 21.

OPCS (Office of Population Censuses and Surveys) (1992) *General Household Survey: Carers in 1990*, OPCS Monitor SS92/2, London: HMSO.

Orr, J. (1987) *Women's Health in the Community*, Chichester. Wiley.

Orros, G. (1988) *The Potential Role of Private Health Insurance. Delivery and Funding of Health Services: Working Paper No. 6*, London: Institute of Health Services Management.

Ovretveit, J. (1993) *Coordinating Community Care. Multidisciplinary Teams and Care Management*, Buckingham: Open University Press.

Owen, D. (1988) *Our NHS*, London: Pan.

Owen, D. (1989) 'Unhealthy prescription for the NHS', *The Daily Telegraph*, 31 January.

Owen, G. (1984) *The Development of Degree Courses in Nursing Education – in Historical and Professional Context*, London: Polytechnic of the South Bank.

Owens, D. (1998) 'Trouble zones?', *Health Service Journal*, **108** (5593) 9.

Packwood, T. and Kober, A. (1995) 'Clinical audit and its relationship to other forms of quality assurance and knowledge generation', in *Making Use of Clinical Audit: A guide to practice in the health professions*, Kogan, M. and Redfern, S. (eds) Buckingham: Open University Press.

Pallot, P. (1989) 'Chorus of critics led by nurses', *The Daily Telegraph*, 1 February.

Parker, G. (1985) *With Due Care and Attention*, London: Family Policy Studies Centre.

Parker, G. and Lawton, D. (1994) *Different Type of Care, Different Type of Carer*, London: HMSO.

Paton, C. (1992) *Competition and Planning in the NHS: The Dangers of Unplanned Markets*, London: Chapman & Hall.

Paton, C. (1995) 'Present dangers and future threats: some perverse incentives in the NHS reforms, *British Medical Journal*, **310** (1), 1245–8.

Paton, C. (1998) *Competition and Planning in the NHS*, second edition, Cheltenham: Stanley Thornes.

Paxton, F., Porter, M. and Heaney, D., (1996) 'Evaluating the workload of practice nurses: a study' *Nursing Standard*, **10** (21) 33–8.

Payling, L., Bowen, T. and Briggs, I. (1987) 'PIs become crystal clear', *Health Service Journal*, **97** (5048) 502–3.

Peaker, C. (1988) *Who Pays? Who Cares? The Future Funding of Residential Care*, London: National Council of Voluntary Organisations.

Peck, E. (1998) 'Share of the action', *The Guardian*, 25 February.

Peckham, S. (1998) 'The missing link', *Health Service Journal*, **108** (5606) 22–3.

Peet, J. (1988) *Healthy Competition: How to Improve the NHS*, London: Centre for Policy Studies.

PEP (Political and Economic Planning) (1937) *Report on the British Health Services*, London: PEP.

Petchey, R. (1986) 'The Griffiths reorganisation of the National Health Service: Fowlerism by stealth?; *Critical Social Policy*, 17, Autumn, 87–101.

Pfeffer, N., Quick, A. (1988) *Infertility Services: A Desperate Case*, London: The Greater London Association of Community Health Councils.

Phillips, A. (1999a) 'Fair game', *Health Service Journal*, **109** (5655) 26–7.

Phillips, M. (1999b) 'They won't admit the truth about the NHS', *The Sunday Times*, 18 July.

Pietroni, P. (1996) *A Primary Care-Led NHS: Trick or Treat?*, London: University of Westminster Press.

Pittilo, M. and Ross, F. (1998) 'Policies for Interprofessional Education: Current Trends in the UK', *Education for Health*, **11** (3) 285–95.

Pollock, A. (1992) 'Local Voices: The bankruptcy of the democratic process', *British Medical Journal*, 305, 535–6.

Pollitt, C., Harrison, S., Hunter, D. and Marnoch, G. (1988) 'The reluctant managers: Clinicians and budgets in the NHS, *Financial Accountability and Management*, 4 (3) 213–33.

Porritt Report (1962) *A Review of the Medical Services in Great Britain: Report*, Medical Services Review Committee, London: Social Assay.

Poulton, B. and West, M. (1999) 'The determinants of effectiveness in primary health care teams', *Journal of Interprofessional Care*, 13 (1) 7–18.

Powell, M. (1997) *Evaluating the National Health Service*, Buckingham: Open University Press,

Powell, M. (1998) 'Policy evaluation in the past, present and future of the National Health Service', in *Fifty Years of the National Health Service: continuities and discontinuities in health policy*', Skelton, R. and Williamson, V. (eds) University of Brighton: Health and Social Policy Research Centre.

Power, M. (1997) *The Audit Society: Rituals of Verification*, Oxford: Oxford University Press.

Poxton, R. (1994) *Joint Commissioning: The Story so Far*, London: King's Fund Centre.

Poxton, R. (1996) 'Bridging the gap: joint commissioning of health and social care' in *Health Care UK 1995/6*, Harrison, A. and New, B. (eds) London: King's Fund.

Pratt, K. (1999) 'When a dentist's bill is a bridge too far', *The Sunday Times*, Money Section, 21 February.

Prigg, M. (1999) 'Teeth regrow to order', *The Sunday Times*, Innovation Section, 28 February.

Propper, C. (1993) 'Quasi-Markets and Regulation', in *Quasi-Markets and Social Policy*, Le Grand, J. and Bartlett, W. (eds) London: Macmillan.

Pryce, A. (1996) 'Details of the exploratory evaluation of a multidisciplinary education module for medical, dental and nursing students', *CAIPE Bulletin*, 11, Summer, 23.

Radford, T. (1998) 'The human cells that will revolutionise medicine', *The Guardian*, 6 November.

Rafferty, A. (1999) 'Practice makes perfect', *The Guardian*, Higher Education Section, 26 January.

Ranade, W. (1994) *A Future for the NHS? Health Care in the 1990s*, First Edition, London: Longman.

Ranade, W. (1997) *A Future for the NHS? Health care for the Millennium*', Second Edition, London: Longman.

Ranger, C. (1994) 'King's evidence', *Health Service Journal*, 104 (5394) 22–3.

Rashid, A., Watts, A. and Lenehan, C. (1996) 'Skill-mix in primary care: sharing clinical workload and understanding professional roles', *British Journal of General Practice*, November, 639–640.

RCN (Royal College of Nurses) (1988) *The Health Challenge*, London RCN.

Redcliffe-Maud Report (1969) *Royal Commission on Local Government in England*, Cmnd 4040, London: HMSO.

Rees, R. (1998) 'Use of complementary medicine in the UK: A summary using papers held on the CISCOM', (unpublished monograph) London: Research Council for Complementary Medicine.

Rehnberg, C. (1997) 'Sweden', in *Health Care Reform: Learning from International Experience*', Ham, C. (ed.) Buckingham: Open University Press.

Reich, R. (1998) 'Third Way needs courage', *The Guardian*, 21 September.

Revill, J. (1997) 'Cash lottery of test tube baby treatment', *Evening Standard*, 12 February.

Riddell, P. (1998) 'French given a revealing lesson in le Blairisme', *The Times*, 25 March.

Rigge, M. (1994) 'The Patients' dilemma', *The Guardian*, (Society section) 23 November.

Rivett, G. (1998) *From Cradle to Grave: Fifty years of the NHS*, London: King's Fund.

Roberts, C. (1995) 'Rational rather than rationed', *Health Service Journal*, **105** (5463) 17.

Robinson, J. and Strong, P. (1987) *Professional Nursing Advice after Griffiths: An Interim Report*, University of Warwick: Nursing Policy Studies Centre.

Robinson, R. (1988) *Efficiency and the NHS: A Case for Internal Markets*, London: Institute of Economic Affairs Unit.

Robinson, R. (1989) 'New health care market', *British Medical Journal*, **298** (18) 437–9.

Robinson, R. (1994) 'Small Change', *Health Service Journal*, **104** (5388) 31.

Robinson, R., Benzeval, M., Ham, C., Hunter, D. and Judge, J. (1988) *Health Finance: Assessing the Options*, London: King's Fund Institute.

Robinson, R. and Le Grand, J. (1993) *Evaluating the NHS Reforms*, London: King's Fund Institute.

Rodgers, J. (1994) 'Power to the People', *Health Service Journal*, **104** (5386) 28–9.

Rogers, L. (1995) 'Doctors ban elderly patients from expensive heart surgery', *The Sunday Times*, 12 February.

Roemer, M. (1986) *An Introduction to the US Health Care System*, second edition, New York: Springer.

Rowden, R. (1986) 'The Griffiths Report: what might it mean to nursing?', *Journal of Clinical Nursing*, **3**, 272–3.

Rowden, R. (1989) 'What's in it for us?', *Nursing Times*, **85**, (8) 45–6.

Rowntree, S. (1901) *Poverty: A study in town life*, London: Macmillan.

Royal Commission on Mental Illness and Mental Deficiency (1957) *Report*, London: HMSO.

Royal Commission on National Health Insurance (1928) *Report*, Cmnd 2596, London: HMSO.

Ryan, M. and Birch, S. (1988) *Estimating the Effects of Health Service Charges: Evidence on the utilisation of prescriptions*, University of York: Centre for Health Economics.

Sale, D. (1996) *Quality Assurance: For Nurses and Other Members of the Health Care Team*, London: Macmillan.

Salmon Report (1966) *Report of the Committee on Senior Nursing Staff Structure*, Ministry of Health, London: HMSO.

Savage, W. and Widgery, D. (1989) 'Working for Patients?', *New Statesman and Society*, 17 February, 10–11.

Schofield, M. (1996) *The future healthcare workforce: the steering group report*, Manchester: University of Manchester.

Schwartz, F. and Busse, R. (1997) 'Germany' in *Health Care Reform: Learning from Experience*, Ham, C. (ed.) Buckingham: Open University Press.

Scrivens, E. (1988) 'The Management of Clinicians in the National Health Service', *Social Policy and Administration*, **2** (1) Spring, 23–34.

Scrivens, E. (1989) 'Customers have choices', *Health Service Journal*, **99**, (5142) 328–9.

Secretary of State for Health (1995) *The Mental Health Act Commission: Sixth Biennial Report 1993–1995*, London: HMSO.

Secretary of State for Health (1996) *The National Health Service: A Service with Ambitions*, Cm 3425, November, London: The Stationery Office.

Secretary of State for Health (1997a) *A New Partnership for Care in Old Age*, CM 3563, London: The Stationery Office.

Secretary of State for Health (1997b) *Developing Partnerships in Mental Health*, London: The Stationery Office.

Secretary of State for Health (1997c) *The new NHS: Modern – Dependable*, Cm. 3807, London: The Stationery Office.

Secretary of State for Health (1998a) *Our Healthier Nation. A Contract for Health*, A Consultation Paper, Cm. 3852, London: the Stationery Office.

Secretary of State for Health (1998b) *Smoking Kills*, Cm. 4177, London: The Stationery Office.

Secretary of State for Health (1998c) *Modernising Social Services: Promoting independence; Improving protection; Raising standards*, Cm 4169, London: The Stationery Office.

Secretary of State for Health (1999a) *NHS Direct: Statement*, 2 February, London: Department of Health

Secretary of State for Health (1999b) *Saving Lives: Our Healthier Nation*, London: Department of Health.

Secretary of State for Scotland (1997) *Designed to Care. Renewing the National Health in Scotland*, Cm. 3811, December, Edinburgh: The Stationery Office.

Secretary of State for Scotland (1998) *Working Together for a Healthier Scotland*, Cm. 3584, February, Edinburgh: The Stationery Office.

Secretary of State for Wales (1998a) *NHS Wales: putting patients first*, Cm 3841, January, Cardiff: The Stationery Office.

Secretary of State for Wales (1998b) *Better Health, Better Wales*, Cm. 3922, May, Cardiff: The Stationery Office.

Seebohm Report (1968) *Report of the Committee on Local Authority and Allied Personal Social Services*, Cmnd 3703, London: HMSO.

Seedhouse, D. (1988) *Ethics: The Heart of Health Care*, Chichester: John Wiley.

Shackley, P. and Ryan, M. (1994) 'What is the role of the consumer in health care', *Journal of Social Policy*, 23 (4) October 517–42.

Shaw, C. (1987) 'Quality assurance: whose role to define quality?', *Health Service Journal*, 97 (5050) 528.

Shaw, T. (1999) 'Ruling on woman's care may save NHS millions', *The Daily Telegraph*, 17 July.

Sheldon, T. (1992) 'More bricks in the wall', *Health Service Journal*, 102 (5309) 26–8.

Sherman, J. (1985) 'After the honeymoon is over', *Health and Social Service Journal*, 13 June, 734–5.

Sherman, J. (1999) 'Dobson's £96m crusade to help poor live longer', *The Times*, 7 July.

Sheuer, M. (1991) 'Street Plans', *Health Service Journal*, 101 (5277) 21–3.

Sheuer, M., Black, M., Victor, C., Benzeval, M., Gill, M. and Judge, K. (1991) *Homeless and the Utilisation of Acute Hospital Services in London*, Occasional Paper 4, October, London: King's Fund Institute.

Shiner, P. and Leddington, S. (1991) 'Sometimes it makes you frightened to go to hospital ... they treat you like dirt', *Health Service Journal*, 101 (5277) 21–3.

Short Report (1980) *Perinatal and Neonatal Mortality: Second report from the Social Services Committee*, Session 1979–80, London: HMSO.

Short Report (1985) *Community Care: Second report from the Social Services Committee*, Session 1984–85, London: HMSO.

Singleton, J. and McLaren, S. (1995) *Ethical Foundations of Health Care. Responsibilities in Decision Making*, London: Mosby.

SMA (Socialist Medical Association) (1933) *A Socialized Medical Service*, London: SMA.

Small, N. (1988) 'AIDS and social policy', *Critical Social Policy*, Spring, Issue 21, 9–29.

Smith, A. and Jacobson, B. (1988) *The Nation's Health A Strategy for the 1990s*, London: King Edward's Hospital Fund.

Smith, J. (1996) 'The OPCS Longitudinal Study, in *Social Trends 26*, Church, J. (ed.) London: HMSO.

Smith, J., Knight, T. and Wilson, F. (1999a) 'Supra troupers', *Health Service Journal*, **109** (5637) 26–8.

Smith, J., Regen, E. and Shapiro, J. (1999b) 'Lending a hand', *Health Service Journal*, **109** (5656) 24–6.

Smith, R. (1987) *Unemployment and Health: A disaster and challenge*, Oxford: Oxford University Press.

Smith, R. (1994) 'Room at the top', *Health Service Journal*, **104** (5430) 28–9.

Snell, J. (1997) 'Action team appointed to tackle rising waiting lists', *Health Service Journal*, **107** (5580) 4.

Snell, J. (1998) 'A force to reckon with', *Health Service Journal*, **108** (5597) 24–6.

Snell, J. (1999) 'A year down the line', *Health Service Journal*, **109** (5647) 20–2.

Snowden, R. (1985) *Consumer Choices in Family Planning: The Clinic and the GP: Cooperation or competition?* London: Family Planning Association.

Social Exclusion Unit (1998) *Bringing Britain Together: a national strategy for neighbourhood renewal*, London: The Stationery Office.

Social Services Committee (1984) *Griffiths NHS Management Inquiry Report, First Report*: Session 1983–4, London: HMSO.

Social Services Committee (1988a) *The Future of the National Health Service*, London: HMSO.

Social Services Committee (1988b) *Resourcing the National Health Service: Short-term issues*, Vol. 1, London: HMSO.

Solomon, M. (1992) 'Happy Now? *Health Service Journal*, **102** (5324) 24–5.

Stocks, M. (1960) *A Hundred Years of District Nursing*, London: Allen & Unwin.

Storrie, J. (1992) 'Mastering interprofessionalism – an enquiry into the development of Masters Programmes with an interprofessional focus', *Journal of Interprofessional Care*, **6** (3) 253–60.

Strong, P. and Robinson, J. (1988) *New Model Management: Griffiths and the NHS*, University of Warwick: Nursing Policy Studies Centre.

Suppiah, V. (1989) 'Accentuate the positive', *Health Service Journal*, **99** (5135) 109.

Sutherland, S. (1999) *With Respect to Old Age: Long Term Care – Rights and Responsibilities. A Report by The Royal Commission on Long Term Care*, Cm. 4192–1, March, London: The Stationery Office.

Taylor, D. (1984) *Understanding the NHS in the 1980s*, London: Office of Health Economics.

Taylor, H. (1989) 'A tale of three health services', *The Times*, 17 February.

Taylor-Gooby, P. (1985) *Public Opinion, Ideology and State Welfare*, London: Routledge & Kegan Paul.

The Cabinet Office (1999) *The government's annual report 98/99*, Cm 4401, London: The Stationery Office.

The Health Services (1983) 'Cooperation between the NHS and the private sector at district level', 3 June.

The Guardian (1997a) 'A Political Earthquake', 2 May.

The Guardian (1997b) 'Mr. Brown's tour de force. But is it enough to cool consumer spending?', 3 July.

The Guardian (1998) 'Smoking to death', 11 December.

The Guardian (1999a) 'Universal vs redistribution: There is a third way', 2 March.

The Guardian (1999b) 'Hackney school deal agreed', 19 June.

The Guardian (1999c) 'NHS funding crisis as debts near £1bn', 12 November.

The *Sunday Times* (1999) 'An unhealthy state', 11 July.

The *Times* (1990) 'A Question of Tolerance', 24 April.

The *Times* (1999) 'A listing service', 7 January.

Times Higher Educational Supplement (1996) 'Dundee nurses an ambition' 17 May.

Thomas, D. (1985) 'Cleaning out the cleaners', *New Society*, 14 March, 414.

Thompson, S. (1999) 'Kiss of life can't come too soon', *Guardian Higher*, 6 July.

Thornley, C. (1997) *The Invisible Workers*, London: Unison.

Thornton, S. (1996) 'Leader of the Pack'. *Health Service Journal*, **106** (5520) 28–9.

Tibbles, I. (1987) 'Five steps to a winning team', *Health Service Journal*, **97** (5027) 187.

Timmins, N. (1988) *Cash, Crisis and Cure: The Independent guide to the NHS debate*, London: Newspaper Publishing PLC.

Timmins, N. (1989a) 'Journey into the unknown', The *Independent*, 2 February.

Timmins, N. (1989b) 'East Anglia leads move to internal NHS market', The *Independent*, 13 February.

Timmins, N. (1989c) 'Is the NHS safe in their hands?', The *Independent*, 9 February.

Timmins, N. (1989d) 'Consultants join opposition to "cut-price" NHS', The *Independent*, 21 March.

Timmins, N. (1991) 'Major spells out his plan for the decade', The *Independent*, 23 July.

Tinker, A. (1997) *Older People in Modern Society*, 4th edition, London: Longman.

Tinsley, R. and Luck, M. (1998) 'Fundholding and the Community Nurse', *Journal of Social Policy*, **27** 471–87.

Titmuss, R.M. (1950) *Problems of Social Policy*, London: HMSO.

Todd Report (1968) *Report of the Royal Commission on Medical Education 1965–1968*, Cmnd 3569, London: HMSO.

Tonkin, B. (1988) 'Strong medicine', *Community Care*, 10 November, 16–18.

Tomlinson Report (1992) *Report on the Inquiry into London's health service, medical education and research*, London: HMSO.

Townsend, P. and Davidson, N. (1982) *Inequalities in Health: The Black Report*, Harmondsworth: Penguin.

Towse, A. (1995) 'Let's get down to brass tax', *Health Service Journal*, **105** (5479) 23.

Toynbee, P. (1999) 'A sense of failure', The *Guardian*, 7 July.

Turnberg, L. (1998) *Health Services in London – A Strategic Review*, London: Department of Health.

Turner, M. (1998) 'Health Services', in *Social Services in Scotland*, English, J.(ed.) fourth edition, Edinburgh: The Mercati Press.

Twigg, J. and Atkin, K. (1994) *Carers perceived: policy and practice in informal care*, Buckingham: Open University Press.

Tyndall, R. (1998) 'Clinical governance. Shift workers', *Health Service Journal*, **108** (5631) 27–9.

UKCC (United Kingdom Central Council for Nursing, Midwifery and Health Visiting) (1984) *Annual Report 1983–1984*, London: UKCC.

UKCC (1986) *Project 2000: A new preparation for practice*, London: UKCC.

UKCC (1987) *Project 2000: Counting the Cost: Is Project 2000 a practical proposal?*, London: UKCC.

van de Ven, W. (1997) 'The Netherlands', in *Health Care Reform: Learning from International Experience*, Ham. C. (ed.) Buckingham: Open University Press.

Vorster, M. (1999) 'Behind the lines', *Health Service Journal*, 109 (5655) 24–5.

Wagner Report (1988) *Residential Care: A Positive Choice*, London: National Institute for Social Work.

Walker, M. (1996) 'Happy Birthday, Mr. President', *The Guardian*, 19 August.

Wall, A. (1995) 'Every Manager's Nightmare', *Health Service Journal*, 105 (5480) 24–6.

Wall, P. (1991) 'Health and homelessness', *Health Service Journal*, 101 (5245) 16–17.

Walshe, K. (1995) *Public Services and Market Mechanisms*, London: Macmillan.

Walshe, K. (1997) 'Indicators won't turn the tables' *Health Service Journal*, 107 (5562) 24.

Wandsworth Social Services Department (1993/4) *Draft Community Care Plan for Wandsworth 1993/4* (produced by Wandsworth Borough Council, Wandsworth District Health Authority, Richmond, Twickenham and Roehampton District Health Authority and Merton, Sutton and Wandsworth Family Health Service Authority) Wandsworth: Wandsworth Social Services Department.

Ward, S. (1999) 'Skimping on Himps', *The Guardian*, Society section, 14 July.

Warner, N. (1994) *Community Care: Just a Fairy Tale?* London: Carers National Association.

Warnock Report (1984) *Report of the Committee of Inquiry into Human Fertilisation and Embryology*, Cmnd 9314, London: HMSO.

Watts, A. and Lenehan, C. (1997) *Towards 2000 – Education for Collaboration and Partnership*, London: Royal College of General Practitioners/Royal College of Nursing.

Watts, G. (1999) 'Cases in need of evaluations', *The Times Higher*, 2 July.

Webb, A. and Wistow, G. (1986) *Planning, Need and Scarcity, Essays on the Personal Social Services*, London: Allen & Unwin.

Webster, C. (1988) *The Health Services since the War, Volume I. Problems of Health Care: The National Health Service before 1957*, London: HMSO.

Webster, C. (1998) *The National Health Service: A Political History*, Oxford: Oxford University Press.

Webster, C. (1998/9) 'The very long history of the PCG', *Health Matters*, Issue 35, Winter, 5.

Webster, P. (1997) 'Blair pledges shake up for welfare state', *The Times*, 15 May.

Weinberg, R. (1999) 'The suicide weapon', *The Guardian*, Online, 14 January.

Welsh Institute for Health and Social Care (1998) *Local Health Groups: What are they used for?* Commentary number five, Pontypridd: University of Glamorgan.

Welsh Office (1993) *Protocol for Investment in Health Gain: Mental Health*, Cardiff: Welsh Office.

Welsh Office, (1998) *Involving the Public*, Cardiff: Welsh Office.

Weston, C. (1997) 'Bones of contention', *Health Service Journal*, 107 (5568) 26–7.

White, M. (1999a) 'Frankly, a magic Moment as nurses stand and cheer', *Health Service Journal*, 109 (5646) 17.

White, M. (1999b) 'PM's deadline to end child poverty', *The Guardian*, 19 March.

White, M. and Hencke, D. (1998) 'Goodbye ... for now', *The Guardian*, 24 December.

Whitehead, M. (1987) *The Health Divide: Inequalities in health in the 1980's*, London: Health Education Council.

Whitehead, M. and Drever, F. (1997) *Health Inequalities*, London: HMSO.

Whitfield, D. (1995/6) 'Is this a good investment?', *Health Matters*, Issue 24, 10–11.

Whitfield, L. (1998a) 'Welsh White Paper outlines different GP structure plus role for Assembly', *Health Service Journal*, **108** (5588) 7.

Whitfield, L. (1998b) 'Mixed welcome for radical Welsh trust cuts proposals', *Health Service Journal*, **108**, (5599) 8.

Whitfield, L. (1998c) 'Paved with good intentions', *Health Service Journal*, **108** (5599) 9.

Whitfield, L. (1999) 'Cost pressures bring threat to HImP work', *Health Service Journal*, **109** (5653) 4.

Whiteside, N. (1988) 'Unemployment and ill health: an historical perspective', *Journal of Social Policy*, **17** (2) 177–94.

Whitney, R. (1988) *National Health Crisis: A Modern Solution*, London: Shepheard Walwyn.

WHO (World Health Organization) (1981) *Global Strategy for Health for All by the year 2000*, Geneva: WHO.

WHO (1984) *Health for All 2000*, Copenhagen: WHO Regional Office for Europe.

WHO (1985) *Targets for Health for All: Targets in support of the European regional strategy for health for all*, Copenhagen: WHO Regional Office for Europe.

Wickings, I. (1983) 'Consultants face the figures', *Health and Social Service Journal*, 8 December, 1466–7.

Widgery, D. (1988) *The National Health: A Radical Perspective*, London: Hogarth Press.

Wilcox, R. (1999) 'Missed: a motivator', *Health Service Journal*, **109** (5631) 21.

Willcocks, A. (1967) *The Creation of the National Health Service*, London: Routledge & Kegan Paul.

Willetts, D. (1989) 'The NHS remedy – to be taken internally', *The Guardian*, 1 February.

Willetts, D. and Goldsmith, M. (1988a) *A Mixed Economy in Health Care – More Spending, Save Taxes*, London: Centre for Policy Studies.

Willetts, D. and Goldsmith, M. (1988b) *Managed Health Care: A new system for a better health service*, London: Centre for Policy Studies.

Williams, A. (1997) 'Rationing health care by age: the case for', *British Medical Journal*, 314 820–2.

Williams, D., Carruthers, J., Clark, J. and Davey, W. (1985) 'Piecing together the jigsaw'. *Health and Social Service Journal*, 30 May, 668–70.

Williams, G. and Wilson, S. (1998) *The Collaborative Imperative: Overcoming Barriers in Health and Social Care*, St Catherine's Conference Report No. 66, Egham: The King George VI and Queen Elizabeth Foundation of St. Catherine's.

Williams, J. (1987) 'Tempting clinicians across the divide', *Health Service Journal*, **97** (5056) 731.

Wilson Committee (1994) *Being Heard*, London: Department of Health.

Wilson, J. (1999) 'Grow your own eyes' operation to save sight', The *Guardian*, 18 March.

Wistow, G. and Fuller, S. (1986) *Collaboration since Restructuring: The 1984 CRSP/ NAHA Survey of Joint Planning and Joint Finance*, Birmingham: The National Association of Health Authorities.

Witney, B. and Moody, D. (1992) 'Health for all', *Health Service Journal*, **102** (5304) 25.

Woods, K. (1998) *Priorities and Planning Guidance for the NHS in Scotland 1999–2002*, Management Executive Letter, Performance Management Division within the NHS Management Executive, Edinburgh: Department of Health, Scottish Office.

Women's National Commission (1985) *Women and the Health Service*, London: Women's National Commission.

Working Group on Specialist Medical Training (1993) *Hospital Doctors: Training for the Future: The Report of the Working Group on Specialist Medical Training*, London: Department of Health.

World Federation for Medical Education (1988) *The Edinburgh Declaration*, Edinburgh: World Health Organization.

Wright, P. (1987) 'Top doctors in NHS Revolt', *The Times*, 7 December, 108–9.

Wynn Davies, P. (1993) 'People 'ignorant of Citizen's Charter', *The Independent*, 18 February.

Young, H. (1997) 'The people's triumph', *The Guardian*, 2 May.

Young, K. and Haynes, R. (1993) 'Assessing population needs in primary health care: the problem of GP attachment', *Journal of Interprofessional Care*, 7 (1) 15–28.

INDEX